CHILD, YOUTH AND FAMILY HEALTH

Strengthening communities

CHILD, YOUTH AND FAMILY HEALTH

Strengthening communities

2nd edition

EDITED BY
MARGARET BARNES
JENNIFER ROWE

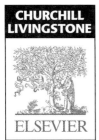

CHURCHILL
LIVINGSTONE

ELSEVIER

Sydney   Edinburgh   London   New York   Philadelphia   St Louis   Toronto

Churchill Livingstone
is an imprint of Elsevier

Elsevier Australia. ACN 001 002 357
(a division of Reed International Books Australia Pty Ltd)
Tower 1, 475 Victoria Avenue, Chatswood, NSW 2067

ELSEVIER

National Library of Australia Cataloguing-in-Publication Data

Child, youth and family health : strengthening communities / edited by Margaret Barnes,
  Jennifer Rowe.

  2nd ed.
  9780729541558 (pbk.)
  Includes index.

Child health services – Australia.
Medical care – Australia.
Family nursing – Australia.

  Barnes, Margaret (Margaret I.)
  Rowe, Jennifer.

362.70994

Publisher: Libby Houston
Developmental Editor: Elizabeth Coady
Project Managers: Natalie Hamad and Nayagi Athmanathan
Edited by Linda Littlemore
Proofread by Tim Learner
Permissions editor: Sarah Johnson
Cover and internal design by Tania Gomes
Index by Robert Swanson
Typeset by Toppan Best-set Premedia Limited
Printed in China by 1010 Printing Int'l Ltd.

CONTENTS

FOREWORD
by Jeanine Young

I am honoured to have been asked to prepare a foreword for the new edition of this absorbing text for health professionals who care for infants, children, young people and their families across a wide range of health contexts and life stages.

A child's health and wellbeing depends on what happens to them as individuals, as part of a family unit, as members of communities and as a member of the greater society as a whole. Evidence shows that the most effective way to protect and nurture children so that they have the chance to flourish is to strengthen their families and develop communities so that children can expect to grow up in an environment that meets their developmental needs.

The majority of our children grow up happy and healthy. Recent reports, however, have suggested that our young people are at a crossroads; with drug use, antisocial behaviour, depression, anxiety, suicide and other mental health issues on the rise. Some stress is brought on due to societal trends – the rise of individualism and consumerism; a decline in the sense of the community and of the importance of the family unit – with each of these trends potentially impacting mental health.

These trends have created a greater focus on the quality of family life and the health and wellbeing of family members, producing a significant demand for assistance as families and communities seek external support to assist them in achieving and maintaining a reasonable standard of living, health and wellbeing.

The intent of this book reminded me of the wise words of Franklin D. Roosevelt:

'We cannot always build the future of our youth, but we can build our youth for the future'.

The approach used in this text is a strengths-based model. Both a philosophy of practice and a specific set of tools and methods, the strengths model is designed to facilitate a collaborative partnership between the child, the young person and their family and the health professional caring for them, by working with families where they are and with the strengths they have. Such an approach fosters resilience in the child, young person and their family which will enable them to cope with and bounce back from risks and adversity that they are very likely to face in our dynamic and rapidly changing society.

This text reveals the broad knowledge and skill base shared by the editors and contributors, which are essentials to practice in meeting the challenges faced by families today. The range of topics across the infant, child and youth continuum is impressive; and always firmly placed on the child and their family.

Fresh, contemporary content included in this revision highlight the progress made and the challenges we continue to face in the care of children in contemporary society. Chapter 5 addresses effective communication strategies using the family strengths model which, if used effectively, may operationalise family-centred-care approaches to actively engage children in decision-making about their own health care. Highlighted in Chapter 8 is the need for partnerships between health, education and community services that create integrated service models in early childhood support in order to achieve optimal life and learning outcomes for children. The unique issues and challenges faced during middle childhood and the role of child-centred care within family-centred frameworks are illustrated in Chapter 9 through scenarios that address acute management and common causes of injury and illness.

The contributors to this valuable text have succeeded in asking key questions relating to current family support systems and approaches, and whether these are meeting the needs of families. Embedded in the chapters is the message that we need to invest more time and energy in the continuing process of constructing shared frameworks of goals and values, and in developing a shared understanding of where we want to go. Health professionals, and particularly nurses and midwives as key health professionals working with families, are charged with taking up proactive leadership roles in providing direction to that process through effective policy, responsive service and program initiatives, research and evaluation and in the encouragement of a wide range of players to innovate and learn better ways to achieve those objectives.

Congratulations to the editors and to their colleagues who have shared their collective knowledge. This book demonstrates admirably the growing evidence base of our professions and signals the skills, growing maturity and professionalism of infant, child and youth services that strengthen and support families.

Professor Jeanine Young
FACN, PhD, BSc Nursing (1st Class Honours), Adv Dip of Nursing Care
Registered Nurse, Registered Midwife, Neonatal Nurse

CONTRIBUTORS

Margaret Barnes PhD, RM, RN
  Associate Professor, School of Nursing and Midwifery, University of the Sunshine Coast, Qld
Rachel Cole PhD (PubHlth), M (Epi), BSc (HonsPubHlth), BScAppl (HMS)
  Lecturer Health Promotion, University of the Sunshine Coast, Qld
Jon Darvill RN, MN, GCert in Higher Ed
  Professional Associate, Nursing and Midwifery, Faculty of Health, University of Canberra, ACT
Karen Ford RN, MN, Cert Paed Nursing, PhD
  ADON Research & Practice Development, Practice Development Unit – Nursing & Midwifery, Royal Hobart Hospital
  Senior Clinical Lecturer, School of Nursing and Midwifery, University of Tasmania
Elizabeth Forster RN, BN, MN, GradCert Higher Ed PhD, Centaur Fellow
  Lecturer, School of Nursing Queensland University of Technology, Qld, Australia
Jennifer Fraser RN, PhD
  Associate Professor, Sydney Nursing School, The University of Sydney
Jane Gregg PhD (HlthProm), MHlthProm, GDIntHlth
  Lecturer in Public Health, Faculty of Science, Health, Education and Engineering, University of the Sunshine Coast, Sippy Downs, Qld
Christine Handley RN, BaAppSci, MEd; FANZCMHN, FCNA
  Senior Lecturer (SNM/UTAS), Hobart, Tas
  ADON (CAMHS) and Statewide coordinator of the mental health specialist stream of the Graduate Diploma of Nursing (SNM/UTAS)
Penelope Harrison BA (Hons), BHlthNurs
  Associate Lecturer, School of Nursing and Midwifery, University of the Sunshine Coast, Sippy Downs, Qld
Evelyn Hikuroa RN, MPH (Hons)
  Senior Lecturer, Faculty of Nursing and Health Studies, Manukau Institute of Technology, Auckland, New Zealand
Vicki Holliday RN, GradDip Indig Hlth, MA Indig Hlth, GradCert Ed
  Lecturer, Discipline of Indigenous Health, School of Medicine and Public Health, University of Newcastle, NSW

Margaret McAllister RN, Ed D, FACHMN, FACN
Professor of Nursing, CQ University, Centre for Mental Health Nursing Innovation, Noosa, Qld

Karen McBride-Henry RN, PhD
Senior Lecturer, Graduate School of Nursing, Midwifery & Health, Victoria University of Wellington, NZ
Member College of Nurses Aotearoa New Zealand (MCNANZ)

Judith Murray BA (Hons), DipEd, BEdSt, PhD, BNurs
Associate Professor, Counselling and Counselling Psychology, The University of Queensland, Brisbane, Qld
Registered Nurse, Princess Alexandra Hospital, Brisbane, Qld

Rachel Reed BSc (Hons), RM
Lecturer, School of Nursing and Midwifery, University of the Sunshine Coast, Qld

Avril Rose MEd, B Ed, DipT (ECE)
Lecturer, Early Childhood Education, School of Science & Education, University of the Sunshine Coast, Qld

Jennifer Rowe PhD, MPhil, Grad Dip Ed (Nurs), BA, Dip Ed, RN
Associate Professor, Nursing, School of Nursing and Midwifery and Associate Dean, Learning and Teaching, Faculty of Science, Health, Education and Engineering, University of the Sunshine Coast, Qld

Lindsay Smith PhD, RN, MACN, BHlthSc (Nurs), MNS, GradCertUniL&T
Graduate Research Coordinator and Lecturer School of Nursing & Midwifery, University of Tasmania, Tas

Helen Stasa PhD, BA (Hons)
Post-doctoral Research Fellow, Sydney Nursing School, University of Sydney, NSW

Kay Thomas RN, GCert Paediatric, Child and Youth Health Nursing
Assistant Director of Nursing Neonatology, Centenary Hospital for Women and Children, Canberra, ACT

Anne Tietzel DipT (ECE), BA, BEd, TAA
Lecturer Early Childhood Education, University of the Sunshine Coast, Qld

Anne Walsh PhD, MHSc, GradDip (HPro), BA (Psych), DipAppSci, EM, RN
Lecturer, School of Nursing, Queensland University of Technology, Qld

REVIEWERS

Michelle Adams MhlthProEd, BHlthSc, RN
  Professional Teaching Fellow, Faculty of Medical and Health Sciences,
  The University of Auckland, NZ
Odette Best PhD, MPhil, BHlthSc, RN
  Senior Lecturer at Oodgeroo Unit, QUT, Qld
Kim Clark BSc, Grad Dip Bus
  Evaluation Consultant, Telethon Institute for Child Health Research, Perth, WA
Jenny Donovan RN, RM, Infant Welfare Cert, DipAppSc, BNg, MSc (Primary
Health Care), A.Mus.A., Cert in Accompanying [Flinders St, Music School, Adelaide]
  Senior Lecturer, Course Coordinator, Graduate Diploma in Child and Family
  Health Nursing [GDCFH], Charles Darwin University, Adelaide, SA
Mandy El Ali MACN, MACCYPN, MANF, MANZAPHE,MN, BHS – Nursing,
Grad Dip Paeds, Grad Cert Paeds
  Lecturer of Nursing – Australian Catholic University, Melbourne, Vic
  Clinical Nurse Specialist – Sunshine Paediatric Ward, Melbourne, Vic
Ginny Henderson RN, DipHE, BN, GradCertHE, MSc
  Associate Centre Member of the Centre for Health Practice Innovation (HPI)
  Lecturer, School of Nursing & Midwifery, Griffith University, Qld
Andrew Gardner RN, BN, MMHN, MBus, Dip Medical Hypnosis
  Lecturer in Nursing, University of South Australia, Adelaide, SA
Robyn Gail Kelly RN, RM, CHN, MIH, PhD Candidate
  Lecturer, School of Nursing and Midwifery, University of Tasmania, Hobart, Tas
Naumai Smith RGON, BA(Ed), MHSc (Hons)
  Head of School, Health Care Practice, Equity Portfolio Holder, Faculty of Health
  and Environmental Sciences, AUT University, Auckland, NZ

ACKNOWLEDGMENTS

Children: they are our past, the present and the future. They are the source of our greatest joy and pleasure, but also our worry and despair. We have been motivated throughout this project by a passion for children and their families – one that has immersed us, professionally and personally, for many years and it is a great pleasure to share this passion.

We have been assisted in this task by a number of people, to whom thanks are due. First, we thank the contributors. New relationships have been forged in the process, as we have communicated the needs of the text through telephone, email and, occasionally, in person. All the authors have drawn on their expertise and experience to write and each has contributed to the richness of the text.

The project has been steered by Liz Coady from Elsevier, who has played a pivotal role in the preparation of this edition. We thank her and all the team at Elsevier who have contributed to the preparation of the text. Feedback from anonymous reviewers of both the initial proposal and individual chapters has been an important influence on the review, revisions and final manuscript preparation and we extend our appreciation to them for their thoughtful comments. Finally we extend our thanks to Karen Watson who has provided valuable research support and assistance.

INTRODUCTION

Margaret Barnes and Jennifer Rowe

It is a great pleasure to introduce the second edition of Child Youth and Family Health. In this edition we provide a foundation for working with children, young people and families across a range of health contexts and life stages. In providing this forum, we highlight the valuable practice undertaken to support and nurture these client groups, across a range of settings. Contemporary policy, practice theory and competencies are discussed in context and all are informed by a strengths approach. In this way practice is constructed in a collaborative and partnership model, centred on working with families where they are and with the strengths they have. The text adopts a critical lens, so as not only to describe practice but also to highlight challenges and issues for readers to consider. Learning for beginning and advanced or specialised practice preparation is supported.

While the foundations of the text set up in the first edition remain, there are a number of additions and revisions. We welcome new contributing authors who have enriched the multi-disciplinary focus. These include Jane Taylor, Rachel Cole, Helen Stasa, Karen Ford, Rachel Reed, Anne Tietzel, Avril Rose, Anne Walsh and Penny Harrison. There are two new chapters in this second edition: Chapter 8 Health Promotion Through Early Childhood; and Chapter 9 Acute Illness: The Child and Their Family. All other chapters have been extensively revised and updated.

The book is organised in two parts. Part A provides an overarching survey of issues facing the health and wellbeing of children and young people and their families. In Chapter 1 the place of family in society, diversity, culture and health influences, as well as healthcare priorities, are discussed. Policy, service and program initiatives, the keys for effective leadership practice, are set out in Chapter 2. In this chapter the principles for sustainable health promotion programs are discussed.

In Chapter 3, there is an emphasis on the particular needs of Indigenous peoples, including a reflection on the social and political circumstance that has led to what continues to be poorer health and wellbeing than the rest of the population in both Australia and New Zealand. In Chapter 4 the reader is challenged to consider the complex and essential ethical and legal dimensions of practice within the overarching imperative of advocacy. Child centred communication with children and their families is the topic of Chapter 5 which also includes Family Strengths framework for healthcare practice.

Part B focuses on contexts of care in which nurses and midwives practise directly or indirectly to improve health outcomes. Chapters 6 and 7 focus upon the developing family, particularly women and parents during pregnancy and the first year of life and the centrality of attachment to infant, child and family. Chapter 8 focuses on health promotion in the early years. The international and national trend towards integrated, multi-sectoral policy and planning is articulated in this chapter, which demonstrates the alignment and synergies among health and education for young children. Chapter 9 addresses care and issues for children with acute illness. The demographic profile, practice settings and responses to illness and injury are discussed. Young people face a number of physical, developmental, psycho-social or behavioural challenges to their health and wellbeing. Further, they are vulnerable to the impacts of alcohol and drug use and abuse, unsafe sexual behaviour, mental health problems and violence. Recognition of the health issues facing young people has led to the development of national policy and strategic directions in Australia and New Zealand. These issues, practice challenges and solutions are set out in Chapters 10 and 12.

Two important and discrete areas of practice form the basis of Chapters 11 and 13. In Chapter 11, chronic illness in childhood is examined. Through two very different scenarios, the reader is taken into the world of the family who has a child with an ongoing health problem. The complexities of service and practice are discussed, showing the multiple, collaborative and partnership basis of effective healthcare. Finally, but not least, in Chapter 13 Grief and Loss are examined and the reader is given the opportunity to understand grief and loss from the position of children of different ages, and family members.

PART A

ISSUES AND CHALLENGES IN CHILD, YOUTH AND FAMILY HEALTH

Chapter 1

LOCATING THE CHILD, YOUNG PERSON AND FAMILY IN CONTEMPORARY HEALTH CARE

Margaret Barnes, Jennifer Rowe

LEARNING OUTCOMES

Reading this chapter will help you to:

» understand the nature of the contemporary family
» appreciate family diversity
» locate the family within contemporary society
» understand the changing nature of the family
» discuss health determinants as they relate to children and young people
» understand the influence of social gradient on child health and the implications for health later in life
» identify current health priorities for children and young people.

Introduction

Families today are conceptualised as the mortar of society. They do, however, face many challenges, replete with risks to the family as it has been known and risks to family and individual health from a widening range of environmental and lifestyle dynamics. Thus, child, youth and family health services seek to strengthen and support families, promote health, prevent illness and manage risks, from both short-term and long-term perspectives.

Health care for the child, young person and family in Australia and New Zealand is publicly funded, with many services delivered through the public sector. At the same time, consumer expectation and interest have motivated a growing private sector providing information, advice and services. Together with information available via the Internet, families are challenged to sift through and interpret the vast array of information and services in searching for helpful support, and to balance the demands of contemporary life and meet their health needs.

Working with children and young people is both rewarding and challenging. Nurses and midwives caring for this client group do so, most commonly, within the context of the family. It is important, therefore, to understand the nature and shape of the family as a mediator and facilitator for children and young people, their health and wellbeing. This chapter situates the child, young person and family in contemporary New Zealand and Australian society and examines the underpinnings of children and young people's health and health care in these countries. As well, we provide an historical overview of the development of nursing as a key healthcare provider for children, young people and families.

As background to this, an overview of how the family is constructed and how it functions today is provided. Societal approaches to capturing health priorities and developing policy to strengthen individual and family health are outlined.

Contemporary impressions of the family and community

Family life has changed over recent decades in Australia and New Zealand with a rise in divorce rates, increasing workforce participation by both parents and single parenting. Such changes have brought into question the quality of family life, especially for children. However, historical analysis tends to point to the importance of a longer term view of family development (Featherstone, 2004). The nature and patterns of family life have changed over time and have probably done so for centuries. An understanding and critique of trends in family life are therefore important, as they influence and shape the way health professionals may view family functioning and child health and, more broadly, how governments prioritise social and health policy and service provision.

Any discussion of the family needs to be prefaced with contemporary definitions. There are a number of definitions of family that can inform thinking about family within the context of child, youth and family health. As families change shape and function over time, so does the definition of family. Family can be thought of in terms of a sense of belonging that is not always linked by legal or biological relationships (Lodge, Maloney & Robinson, 2011).

However, for the purpose of census data collection, the Australian Bureau of Statistics (ABS) (2006) defines a family as a couple with or without resident children; a lone parent with resident children of any age; or related adults, such as brothers and/or sisters, living together where no couple or parent–child relationship exists. In New Zealand, and again in the context of social statistics, Statistics New Zealand differentiates between families and households. A family (or family nucleus) is defined as a couple, with or without child(ren), or one parent and their child(ren), all of whom have usual residence together in the same household. Households, on the other hand, are classified according to the relationships between the people in them (Statistics New Zealand, n.d.).

Discussion about the family within the nursing context requires a broad definition. For example, Wright and Leahey suggest that 'the family is who they say they are' (2005, p. 60). Although definitions of family vary, it is important to understand the social, cultural and political factors that might shape the way family is considered. There may be an ideal image of a family embedded in our thinking about families, but the reality is that the nature and shape of families is dynamic and the result of decades, and centuries, of social change. Family diversity, then, is a response to changing times.

Gilding (2001) observed that there have been a number of distinct eras in family structure in postcolonial Australia. The first was the era of federation, over a century ago, when families were enmeshed in wider relationships. They may have produced a variety of goods and services in the home and opened their home to guests and extended family. Middle class households employed servants (domestic service being the main source of employment for women). For the working class family, households were commonly overcrowded, experiencing difficult economic circumstances. This was a time of declining birthrate, one of the responses to which was the infant welfare movement. The declining birthrate was blamed on the 'selfishness' of women who preferred the luxuries of life over rearing children (Royal Commission, 1904, p 17, cited in Gilding, 2001). This decline was the cause of a moral panic about the population and about women's role in the family and society. In addition, the declining birthrate was a concern in both countries as each sought to develop a labour force. The effect was increased surveillance of mothering and an increasing separation of the domestic and the private from commercial and public space.

The postwar decades of the 1950s and 1960s saw the predominance of the nuclear family and the dominance of western values, despite the increasing ethnic diversity in each country. Women became 'housewives' as fewer servants were employed and households were more likely to be a single family and as the growth of the welfare state meant that financial support was more readily available (Gilding, 2001). This era promoted marriage and the family and is often reflected upon as the time of the 'traditional' family (Gilding, 2001).

During the following decades significant change was occurring to the family. In the 1970s and 1980s there was growing diversity: women increasingly entered the workforce, children stayed at home and at school longer and it was the age of sexual liberation. There were fewer marriages, more de facto relationships, more divorces and fewer children (Gilding, 2002). There was also increasing diversity in migrant families, and therefore ethnicity (Poole, 2005), as Australia became a multicultural society. For some, the family had undergone irreparable change.

Over a century of change, diversity and panic about the family might lead to a perception that the family is in decline. However, the majority of the population in Australia and New Zealand live within a family household. So the family is not in decline as such, but the characteristics of the family have changed. For example, the family of the twenty-first century is characterised by the activities and products of a technological age (Gilding, 2002).

Comparing the shape of Australian families between 1980 and 2010, the Australian Institute of Family Studies (AIFS) (2010) identifies a number of trends, including a reduction in the size of families, an increase in the age at which women are having their first child and a continuing rise in full-time and part-time employment for mothers with dependent children. Despite these changes, over time the family has remained the basic unit of society and where most children are raised (AIFS, 2010).

Similarly, an analysis of family change in New Zealand over the past 60 years notes change and increased diversity. Although generational change in family function has been seen as a demise of family life, the core functions of the family are as important today as ever, even if some activities are undertaken outside the family (Cribb, 2009).

The Families Commission (2008) provides a useful summary of four core functions of families:

1. nurturing, rearing, socialisation and protection of children
2. maintaining and improving the wellbeing of family members by providing them with emotional and material support
3. psychological 'anchorage' of adults and children by way of affection, companionship and a sense of belonging and identity
4. passing on culture, knowledge, values, attitudes, obligations and property from one generation to the next.

Understanding families within the above definitions and frameworks is critical as health professionals practise within family contexts, which are in turn influenced by community, culture and the environment.

Family diversity – the new normal

Families are increasingly becoming more diverse and complex as a result of social change. Often our view of family life is based on assumptions about what a 'normal family' is – and deviations from this view are somehow considered abnormal or pathological. Family types today comprise any of the following: couples with or without children, lone parents with children, couple families, step and blended families and grandparent families. This exemplifies the wide range of diversity across family life.

Walsh (2012) contends that the notion of a 'normal' family is socially constructed and that it is important to continue to challenge this notion as families become increasingly complex and diverse, suggesting that:

> As families have become increasingly varied over a lengthening life course, our conceptions of normality must be examined and our very definition of 'family' must be expanded to encompass a broad spectrum and fluid

---

Box 1.1 Research highlight

Assumptions are often made about the characteristics of different family groups. For example, adolescent women are often stereotyped as less able mothers. In a study by Farnell, Jones, Rowe and Sheeran (2012), the researchers examined how preterm birth affected the psychological wellbeing of adolescent mothers. They compared mothers' wellbeing, stress in terms of how women perceived their situation and social support before and after the preterm infant's discharge from a special care nursery. Young mothers reported experiencing less psychological distress and similar perceptions of control to adult mothers when their infant was in hospital. Further, and contrary to the researchers' expectations, adolescent mothers were adjusting well to motherhood 3 months after discharge and had limited but helpful sources of social support available to them. It could be that young mothers have different or fewer expectations around birth and parenting when compared with adult women and that this functions to protect their wellbeing in the face of the stressful situation presented by the birth of a preterm infant. Their experience can be normalised by health professionals who take these factors into consideration.

---

reshaping of relational and household patterns. This is the 'new normal'. (Walsh, 2012, p. 3).

For health professionals working with families it is important to challenge our assumptions and reconsider what is now considered family, as our world view can influence policy and practice development. See Box 1.1 for a research example that challenges our thinking about young mothers.

Health determinants and implications for policy

The importance of the need to provide services for children and families, prioritising prevention, support and early intervention, is well recognised (Australian Institute of Health and Welfare, 2011; NZ Ministry of Health, 2010; Siddiqi, Hertzman, Irwin & Hertzman, 2011). This approach has coincided with international recognition that children's health is not just a matter of providing services responsive to illness, but that early childhood experiences and development are fundamental to health, happiness and success during the life course (Hertzman & Boyce, 2010).

The New Zealand Well Child Tamariki Ora Framework, for instance, sets out the following agenda:

> … the primary objective … is to support families/whanau to maximise their child's developmental potential and health status from birth to five years to establish a strong foundation for ongoing healthy development. (Ministry of Health New Zealand, 1998).

A number of individual, family, community and societal characteristics need to be accounted for to meet these policy imperatives. Increasingly, the relationship between social gradient and the health of children is being recognised. Siddiqi et al. (2011)

suggest that this gradient effect implies that, with each improvement (however small) in socioeconomic resources, there is an improvement in both health and early childhood development. The authors stress the importance of early childhood development to health across the lifespan in that 'equity in early child development is imperative for bringing about health equity along the entire lifespan' (Siddiqi et al., 2011, p. 115).

Disadvantage influences health in childhood but, importantly, such disadvantage early in life is increasingly being linked with later adult health. As Graham and Power (2004, p. 673) describe it, 'childhood origins shape adult destinations', and underlying these generational continuities are the educational and social trajectories along which children steer their way to adulthood. The lifecourse framework described by Graham and Power (2004) for considering childhood disadvantage and later adult health includes the important factors of social identity, cognition and education, health behaviour and physical and emotional health.

The evidence suggests that the link between childhood disadvantage and poor adult health can be described as having four elements and is a dynamic and interactive process. The four elements are: poor childhood circumstances, a set of interlocking child-to-adult pathways, poor adult circumstances and poor adult health (Graham & Power, 2004).

One tool that synthesises the most nurturant environmental conditions for early child development is the Total Environment Assessment Model of Early Child Development (TEAM–ECD; see Figure 1.1). TEAM-ECD (Irwin et al., 2007) is rooted in Bronfenbrenner's ecological model of child development (1979) but extends this to explicate by micro (family and community) and macro (regional, national and global) environments. The model acknowledges multiple influences on early child development and the direct relationships of family out to the global environment.

The model acknowledges that early childhood development is the result of interactions between biological and environmental factors and that successful early childhood development occurs when the environment setting is nurturant (MacLeod & Betker, 2012). The AIHW also make the point that when a child has close family relationships, particularly with at least one parent, this can be protective of the risks associated with lower social gradient and economic disadvantage (AIHW, 2011). Further, MacLeod and Betker (2012) suggest that the use of an equity-based approach to providing nurturant environments can address inequalities in socioeconomic resources and that any socioeconomic gains for a family result in gains in children's developmental outcomes.

In essence, a complex set of interactions among risk and protective factors influences health, development and wellbeing and is also able to be identified at the individual, micro and macro system levels. We have mapped some of these factors in Table 1.1 in order to provide a visual display of some of the characteristics and dynamics among them that require consideration in policy and service development. You can see the interplay among a diverse range of factors in the family, and also the community beyond the family, as they potentially influence a child's health and wellbeing. You can see also the multitudinous, complex and interdependent nature of these factors. For each family a specific map could be developed. In each map some factors would have more prominence than others. Some would represent significant mechanisms of protection. Some risks would be more modifiable than others.

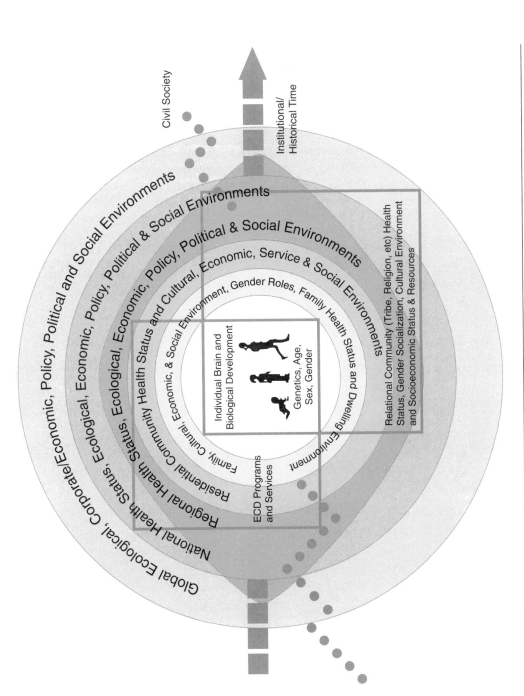

FIGURE 1.1 Total Environment Assessment Model of Early Child Development (TEAM-ECD)

Source: Irwin, Siddiqi, Hertzman Early Child Development: A Powerful Equalizer http://www.who.int/social_determinants/resources/ecd_kn_report_07_2007.pdf, page 17, 2007. HELP.

TABLE 1.1 Risk and protective factors

TEAM-ECD (Irwin et al, 2007)	RISK FACTORS FOR CHILD HEALTH, DEVELOPMENT AND WELLBEING (Compiled from a range of evidence*)	PROTECTIVE FACTORS FOR CHILD HEALTH, DEVELOPMENT AND WELLBEING	HEALTH INDICATORS FOR CHILDREN'S HEALTH, DEVELOPMENT AND WELLBEING (AIHW, 2011)
Individual brain and biological development	Young maternal age Low birthweight Prematurity Birth injury/trauma Neonatal and childhood illness Maternal illness Poor attachment and inconsistent caregiving	Secure attachment Good maternal health and nutrition Antenatal care and screening Uncomplicated birth Breastfeeding exclusively for 6 months with addition of complementary food and continued breastfeeding into the second year Continuity in and nurturing primary care givers Immunisation	Health indicators: • Smoking in pregnancy • Birthweight • Infant mortality • Breastfeeding Immunisation
Genetics	Congenital anomalies Chromosomal abnormalities		
Family cultural, economic and social environment, family health status	Prone sleeping Smoke-filled environment Lower parental education High parity, child spacing Family violence, stress and ineffective coping Single parent family Family breakdown Unstable family Death of a family member	Stable home/family Middle to higher social gradient Parent education Effective coping strategies for stressors Adequate support networks Spacing of any siblings >2 years Access to early education	Health priorities: • Oral health • BMI • Aspirational – social and emotional wellbeing Family/community priorities: • Child abuse and neglect • Aspirational – social network

			Family/community priorities: • Family income and housing
Residential community health status and cultural, economic, service and social environment/housing environment	Inadequate housing, sanitation and water supply Overcrowding Limited green space	Good community cultural identity Community health and social infrastructure, good balance of built and natural environment Adequate housing, sanitation and water supply	
Regional health status, ecological, economic, policy, political and social environments	Family isolation, poor access to health care Pollution	Geography and access to health care	
National health status, ecological, economic, policy, political and social environments	Poor national health policy, lack of health and social services	Strong national health policy Provision of universal health services	
Global ecological, corporate/economic, policy, political and social environments	War/natural disasters Economic instability	Peace and stability Global economic stability	

*Developed from Blum, McNeely & Nonnemaker (2002), National Health and Medical Research Council (NHMRC) (2002), Child and Youth Health Intergovernmental Partnership (CHIP) (2005), Prevatt (2003) and Spencer (2000).

Health priorities

Given these complex and interdependent environments influencing the health of children, it is clear that improving child health is a priority in the goal of improving health, overall. The AIHW argues that there is ample evidence for the importance of providing 'the best possible early start' investing in human capital because of the long-term impacts on the health and wellbeing of individuals and communities (2011, p. 1). However, as discussed, the greatest challenge is to address the inequalities and disadvantages that influence child health. If such disadvantages were addressed, the overall health of a society would be positively impacted. With ample evidence pointing to the importance of child health, beginning with a healthy pregnancy and maternal health, national policy and strategy is developed to provide a framework for the development of services, infrastructure support and inter-sectoral collaboration.

The Australian context

Australia began the 21st century with a public health strategic framework for children, grounded in primary healthcare principles to prevent illness, promote health and address inequalities and focused on capacity building in the healthcare sector (National Public Health Partnership, 2005). At the time of writing the chapter, policy directions remain consistent with this framework and are informed through the lens of the *Headline indicators for children's health, development and wellbeing* (AIHW, 2011). It provides a framework and system for articulating priorities that are indicative of the health, development and wellbeing of children aged 0–12 years in a database of evidence-based and measurable indicators, for the purpose of monitoring trends and change or responses to risks at national and state levels. It draws on Bronfenbrenner's model (1979) in an effort to look within and across systems that influence health, development and wellbeing. The indicators are presented in three sections: 'Health' priorities, 'Early learning and care' priorities and 'Family and community' priorities. It does not include political, ecological or global aspects of macro system thinking, rather stopping at the level of family and community.

The New Zealand context

New Zealand continues to base its policy and service development on the *New Zealand Child Health Strategy* released in 1998 by the Ministry of Health. Originally a 10-year plan, the strategy was developed to reflect the child health community's views about what was needed to improve health outcomes for children/tamariki and their families and whanau in New Zealand.

The future directions outlined in the strategy included:

- a greater focus on health promotion, prevention and early intervention
- better coordination
- the development of a national child health information strategy
- child health workforce development

Box 1.2 Practice highlight: Using TEAM-ECD in practice

1. How do you imagine the 'family' within your own social, cultural or practice context?
2. What and who has influenced your family picture?
3. To what extent does understanding of the family contribute to nursing and midwifery practice?
4. How might the TEAM-ECD model inform the way you work with children, young people and families?

Social mapping

Try to map your family and relationships, drawing on the concepts included in the Total Environment Assessment Model of Early Child Development (TEAM-ECD) described above, and try to imagine and indicate the mechanisms for getting and giving support to members of your social map.

- improvements in child health evaluation and research
- leadership in child health.

At the time of writing the chapter, this policy is under review. Limited information about likely policy and service direction is available via the Well Child homepage (www.moh.govt.nz/wellchild). However, the future directions as outlined are consistent with contemporary approaches to child health and wellbeing.

To explore your understanding of 'family', consider the critical questions and reflections in Box 1.2.

Nursing within the child, youth and family context

The involvement of nurses in the care and health of children, young people and their families has a long history in Australia, New Zealand and other parts of the world. The infant welfare movement in Australia, of which nurses were central service providers, developed in the early twentieth century in response to concerns about high infant mortality, which, together with declining fertility rates, threatened population growth (Mein Smith, 1997). Strategies aimed to educate women and to replace traditional childrearing practices with scientific rationality, a newly found concept successful in industry, now applied to the domestic sphere (Ritson, 1997; Selby, 1992). In New Zealand, Dr Truby King was most influential in the area of maternal and child welfare. A paediatrician, in 1907 he founded the Royal New Zealand Society for the Health of Women and Children, known as the Plunket Society (www.plunket.org.nz). Dr King believed that scientific doctrines regarding nutrition were the only key to reducing the death rate among children and to improving the health of the nation. As with the Australian maternal and child welfare system, his health regimen was based on the education and support of mothers and reliance on 'expert' advice from health professionals, specifically child health nurses.

There has been significant development in the discipline since these practice beginnings and recent research indicates that the essence of community child health nursing remains grounded in health promotion and education and support for maternal wellness and child health assessment (Borrow et al., 2011). In the following chapters the way in which nurses and others contribute to the health of children, young people and their families will be explored, and you will find the concepts presented here are applied in a number of ways.

In the contemporary context, child health services are developed in response to policy and strategy at the national or local level, and are based on priority health areas, with varying levels of input from nurses and midwives into this process. The shopfront of practice is diverse, from community and outreach centres and hospitals to telephone, telemedicine and internet bases. In these settings, nurses are challenged by the question of how to occupy the space between service agendas and family needs – that is, how to maintain a focus on the individual, while also providing targeted, population-based practice (Barnes, Courtney, Pratt & Walsh, 2003; Borrow, Munns & Henderson, 2011).

Increasingly, the work of nurses and midwives is that of knowledge worker, helping families make sense of the vast amount of information readily available. Consumers often come to a health activity informed and aware – this has necessitated a shift in health professionals' perspective from that of an 'expert' to one of health partner – and practice has needed to change accordingly. Frameworks for practice emphasise the care partnership, are strengths-based and solution-focused and demonstrate this shift.

Conclusion

In this chapter, we have outlined the way in which the family is perceived today. In doing this, contemporary definitions of family are provided, and the dynamic and changing nature of the family discussed. Importantly, discussion of child health priorities is underpinned by an understanding of the influence of social gradient on child health as well as health in later life. Understanding these concepts is essential to practice where policy and programs are driven by epidemiological and demographic data.

Working with children, young people and families requires an understanding of the interplay between social, community and family influences; biology and the environment; and risk or protective factors for health, development and wellbeing. Understanding risk and protective factors informs approaches to program development, service delivery and individual interactions, and can be applied to partnership and strengths-based practice frameworks.

KEY POINTS

» The contemporary family is changing and dynamic.
» Your view of what constitutes 'family' may be different from that of others.
» There is significant social and cultural diversity in families.
» A number of interdependent individual, family and community factors serve risk and protective functions for the developing child's health and wellbeing.

» Social gradient influences child health.

» Childhood disadvantage influences adult health.

» Health priorities and targets are determined at international, national and local levels.

» Strengths-based family assessment approaches provide skills for nurses to work in partnership with families to shape family function, help families meet their healthcare needs and increase resilience.

CRITICAL QUESTIONS AND REFLECTIONS

As you work through the chapters in this text a number of frameworks will be introduced, for example in Chapter 5, *The Australian Family Strengths Nursing Guide*. Other frameworks you may like to explore further as you work through the text include:

1. *Solution focused nursing* (McAllister, 2007)

2. the Family Partnership model, implemented in both Australia and New Zealand, developed by Hilton Davis and Crispin Day from the UK Centre for Parent and Child Support

3. the Australian Nurse–Family Partnership Program model, based on the work of David Olds (http://www.anfpp.com.au/).

USEFUL RESOURCES

Australian Bureau of Statistics: www.abs.gov.au

Australian Institute of Family Studies: www.aifs.gov.au

New Zealand Government, *New Zealand Families Today*: http://www.msd.govt.nz/about-msd-and-our-work/publications-resources/research/nz-families-today/index.html

References

Australian Bureau of Statistics (ABS). (2006). *Census Dictionary Reissue*. Retrieved from http://www.abs.gov.au/Ausstats/abs@.nsf/0/014F8C1E2D27DFF8CA25720A0010F03D?opendocument (accessed 14 October 2012).

Australian Institute of Family Studies. (2010). *Families then and now 1980–2010*. Melbourne: Commonwealth of Australia.

Australian Institute of Health and Welfare (AIHW). (2011). *Headline indicators for children's health, development and wellbeing 2011* [Cat. no. PHE 144]. Canberra: AIHW.

Barnes, M., Courtney, M., Pratt, J., & Walsh, A. (2003). Contemporary child health nursing practice: services provided and challenges faced in metropolitan and outer Brisbane areas. *Collegian, 10*(4), 14–19.

Blum, R. W., McNeely, C., & Nonnemaker, J. (2002). Vulnerability, risk and protection. *Journal of Adolescent Health, 31S*, 28–39.

Borrow, S., Munns, A., & Henderson, S. (2011). Community-based child health nurses: an exploration of current practice. *Contemporary Nurse, 40*(1), 71–86.

Bronfenbrenner, U. (1979). *The ecology of human development: Experiments by nature and design*. Boston: Harvard College.

Cribb, J. (2009). Focus on families: New Zealand families of yesterday, today and tomorrow. *Social Policy Journal of New Zealand, 35*, 4–16.

Child and Youth Health Intergovernmental Partnership (CHIP). (2005). *The strategic framework, healthy children – Strengthening promotion and prevention across Australia. National Public Health Strategic Framework for Children 2005–2008*. Retrieved from http://www.nphp.gov.au/workprog/chip/cyhactionplanbg.htm (accessed 22 January 2013).

Families Commission. (2008). *The Kiwi nest: 60 years of change in New Zealand families*. Wellington: Families Commission.

Farnell, L., Jones, L., Rowe, J., et al. (2012). Effects of age and the preterm birth of an infant on adolescent mothers' psychological adjustment. *Children's Health Care, 41*(4), 302–321.

Featherstone, B. (2004). *Family life and family support. A feminist analysis*. Houndmills, UK: Palgrave.

Gilding, M. (2001). Changing families in Australia 1901–2001. *Family Matters, 60*, 6–11.

Gilding, M. (2002). Families of the new millennium. Designer babies, cyber sex and virtual communities. *Family Matters, 62*, 4–10.

Graham, H., & Power, C. (2004). Childhood disadvantage and health inequalities: a framework for policy based on lifecourse research. *Child: Care, Health and Development, 30*(6), 671–678.

Hertzman, C., & Boyce, T. (2010). How experience gets under the skin to create gradients in developmental health. *Annual Review of Public Health, 31*, 329–347.

Irwin, L., Siddiqi, A., & Hertzman, C. (2007). *Early child development: A powerful equalizer. Final report for the World Health Organization's Commission on the Social Determinants of Health*. Vancouver: Human Early Learning Partnership (HELP).

Lodge, J., Moloney, L., & Robinson, E. (2011). *Domestic and family violence: A review of the literature. A report for the Department of Human Services*. Melbourne: Australian Institute of Family Studies.

MacLeod, A., & Betker, C. (2012). *Antoinette's story: An introduction to an early child development model of care and post-natal home visiting scenario*. Vancouver: Human Early Learning Partnership with the National Collaborating Centre for Determinants of Health.

McAllister, M. (2007). An introduction to solution-focused nursing. In M. McAllister (Ed.), *Solution focused nursing. Rethinking practice* (pp. 49–62). Houndmills, UK: Palgrave.

Mein Smith, P. (1997). *Mothers and king baby: Infant survival and welfare in an imperial world: Australia 1880–1950*. London: Macmillan.

Ministry of Health New Zealand (MOH NZ). (1998). *Child health strategy*. Wellington: MOH NZ. Retrieved from http://www.health.govt.nz/publication/child-health-strategy (22 January 2013).

National Health and Medical Research Council (NHMRC), Child and Youth Health Intergovernmental Partnership (CHIP). (2002). *Child health screening and surveillance: A critical review: Supplementary document-context and next steps*. Canberra: NHMRC.

National Public Health Partnership. (2005). *Healthy children — Strengthening promotion and prevention across Australia. National Public Health Strategic Framework for Children 2005–2008*. Retrieved from http://www.nphp.gov.au/workprog/chip/documents/chip_backgrd_paper_sep.pdf (accessed 31 January 2013).

NZ Ministry of Health. (2010). *Changes to the well child/tamariki ora framework*. Wellington: Ministry of Health. Retrieved from http://www.health.govt.nz/publication/changes-well-child-tamariki-ora-framework (accessed 22 January 2013).

Poole, M. (2005). Changing families, changing times. In M. Poole (Ed.), *Family: Changing families and changing times* (pp. 1–19). Sydney: Allen & Unwin.

Prevatt, F. (2003). The contribution of parenting practices in a risk and resiliency model of children's adjustment. *British Journal of Developmental Psychology, 21*, 469–480.

Ritson, R. (1997). The birth of the clinic. *Transition, 54*(55), 42–53.

Selby, W. (1992). Motherhood in Labor's Queensland 1915–1957. Unpublished PhD thesis. Griffith University, Nathan, Queensland.

Siddiqi, A., Hertzman, E., Irwin, L., et al. (2011). Early child development: a powerful equalizer. In J. Lee & R. Sadana (Eds.), *Improving equity in health by addressing social determinants*. The Commission on Social Determinants in Health Networks, Geneva: WHO.

Spencer, N. (2000). Social gradients in child health: why do they occur and what can paediatricians do about them? *Ambulatory Child Health, 6*, 191–202.

Statistics New Zealand. (n.d.). Retrieved from www.stats.govt.nz (accessed 19 September 2012).

Walsh, F. (2012). The new normal: diversity and complexity in 21st century families. In F. Walsh (Ed.), *Normal family processes* (4th ed.). New York: Guilford Publications.

Wright, L., & Leahey, M. (2005). *Nurses and families: a guide to family assessment and intervention* (4th ed.). Philadelphia: FA Davis.

Chapter 2

DEVELOPING HEALTHCARE PROGRAMS FOR THE CHILD, YOUNG PERSON AND FAMILY

Karen McBride-Henry, Jane Gregg, Rachel Cole

LEARNING OUTCOMES

Reading this chapter will help you to:

» understand how policy influences healthcare programs

» identify current global and national health-related policies that influence healthcare programs for the child, young person and family at the regional and local levels

» discuss the role of nurses and midwives as change agents through their participation in health policy processes and healthcare programs

» understand how to use health promotion to develop sustainable healthcare programs, including needs assessment, planning, implementation and evaluation

» discuss the importance of collaborative partnerships in developing healthcare programs for the child, young person and family.

Introduction

There has been an increase over recent years in health-related policy and healthcare programs globally and nationally focused on the health and wellbeing of the child, young person and family. This focus is important because it influences the day-to-day practice of nurses and midwives who work with children, young people and families. Nurses and midwives play a key role in translating policy into practice through the development of healthcare programs as well as being involved in the policy-making process at regional and local levels.

The World Health Organization (WHO) has a long-standing definition of a program as 'an organized aggregate of activities directed towards the attainment of defined objectives and targets' (1984a, p. 4). Objectives and targets are reflected in health policies and/or strategies established by international organisations, national and state governments and regional health service providers. Healthcare programs are the mechanism through which such policies are implemented; therefore, they need to address policy aims as well as serving the needs of the community for whom they are intended.

This chapter explores healthcare program development as it relates to midwives and nurses working with children, young people and families. It discusses how government health policies set the context in which such programs exist, and presents a health promotion framework for developing, implementing and evaluating sustainable healthcare programs, using examples drawn from the authors' experience in Australia and New Zealand.

Understanding the policy context

Nurses and midwives working in the community have many opportunities to become involved in the public policy-making process that can lead to the development, implementation and evaluation of healthcare programs. The majority of nurses and midwives are involved in translating policy into practice (Armstrong, Waters, Dobbins et al., 2011; Waters, Armstrong, Swinburn et al., 2011). A recent example of the key role nurses and midwives can play was the development of the policy guidelines *Improving Maternity Services: Working Together Across WA* (Department of Human Services, 2007) by a multidisciplinary team of policymakers, medical doctors, maternal and child health nurses and midwives. These guidelines were developed to support the provision of quality care for women, infants and young children, with a focus on issues such as safety, child development and workforce needs. They were also designed to ensure continuity of care across the full spectrum of maternity and child health services. The protocols were launched in Western Australia in 2007 (Department of Human Services, 2007), and are now being used across the state by public hospitals and the Maternal and Child Health Service. Although program implementation may be quite removed from their day-to-day activities, nurses and midwives need to understand that they have a significant influence on health priorities, and the availability of funding for healthcare programs, at regional and local levels.

Many early childhood programs have been developed in New Zealand and Australia over the past decade, reflecting the integral role that successful early childhood policy has played in the development of new programs. See Table 2.1 for

TABLE 2.1 Linking policy to program development

GLOBAL POLICY LEVEL	GOVERNMENT OR SECTOR POLICY LEVEL	PROGRAM LEVEL
	New Zealand examples	
Ten steps to successful breastfeeding (World Health Organization & UNICEF, 1989)	The Ministry of Health New Zealand (MOH NZ) subsequently developed Breastfeeding: A guide to action (2002) to support and improve breastfeeding rates. It was intended that the action plan would assist healthcare professionals to achieve Baby Friendly Hospital status, based on the Ten steps to successful breastfeeding. In 2007 the MOH NZ identified the importance of breastfeeding by making it one of the country's health targets, which aims to improve the breastfeeding initiation and duration rates.	Different district health boards (DHBs) and small maternity hospitals are now required to demonstrate how they are working to improve breastfeeding rates. In addition, Baby Friendly Hospital accreditation must be gained and/or maintained.
Ottawa Charter for Health Promotion (World Health Organization, 1986)	The Primary Health Care Strategy created by MOHNZ (2001), is still guiding the provision of health care in 2012. Its key aims are to provide population-based health care and promote the role of the community in health promotion and preventive care. DHBs respond by adjusting organisational visions and aligning planning and funding with the policy.	A policy and guidelines group in a child health service embraces a philosophy of 'seamless care', which emphasises integrated, interdisciplinary collaboration to improve healthcare delivery. This results in a program that crosses traditional tertiary and community healthcare boundaries (see Box 2.1, Practice highlight).

GLOBAL POLICY LEVEL	GOVERNMENT OR SECTOR POLICY LEVEL	PROGRAM LEVEL
	Australian examples	
Adelaide Statement of Health in All Policies (HiAP): Moving Towards a Shared Governance for Health and Well-being (Government of South Australia, 2009 and WHO, 2010) The aim of this policy is to address social determinants of health through the policies of all government departments and reduce health inequity. HiAP is based on a whole-of-government approach. Areas of focus include education and early life.	The South Australian (SA) Government endorsed the application of HiAP across government in 2007. The SA HiAP model was subsequently developed to support its implementation. The SA HiAP model has two key components: a centralised governance structure and the Health Lens Assessment process.	Priority policies across government are identified annually by the SA Department of Health (DoH) in collaboration with the Department of the Premier and Cabinet. Lead agencies for these policies are invited to work with the DoH to implement the Health Lens Assessment process (similar to a Health Impact Assessment) prior to a policy being developed. An example of the application of the Health Lens Assessment has been in the area of improving education outcomes in low socioeconomic status communities in partnership with the Department of Education and Children Services.
Closing the Gap in a Generation: Health equity through action on the social determinants of health 2008 (WHO, 2008 and Commission on the Social Determinants of Health) This policy provides recommendations for action to address inequities within and between countries within a generation. It calls on all governments of member state countries, which include New Zealand and Australia, to respond to these recommendations at the national level.	The Closing the Gap initiative of the Council of Australian Governments (COAG) is a commitment by national and state/territory governments to close the life expectancy gap between Indigenous and non-Indigenous Australians within a generation. The targets of the policy are to halve: the mortality rate of Indigenous children under 5 years; the gap in reading, writing and numeracy achievements within a decade; and the gap for Indigenous students in year 12 attainment rates by 2020; and to ensure access to early childhood education for all Indigenous 4-year-olds in remote communities within 5 years. Over 40 organisations are working together on programs in the areas of early childhood, schooling, health, economic participation, healthy home, safe communities and governance and leadership to achieve these targets.	The Queensland Government has produced the Making Tracks Towards Closing the Gap in Health Outcomes for Indigenous Queenslanders by 2033 – Policy and Accountability Framework (Queensland Health, 2010b). Focus areas of this framework include: a healthy and safe start to life; reducing modifiable chronic disease risk factors; improving living environments; developing cultural competence of the health workforce; and working with the Aboriginal and Torres Strait Islander controlled health sector. Subsequently, Making Tracks Toward Closing the Gap in Health Outcomes for Indigenous Queenslanders by 2033: Implementation Plan 2009–10 to 2011–12 was produced and identifies a range of healthcare programs focused on children, women and families (Queensland Health, 2010c).

examples in both countries. These successes have been supported by evidence-based research (Waters et al., 2011) and a response to informed community need (Rohleder & Apatu, 2009). It is important, therefore, that nurses and midwives have an understanding and working knowledge of the international and national policies relevant to their day-to-day practice. Developing, implementing and evaluating healthcare programs generally relies on funding from a local, regional, state and/or national level government agency, and aligns with current healthcare policy directions. Effective policy development requires input and support from frontline staff, for example through the participation of nurses and midwives in multidisciplinary teams. They also require knowledge and skills in the development of healthcare programs.

Developing healthcare programs

Nurses and midwives have an important role in developing programs for the child, young person and family within the healthcare system they work in. They also have a role in influencing programs in other healthcare systems and non-health organisations whose core business impacts the health and wellbeing of the child, young person and family. Child and family healthcare programs in Australia and New Zealand exist within the context of global and national health policies. Such policies determine health priorities, such as improving immunisation rates, vision screening programs for 4-year-olds or enhancing youth mental health. When proposing or establishing a healthcare program, consideration must be given to the relevant health policies that support it. For infants, children and young people, early intervention is vital and there are many more programs now focused on the early years. The development, implementation and evaluation of such programs utilise health promotion knowledge and skills. It is therefore important to review the principles of health promotion, as prevention and early intervention represent the core practice of nurses and midwives who work with children, youth and families.

The following principles of health promotion were originally developed by a World Health Organization (WHO) working party (1984b, p. 20). They highlight the key elements of what constitutes health promotion and are a good starting point when considering the development of any healthcare program:

1. Health promotion involves the population as a whole in the context of their everyday life, rather than focusing on people at risk for specific diseases. It enables people to take control over, and responsibility for, their health as an important component of everyday life, both as spontaneous and organised action for health.

2. Health promotion is directed towards action on the determinants of health. Health promotion action addresses the inter-related individual level and the social, cultural, economic, political, physical and natural environmental determinants of health. As in primary healthcare, health promotion also acknowledges that the majority of health care occurs outside the health sector, therefore, requires cooperation of sectors beyond health services. Governments at local and national levels have responsibility to act appropriately in a timely way to ensure that the 'total' environment, which is beyond the control of individuals and groups, is conducive to health.

3. Health promotion combines diverse, but complementary, strategies and/or approaches, including communication, education, policy and legislation, fiscal measures, organizational change, community development and spontaneous local activities against health hazards. Combinations of these strategies are used to achieve the subsequent Ottawa Charter action areas including: building healthy public policy; developing personal skills; creating supportive environments; strengthening community action; and reorienting health services. (WHO, 1986).

4. Health promotion aims particularly at effective and concrete public participation. This requires the development of problem-defining and decision-making life skills, both individually and collectively.

5. While health promotion is basically an activity in the health and social fields, and not a medical service, health professionals – particularly in primary health care – have an important role in nurturing and enabling health promotion. Health professionals should work outwards developing their special contributions in education and health advocacy.

Principles have also been developed for working in health promotion with Indigenous peoples. One such set of principles, the Iga Warta Principles, states:

1. The project must be sustainable, that is, in funding, leadership, coordination and continuously evaluated.

2. It must have a pro-active/preventative approach, that is, addresses the need to 'get in early'.

3. It must address the environmental determinants of health, that is, food water, housing and unemployment.

4. It must have an Aboriginal community and family approach, that is, it must address the need to empower Aboriginal communities and families and enhance their traditional guiding function over Aboriginal people.

5. It must respect Aboriginal time and space, that is, it should be culturally sensitive.

6. It must address the need for coordination and continuity between regions and cities, that is, strategies must be coordinated with other activities in other sectors, for example, transport, housing, example, transport, housing, education which offer the potential to strengthen health outcomes. (Government of South Australia Department of Health, 2007).

In addition to the above principles, the *Bangkok Charter for Health Promotion in a Globalized World* (World Health Organization, 2005, pp. 4–5) outlines four statements of philosophical intent that should underpin the development of all health promotion programs. They include making the promotion of health central to the global development agenda, a core responsibility for all governments, a key focus of communities and civil society and a requirement for good corporate practice.

More recently, the scope for nurses to enable populations not only at the coalface of delivering healthcare programs but also through active participation in the development of policy and program development is gathering momentum. Edelman and Mandle (2006, p. 613) are of the view that nurses need to consider three principal goals with respect to health promotion and program development:

1. participate in health promotion policy development
2. influence public expectations about health promotion
3. promote equitable access to preventive health care.

These principles underpin global, national and local policies, which in turn inform and underpin all healthcare program development. When actioned, these principles ensure a more integrated, informed and unified approach to health programs, removing the 'silo' nature of health care.

Global health policy perspective

Global health organisations such as the WHO and the United Nations Children's Fund (UNICEF) provide guidance on global health issues, which informs the decision makers in individual countries who are responsible for setting health priorities, policies and programs. These organisations attempt to focus the attention of individual nations on healthcare programs that are considered to be of the utmost importance from a global perspective. One example of a current priority is providing amenities and opportunities for marginalised and impoverished children in urban areas through a range of infrastructure, resourcing and partnership strategies (UNICEF, 2012).

For example, the *United Nations Convention on the Rights of the Child* or UNCROC (1990 article 24) states that supporting nations must 'recognise the rights of the child to the enjoyment of the highest attainable standard of health and to facilities for the treatment of illness and rehabilitation'. It also states that governments should ensure that children be given the right to access appropriate health care, which means that governments must embrace this right when planning child and family health policy and programs at a national level. An example of the flow-through of prioritisation at a global level to national policy and subsequent program initiatives is set out in Box 2.1. This example describes how global policy has influenced national policy and planning of breastfeeding programs in New Zealand.

A common theme running through global health policy is the need for improved health literacy. Health literacy is, therefore, a key aspect of national policies and program development and relevant in the everyday work of nurses and midwives. Health literacy is defined as 'the degree to which individuals have the capacity to obtain, process and understand basic health information and services in order to make informed and appropriate health decisions' (Kickbusch, Wait & Maag, 2005). Leaders in the field of health literacy are providing useful global challenges for us all, with experts arguing for the need to ensure that people have access to community-focused programs and targeted health education. It is only through appropriately targeted programs that health inequalities are minimised and health literacy skills are enhanced (Lynch, Law, Brinkman, Chittleborough & Sawyer, 2010; Peerson & Saunders, 2009).

Going beyond the notion of information dissemination, health literacy seeks to increase the accessibility of information and motivation for engaging in health-seeking behaviours. Health literacy is an issue that nurses and midwives deal with daily and is an important consideration for all healthcare programs.

Box 2.1 Practice highlight: Applying global policy – national programs for promoting breastfeeding in New Zealand

Global policy

In 1990, WHO and UNICEF produced the *Innocenti Declaration: Breastfeeding in the 1990s – a global treatise* (World Health Organization & UNICEF, 1990). In addition, the *Global Strategy for Infant and Young Child Feeding* was released in 2003 (World Health Organization & UNICEF, 2003). These documents aimed to promote breastfeeding globally, enable women to practise exclusive breastfeeding and to pressure governments to implement policies that would support women to breastfeed. The declaration argued the optimal nutritive qualities of breastfeeding for growth and development and its role in reducing infant morbidity and mortality, enhancing women's health and producing economic benefits. It stipulated exclusive breastfeeding for all infants to 6 months of age and that breastfeeding be maintained to age 2 years.

The *Innocenti Declaration* sets out targets for individual countries to achieve, and strategies to help meet the targets. These include:

1. the appointment of a national breastfeeding coordinator
2. the establishment of a multisector national breastfeeding committee
3. ensuring hospitals support the '10 steps to successful breastfeeding', and
4. compliance with the 'International code for the marketing of breast-milk substitutes', and legislation to protect breastfeeding women.

When the *Global Strategy for Infant and Young Child Feeding* was released, the authors recognised that not all of the above steps had been implemented by governments and there was a renewed need for additional work on this important child health issue.

National policy

In New Zealand, the Department of Health (now called the Ministry of Health) signalled its support for the *Innocenti Declaration* (Gordon, 1998; Vogel & Mitchell, 1998), and a meeting was convened in 1991 to reconsider the code's place within New Zealand; however, little action was taken. In 1999, the Ministry of Health established clear breastfeeding definitions and, in, 2002, established national breastfeeding targets and a breastfeeding action plan (Ministry of Health New Zealand, 2002). In 2009 The National Breastfeeding Advisory Committee of New Zealand published a document titled *National Strategic Plan of Action for Breastfeeding 2008–2012 (2009)*, which examined how the New Zealand Government was doing in relation to the WHO and UNICEF strategy documents on breastfeeding.

Programs

In 1998, the New Zealand Breastfeeding Authority (n.d.) was established to coordinate the many breastfeeding stakeholders and oversee the Baby Friendly Hospital Initiative (BFHI) (see Chapter 6 for more information), a program promoted by WHO and known to increase breastfeeding rates. In addition, the MOH has also established the Breastfeeding Peer Counsellor Program, which is an initiative that provides training for women who have breastfed to help others to establish breastfeeding support within their own communities. This program supports Step 10 of the BFHI, the Global Strategy for Infant and Young Child Feeding and the *Innocenti Declaration*.

Outstanding issues

1. No legislation requiring compliance with the code has been developed and monitoring and compliance remain voluntary.
2. Breastfeeding rates have shown little change in the past decade.

The national health policy perspective

New Zealand and Australia both have national mechanisms for developing health policy and programs. Understanding national planning pathways is central to healthcare program development. An overview of healthcare policies for each country follows with a specific focus on child health policy development.

New Zealand

The New Zealand government plans and directs the provision of health care for its citizens through the Ministry of Health (MOH NZ), which is charged with implementing health-related legislation, such as the *New Zealand Public Health and Disability Act* (Ministry of Health New Zealand, 2000a), and the development of nation-wide health strategies and policy. Policy and program development at MOH NZ takes into account the recommendations of WHO and other international organisations, with child healthcare direction based on documents such as the UNCROC.

A number of key national strategies continue to have a significant ongoing effect on healthcare provision for children and their families in New Zealand, despite having been developed over 10 years ago. These include the *Child Health Strategy* (Ministry of Health New Zealand, 1998), which was introduced in Chapter 1, the *New Zealand Health Strategy* (Ministry of Health New Zealand, 2000b) and the *Primary Health Care Strategy* (Ministry of Health New Zealand, 2001). These documents highlight the nation's goals and direction for care provision.

The vision for children's health care set out in *Child Health Strategy* (MOH NZ, 1998) is 'our children/tamariki: seen, heard and getting what they need' (p. vii). The strategy outlines a number of guiding principles for the development of child health programs in New Zealand, including: children's needs are paramount, childcare services should be based on 'international best practice, research and education' (p. 19) and childcare services should be culturally acceptable and safe. It also acknowledges that services require regular review to ensure they continue to meet the changing needs of children and families.

The *New Zealand Health Strategy* is based on similar principles, but highlights the special relationship between Maori and the Crown under the Treaty of Waitangi. It sets out a number of health objectives, based on emergent health determinants, which include improving nutrition, increasing the level of physical activity, reducing obesity, improving oral health and reducing community violence.

The *Primary Health Care Strategy* identifies six key goals that include: working with local communities; identifying and removing health inequalities; improving access to comprehensive services so that health can be improved, maintained and restored; the coordination of care across services; workforce development; and continuous quality improvement.

Australia

The Australian federal government shares responsibility for health services with the states and territories through the Council of Australian Governments (COAG). A subcommittee of COAG is the Standing Council on Health, which includes the Australian Health Ministers' Advisory Council (AHMAC) whose responsibility it is to oversee the achievement of COAG's strategic health themes by establishing funding arrangements and jurisdictional responsibilities (AHMAC, 2012). The three key federal government departments involved with child health and parenting are: the Department of Health and Ageing; the Department of Families, Community Services and Indigenous Affairs; and the Department of Education, Employment and Workplace Relations. A number of other national bodies also influence child health policy and programs, including the Australian Research Alliance for Children and Youth, the National Health and Medical Research Council and the Australian Institute of Family Studies. Key national strategies that impact on the children, young persons and families in Australia include the *Investing in the Early Years – A National Early Childhood Development Strategy* (Commonwealth of Australia, 2009a), *Australia: The Healthiest Country by 2020: National Preventative Health Strategy – The Roadmap for Action* (Commonwealth of Australia, 2009b) and the *National Primary Health Care Strategy 2009* (Department of Health and Ageing, 2008).

The *Investing in the Early Years Strategy* was released in 2009 by COAG and has the vision that by 2020 all children have the best start in life to create a better future for themselves and the nation. The strategy has six focus areas: holistic child development across cognitive, learning, physical, social, emotional and cultural dimensions; whole of early childhood from the antenatal to 8 years; all children with an emphasis on those most in need to reduce social equalities; promoting protective factors, such as secure bonding with a primary carer, good nutrition and stimulating play-based learning, and reducing risks, such as abuse/neglect or poor diet; the whole service system, including universal and targeted across sectors such as maternal, child and family health, support for parents, and play-based learning and care; and respect for diversity and difference to develop a positive sense of self and culture (Council of Australian Governments, 2009).

The *National Preventative Heath Taskforce* was established in 2008 to facilitate the development of the National Preventative Health Strategy (Commonwealth of Australia, 2009b). The strategy was released in June 2009 with the goal of making Australia the healthiest nation by 2020. It focuses on a range of prevention strategies to address the initial priorities of tobacco use, obesity and the excessive consumption of alcohol. All of these areas include specific targets for children and/or young people. States and territories, in turn, are funded to deliver on these priorities via partnership agreements. For example, the state of Queensland has developed *Preventative Health: Strategic Directions 2010–2013*, which includes healthy children and healthy communities as program areas (Queensland Health, 2010a).

The *National Primary Health Care Strategy* was released in 2009 and the subsequent establishment of primary health care organisations, known as Medicare Locals, to increase the capacity of health services to deliver primary health care (Department of Health and Ageing, 2008). These reform initiatives provide direction on delivering frontline care and healthcare programs at the local community level. Focus areas of interest to children, young people and families include rewarding prevention, management of chronic disease and multidisciplinary team-based care.

However, it is important to note that the consideration of child health issues is not restricted to health and community service agencies. Australian governments at the national, state and local levels all recognise the need to consider children and their families when developing any new policies or programs. For example, policy related to road safety integrates research findings on road accidents involving children; similarly, policy on juvenile justice incorporates knowledge of the factors that contribute to young people coming into conflict with the law, such as providing drug diversion programs for minor drug offences. Non-government organisations such as Kidsafe also exist to ensure child health issues are being met. Kidsafe produces resources and works with governments to develop policy to prevent unintentional childhood injuries (Child Accident Prevention Foundation of Australia, 2012).

The local health policy perspective

National policy provides guidance in New Zealand for DHBs and in Australia for state and local government and regional health authorities when planning healthcare program delivery and the distribution of funding, and ensures alignment with national healthcare goals. Local demographics and health determinants are also important influences at the local level and affect and influence program development and uptake by individual DHBs (in New Zealand) or local government authorities and regionalised health services (in Australia). These are the local context issues that might first impress nurses and midwives in their everyday practice and are most likely to influence them when they are developing child and family health programs at the local level.

Policymaking and developing healthcare programs

It is well established that there is a need for integrated approaches to the development of policies and programs to minimise inequalities across populations, including addressing issues such as housing, access to high quality child care and flexible work schedules such as family-friendly work policies as well as traditional health programs (Lynch et al., 2010). Experts have identified challenges in the process of translating policy to practice referred to as a 'translation gap' (Lynch et al., 2010). Translating policy into practice is a key challenge for nurses and midwives in their day-to-day work and requires an understanding of the policy-making and program development processes.

So what does the policy-making process and subsequent program development look like? So far we have looked at the role of policy in determining priority areas of focus at global and national levels, and how these policies influence policies and healthcare programs at the regional and local level. Developing healthy public policy is also a key action area in the Ottawa Charter for Health Promotion and a foundation strategy of any healthcare program. The WHO describe healthy public policy as that which is concerned with health and equity in all policy areas, and accountable for health impact, with the aim of creating social, economic, cultural and physical environments that support people to live healthy lives (WHO, 1988).

Lynch and colleagues (2010) highlight that all those involved in policy development, including healthcare providers, have a role to play in the implementation of policy. This requires that effective healthcare programs are developed and that the 'translation gap' between policy and implementation is minimised. This is achieved through programs that include due consideration to 'governance, accountability, financing, training, consultation and workforce capacity', all of which determine the effectiveness of a program (Lynch et al., 2010, p. 1245).

Research conducted by Edgecombe in 1992 examined the role that nurses and midwives who work with children, youth and families played in a policy-making process in one Australian state over several decades (from the 1950s). Findings provide insight into the complex process of taking policy and applying it in practice through healthcare programs in often complex healthcare systems.

Policy processes are not linear and there are a number of policy-making models used in health promotion to guide the process. Policy-making models follow a similar trajectory that involves the identification of the issue to be addressed, formulation of policy to address the issue, implementation and evaluation of the policy process and outcomes. A commonly used conceptual framework for making healthy public policy is that of Milio (1987). It is useful for nurses and midwives to familiarise themselves with this and other policy-making frameworks. Some aspects of the policy process take place simultaneously, while other policy processes may take years before a program is eventually developed and implemented.

There are a number of processes that must be undertaken prior to establishing any healthcare program. The link between global and national policy as these relate to healthcare programs has been set out above. The importance of understanding this link is critical to planning any healthcare program that targets child and family health. In the following sections we present a framework to guide the development of a nursing or midwifery healthcare program.

There are a number of health promotion frameworks that can be used to guide the development of healthcare programs. The framework adopted in this chapter is presented in Figure 2.1 and includes the following four broad stages: identifying and

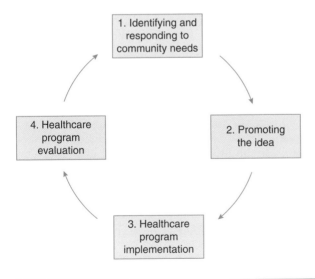

FIGURE 2.1 Healthcare program development framework

responding to community needs; promoting the idea; implementation; and evaluation. A description of each stage including key considerations and activities follows.

Stage one: Identifying and responding to community needs

Stage one, and a prerequisite for establishing any healthcare program, is understanding the health needs and priorities of the community. This is consistent with both the first and second WHO (1984b) principles of health promotion presented earlier that focus on understanding the community as a whole as well as the determinants of health. This process typically requires a community needs analysis, which assesses the demographics, health status, health behaviours and the social, economic, physical, cultural and political determinants and infrastructure of a community. The needs analysis data are collected via a range of sources including existing epidemiological and demographic information, such as *Headline Indicators for Children's Heath, Development and Wellbeing 2011* (AIHW, 2011) and *Children and Youth* (Australian Bureau of Statistics, 2006), and community consultation. A range of methods is used to collect this data including surveys, focus groups and interviews. For example, of interest might be the number and percentage of children in an area, average household income, ethnic make-up, avoidable hospital admission rates, infectious disease rates and reported violence rates as well as morbidity and mortality data.

Ethical consideration needs to be given to the collection of data from multicultural communities such as in Australia and New Zealand. A strategy to ensure data are collected appropriately from people of different ethnic backgrounds is to utilise someone from the same ethnic background. In addition, knowledge of all available primary and secondary health services and resources to address the health issue is important. This information provides essential insight into the health service gaps within the community with attention to where inequities exist.

It is also important to establish working relationships with community groups to help identify the health needs within communities (Harris & Harris, 2011). For example, if you wanted to develop a targeted program for increasing immunisation rates within a certain geographic area, there are a number of ways that community's needs could be assessed. First, it would be important to understand which groups of children are most likely to be fully immunised and which are not. Conducting a comprehensive literature search on successful immunisation initiatives might help you identify appropriate strategies to address the issue. An assessment of services available in the community to support and promote vaccination initiatives, as well as identification of potential barriers to the uptake of vaccinations, would also be key early steps to take. Speaking directly to health professionals, or others, who are working with young families may also give valuable insights, as would focus group discussions with families in the community.

Another method for identifying and responding to community need is a health impact assessment (HIA). This offers a comprehensive approach to identifying the impacts, both positive and negative, of a proposed program on a community prior to its implementation (Public Health Advisory Committee, 2005). An example of an HIA was produced by the Hawke's Bay District Health Board in New Zealand when they were examining how to best implement an oral health strategy (Rohleder & Apatu, 2009). Those involved with the HIA engaged in a four-stage process, which included screening, scoping, appraising/reporting and evaluation (p. 13). To achieve these four phases those involved engaged in activities such as a literature search, community input and meetings with key stakeholders from the community and the Hawke's Bay Regional Council. The outcome of this HIA was a well-developed plan, which the community was involved in building and committed to achieving.

Stage two: Promoting the idea

After the needs analysis has been completed, the next step is to assemble a team of people with an interest in the health issue. For example, a team that emerged through the process of undertaking an HIA may form the basis of a partnership to support and progress the development of a program to address the issue. For an example of how an HIA led to the development of such a partnership, refer to the HIA developed by Rohleder and Apatu (2009). The partnership to progress a children, young people or family health issue may ideally consist of representatives from the health, education and social services sectors who have an interest in the community, and a working knowledge of community strengths and potential service gaps. From this position, the team can assist in determining possible solutions to the issue and develop the healthcare program plan. A healthcare program plan generally specifies the goal, objectives, strategies to be employed, sequence of activities to achieve strategies and resources required, evaluation, a communication strategy, a realistic budget and the identification and engagement of local stakeholders required to deliver the program. A well-developed healthcare program plan will greatly assist the implementation of healthcare programs and most organisations have preferred project planning templates.

The engagement of local stakeholders is especially important and a foundation health promotion principle, as having strong relationships with key community members and groups is essential when advocating for, and gauging the level of support for, a program within the wider community (WHO, 1984). For example, if you are seeking to develop a breastfeeding promotion program, it would be beneficial to develop strong relationships with the community and other key stakeholders such as appropriate women's community groups, community leaders, early childhood education providers, public health nurses, maternal and child health nurses, Plunket nurses (community-owned and governed child health nurses in New Zealand), school nurses and local general practitioners. They will assist you to understand the local culture and provide insight into appropriate community venues to promote the healthcare program. Gaining community support requires that the community actively contribute to program development, a process referred to as the community partnership model. The importance of community partnership in proposed health programs has been highlighted by many nursing and midwifery researchers (Fraenkel, 2006; Kemp & Harris, 2012; Lynch et al., 2010; Rohleder & Apatu, 2009; Subhi & Duke, 2011). This concept can easily be incorporated as a fundamental philosophical tenet in any program; without it, community-focused initiatives will have limited success (Fraenkel, 2006; Lynch et al., 2010; Rohleder & Apatu, 2009). There are partnership models available to assist in establishing and monitoring healthcare program partnerships. For example, VicHealth have developed a tool to guide the development, monitoring and evaluation of the partnership process (VicHealth, 2008).

Stage three: Healthcare program implementation

Stage three, program implementation, involves implementing and monitoring the healthcare program according to the program plan. This is a challenging phase and involves the consideration and operationalisation of multiple components (Lynch et al., 2010). For any program to be successful, issues such as visible senior management commitment and program governance, namely who is responsible for the program as a whole, as well as the healthcare program activities need to be explicitly identified. For example, who will be responsible for leading the entire program, versus those responsible for aspects of the program such as professional workforce standards or financial administration? Another key issue to be considered is workforce readiness; for example, to implement a widespread vaccination program the appropriate numbers of vaccinators are needed.

Implementing a healthcare program will also require that a number of operational issues be addressed. Early steps may include documentation of the program's policies and procedures, such as the processes for tracking client progress and the mechanisms for program evaluation. Infrastructure requirements also need to be considered, which may include provision of computers and associated networks and software, office space and screening equipment, to name just a few.

Community members may have working knowledge of existing resources and their input on the location for a program will be invaluable. Media campaigns may also be needed to publicise the program's launch or, in some cases, to assist in establishing community support. If you have been working with the local community to establish a program, such as a child injury prevention program, this will assist greatly in its implementation. It is also an approach that builds on the key principles for health promotion, which require the involvement of local communities and the use of diverse strategies for health promotion action (WHO, 1984).

Workforce development is another key aspect of program implementation. Providing sufficient training to enable staff to obtain the clinical skills to successfully deliver interventions aimed at promoting health and wellness for children and their families is of the utmost importance. To this end, to better support workforce development in the primary sector, the Health Promotion Forum of New Zealand have developed practice competencies for those seeking to work in primary care (2012). In Australia a national set of health promotion competencies has also been developed, was endorsed by the Australian Health Promotion Association in, 2009 and is used by a range of organisations to develop the competency of the health workforce to deliver health promotion programs (Australian Health Promotion Association, 2009). These documents provide an excellent overview of the skills needed for the primary care workforce. In addition to knowledge of specific competencies, sharing the health promotion principles that underpin the program that has been developed will provide vision and help emphasise the importance of the healthcare program. Using the oral health promotion program for Hawke's Bay in New Zealand as an example, awareness of global policies such as the *Ottawa Charter for Health Promotion* (World Health Organization, 1986) and the document *Early Childhood Oral Health* (MOH NZ, 2008) would help staff understand and support the program to be implemented at the local level. Staff also need to be aware of the local policies and procedures that underpin the program, and keep up to date on changes to these.

Stage four: Healthcare program evaluation

Historically, nurses and midwives have conducted a wide range of exciting, innovative healthcare programs; however, these have often been set up without appropriate mechanisms for evaluating health outcomes, in this way undermining a program's effectiveness. It is important that effective evaluation mechanisms be built into any program from the outset. The World Health Organization has also recognised the importance of evaluation of health programs and published a document titled *Evaluation in health promotion: Principles and perspectives (2001)*, which provides policymakers and health practitioners with wide-ranging guidance on program evaluation.

As identified in stage two, evaluation plans need to be established prior to a program commencing and are subsequently implemented across the lifespan of a program. The central evaluation question(s) relates to whether a program worked and achieved its intended changes. Key reasons for evaluating programs include: understanding the program processes, strategies and activities, and how they did or did not work; determining the shorter term impacts and longer term outcomes resulting from the implementation of a program; generating knowledge that can be used to influence policy and the distribution of resources for public good; contributing to the knowledge and theoretical basis of a discipline; and ensuring public accountability for the expenditure of public resources (Nutbeam & Bauman, 2006; Tones & Tilford, 2001).

There are multiple evaluation approaches, models and frameworks used to evaluate programs. These frameworks provide guidance on how to develop evaluation questions, indicators and data collection and analysis methods to evaluate a program's strategies, objectives and goal(s). Commonly used is the process, impact and outcome evaluation framework developed by Hawe, Degeling and Hall (2007). Process evaluation assesses program strategies including participant satisfaction, reach, implementation, quality and the political, social and cultural context. Impact evaluation assesses program objectives and determines the immediate or shorter term impacts of a program such as changes in knowledge, attitudes, beliefs, legislation, public opinion and community participation. Outcome evaluation assesses the program goal(s) and determines the longer term outcome(s) of a program in relation to changes in the broader determinants of health, for example, behaviour changes, social conditions, access to service provision, economic changes and health outcomes such as quality of life, dimensions of health status, population health inequities, morbidity and mortality.

Issues such as the communities' attendance at, or uptake of, a program are an important measure of its success. In addition, any evaluation has to attend to a program's ability to be sustainable over time, which takes into account issues such as financial viability and workforce development. Finally, one of the key aspects to evaluation is the extent of the health improvements in the health of the community (Draper, Hewitt & Rifkin, 2010).

Common evaluation methods include survey questionnaires, focus groups, participant observation, key stakeholder interviews and document reviews. An example of evaluating community participation in a child nutrition promotion program has been described by Draper and colleagues (2010). In their 2010 article titled 'Chasing the dragon: Developing indicators for the assessment of community participation', they offer multiple practical examples of how to measure participation that are useful for those seeking to evaluate health promotion programs that have involved the community as an integral part of the process.

In addition to measuring a community's participation in a health program, a particularly useful method during an evaluation cycle is the client or patient satisfaction survey. Well-developed patient satisfaction surveys can provide important information about how children and their families experience the service (see, for example, Wood, McCaskill, Winterbauer et al. [2009] and Chin and Amir [2008]). They can also provide valuable insights into operational issues, such as the usefulness of program venues or associated materials.

The collection of evaluation data must be well thought through ahead of time, so that data collected will give maximum benefit. Lynch and colleagues (2010) have discussed the importance of this issue for the success of child health programs. They highlight how many programs fail to meaningfully measure the effectiveness of the program, which ultimately undermines the success and continuation of what might be a valuable program. The process of evaluation also needs to consider how evaluation data will be stored and, although this may seem like a trivial part of the process, it facilitates ease of access and data analysis as well as consideration of ethics and data confidentiality. This also has the added benefit of requiring senior management support and development of administrative processes to support the program right from the start.

Many policy documents provide guidance on program development processes (e.g. *A Guide to Developing Public Health Programs: A Generic Program Logic Model*, published in 2006 by the MOH NZ). Some universities offer the services of research statisticians who can evaluate approaches to data collection and analysis at minimal cost, which may be invaluable during the planning phase of program evaluation.

Working with a local research centre for child and family research is ideal where they exist. Such centres are usually linked to or based within a university and provide regular research seminars where research findings are presented. A large research team has recently participated in a New Zealand project called Evaluation of the Diabetes Nurse Specialist Prescribing Project (Wilkinson, Carryer, Adams & Chaning-Pearce, 2012). This document highlights how the evaluation was conducted, including issues of setting up a nationally run research study, data collection methods and the lessons learnt from undertaking the evaluation. Similarly, in Australia the Children's Research Centre conduct extensive research on the health of Australian children and have produced reports such as the national survey results of mental health and wellbeing of young people in Australia (The University of Adelaide, 2011).

Managing change

New child health policies and programs are being developed in Australia and New Zealand and will change aspects of midwifery and child and family nursing practice. Nurses and midwives in both countries have a long history of effectively adapting their practice to meet family needs. However, change can be difficult to manage if it has not been carefully considered during policy and program development. Successful programs have considered the effects of change on the people involved throughout the development process, recognising that keeping people informed of changes and the reasons why change is occurring is crucial to effective change management (Heward, Hutchins & Keleher, 2007; Kemp & Harris, 2012; Mathena, 2002). For research findings into managing change during program development, see Box 2.2.

> ### Box 2.2 Research highlight: Managing change during program development
>
> Research by Heward and colleagues (2007) examined the process of managing change across several different phases of implementing a health promotion program in Victoria, Australia. The authors describe how leadership skills and change management frameworks are crucial for implementing such programs and are key to the development of successful health promotion programs.

Working with communities as partners in health promotion programs also ensures that those potentially affected by change can participate in the process of redefining and reorienting services according to community need.

Ford, Boss, Angermeier, Townson & Jennings (2004) argue the need for change to be managed through a process of participative–democratic practices, which involves three distinct principles: 'creating space for new communicative interaction, safeguarding a credible and open process and reclaiming suppressed views' (p. 21). Creating space for communication means prioritising opportunities to communicate how changes will occur. Safeguarding processes involves dealing with the difficult issues and developing action plans to deal with them as they arise. Finally, reclaiming suppressed views involves taking the time to listen to concerns about former processes and incorporating solutions into future program planning. Stripped down, this change process means involving staff in the process of change through transparent lines of communication between those directing change and those who are being affected by the change.

It is important that nurses and midwives are involved in all aspects of program development – from the formation of policy to locally embedded practice development initiatives. Historically, they have taken a back seat in driving such initiatives, instead taking the lead from other professional groups. It is important to harness the knowledge they have gained through working alongside communities and use this to shape policy and subsequent development of programs (Mathena, 2002). In addition to this, they also need to become active change agents through practice development methodologies, which require them to focus on achievable, community-centred initiatives. In these actions they will create sustainable and useful programs, which are based upon appropriate health promoting principles.

Conclusion

Nurses and midwives in Australia and New Zealand have a long history of involvement in developing, implementing and evaluating healthcare programs to improve health outcomes for children, young people and families. This process is influenced by global and national policy, which drives healthcare priorities and the availability of funding for programs. Examples presented in this chapter have illustrated the need to address policy considerations during program development, while at the same time meeting the needs of local communities.

Guiding principles for developing healthcare programs have also been discussed in this chapter, as has the need to effectively plan, implement and evaluate healthcare programs that contribute to enhanced health outcomes for children, young people and their families. This chapter has also highlighted the importance of the role of nurses and midwives in creating structures that provide flexibility to manage change, so programs continue to meet the needs of children, young people and their families.

KEY POINTS

» Stay up to date with the latest research and practice developments relevant to children, young people and their families.

» Be familiar with the global and national policies that impact on children, young people and their families to guide the development of healthcare policy and programs.

» Know the health goals and targets in your country for children, young people and their families.

» Develop relationships with members of the community in which healthcare programs will be implemented.

» Develop knowledge, skills and confidence in assessing community needs, and designing, implementing and evaluating health promotion programs.

» Understand your role as a nurse or midwife in translating policy into practice.

CRITICAL QUESTIONS AND REFLECTIONS

1. Identify examples from your practice where a specific nursing program could improve child, young people and family health outcomes.
2. Identify current child health-related policy in your country and region, and how it might relate to the development of your proposed program.
3. Develop a program plan to address your issue including a goal, objectives, strategies, communication plan and evaluation.
4. What issues would you need to address to make the program a reality?

USEFUL RESOURCES

There are numerous websites that provide information about programs for children, young people and families. A selection of these appears below:

Australian Indigenous Health InfoNet: http://www.healthinfonet.ecu.edu.au/population-groups/infants

Australian Institute of Family Studies: www.aifs.gov.au/institute/links.html

Child and Youth Health: www.cyh.com/Default.aspx?p=1

kidshealth.org.nz: www.kidshealth.org.nz/

Ministry of Health New Zealand: http://www.health.govt.nz/

Plunket New Zealand: www.plunket.org.nz/

South Australian Council of Social Service, Evaluation Principles and Frameworks: http://www.sacoss.org.au/online_docs/081001%20Evaluation%20principles%20 and%20frameworks.pdf

The Paediatric Society of New Zealand: www.paediatrics.org.nz/

Victorian Department of Human Services: www.dhs.vic.gov.au/for-individuals/ children,-families-and-young-people

Health promotion links include:

Australian Health Promotion Association: http://healthpromotion.org.au/

COAG meeting, 2 July 2009: http://www.coag.gov.au/node/66

VicHealth: www.vichealth.vic.gov.au

WHO Health promotion: http://www.who.int/healthpromotion/en/

WHO Milestones in health promotion: http://www.who.int/healthpromotion/ milestones/en/index.html

References

Armstrong, R., Waters, E., Dobbins, M., et al. (2011). Knowledge translation strategies for facilitating evidence-informed public health decision making among managers and policy-makers. *The Cochrane Collaboration*, 6, 1–12.

Australian Bureau of Statistics (ABS). (2006). *Children and youth*. ABS. Retrieved from http://www.abs.gov.au/websitedbs/c311215.nsf/20564c23f3183fdaca25672100813ef1 /93f51a7925f6d465ca256fc60026081e!OpenDocument (accessed 27 October 2012).

Australian Health Ministers' Advisory Council (AHMAC). (2012). *Terms of Reference of the COAG Standing Council on Health*. AHMAC. Retrieved from http:// www.ahmac.gov.au/site/home.aspx (accessed 27 October 2012).

Australian Health Promotion Association. (2009). *Core competencies for health promotion practitioners*. Australia: Australian Health Promotion Association, retrieved from http://www.healthpromotion.org.au/issues/91-news-item-headline-2 (accessed 28 June 2012).

Australian Institute of Health and Welfare (AIHW). (2011). *Headline indicators for children's health, development and wellbeing 2011*. Australian Government AIHW. Retrieved from http://www.aihw.gov.au/publication-detail/?id=10737419587&li bID=10737419586 (accessed 27 October 2012).

Child Accident Prevention Foundation of Australia (CAPFA). (2012). *Kidsafe*. CAPFA. Retrieved from http://www.kidsafe.com.au/links.html (accessed 27 October 2012).

Chin, L., & Amir, L. (2008). Survey of patient satisfaction with the Breastfeeding Education and Support Services of The Royal Women's Hospital, Melbourne. *BMC Health Services Research*, 8(83). doi:10.1186/1472-6963-8-83

Commonwealth of Australia. (2009a). *Investing in the early years – A National Early Childhood Development Strategy*. Canberra: Commonwealth of Australia. Retrieved from http://www.coag.gov.au/node/205 (accessed 29 January 2013).

Commonwealth of Australia. (2009b). *Australia: The healthiest country by 2020 – National Preventative Health Strategy – The roadmap for action.* Canberra: Commonwealth of Australia. Retrieved from http://www.preventativehealth.org.au/internet/preventativehealth/publishing.nsf/Content/national-preventative-health-strategy-1lp (accessed 28 June 2012).

Council of Australian Governments. (2009). *Investing in the early years – A National Early Childhood Development Strategy.* Canberra: Commonwealth of Australia. Retrieved from http://www.deewr.gov.au/EarlyChildhood/Policy_Agenda/Pages/EarlyChildhoodDevelopmentStrategy.aspx (accessed 28 June 2012).

Department of Health and Ageing. (2008). *National Primary Health Care Strategy.* Canberra: Department of Health and Ageing, Australian Government. Retrieved from http://www.yourhealth.gov.au/internet/yourhealth/publishing.nsf/Content/report-primaryhealth (accessed 28 June 2012).

Department of Human Services (DHS). (2007). *Improving maternity services: Working together across Western Australia.* Perth: Government of Western Australia DHS. Retrieved from http://www.healthnetworks.health.wa.gov.au/docs/Improving_Maternity_Choices-A_Policy_Framework.pdf (accessed 22 January 2013).

Draper, A., Hewitt, G., & Rifkin, S. (2010). Chasing the dragon: developing indicators for the assessment of community participation in health programs. *Social Science in Medicine, 71*(6), 1102–1109.

Edelman, C. L., & Mandle, C. L. (2006). *Health promotion throughout the lifespan* (6th ed.). St Louis, Missouri: Elsevier Mosby.

Edgecombe, G. (1992). Critical ingredients for public policy: a study of public health nursing policy process in Western Australia. Unpublished thesis, University of Western Australia.

Ford, R., Boss, W., Angermeier, I., Townson, C., & Jennings, T. (2004). Adapting to change in health care: aligning strategic intent and operational capacity. *Hospital Topics: Research and Perspectives on Healthcare, 82*(4), 20–29.

Fraenkel, P. (2006). Engaging families as experts: collaborative family program development. *Family Process, 42*(2), 237–257.

Gordon, R. (1998). The role of La Leche League in the promotion and support of breastfeeding. In A. Beasley & A. Trlin (Eds.), *Breastfeeding in New Zealand: Practice, problems and policy* (pp. 127–139). Palmerston North: Dunmore Press.

Government of South Australia Department of Health. (2007). *South Australia Health: Preparing an Aboriginal health impact statement.* Adelaide: Government of South Australia Department of Health. Retrieved from http://aboriginalhealth.flinders.edu.au/Newsletters/2010/Downloads/preparing%20an%20aboriginal%20impact%20statement-.pdf (accessed 29 January 2013).

Government of South Australia. (2009). *Health in All Policies: The South Australian approach.* Adelaide: Health in All Policies Unit, Public Health Government of South Australia. Retrieved from http://www.sahealth.sa.gov.au/wps/wcm/connect/public+content/sa+health+internet/health+reform/health+in+all+policies (accessed 22 January 2013).

Harris, M., & Harris, E. (2011). Partnerships between primary health care and population health preventing chronic disease in Australia. *London Journal of Primary Care, 194*, 188–191.

Hawe, P., Degeling, D., & Hall, J. (2007). *Evaluating health promotion: A health worker's guide*. Sydney: MacLennan and Petty.

Health Promotion Forum of New Zealand. (2012). *Nga Kaiakatanga Haoura mo Aotearoa health promotion competencies for Aotearoa–New Zealand*. Auckland: Health Promotion Forum of New Zealand. Retrieved from http://www.hpforum.org.nz/assets/files/Health%20Promotion%20Competencies%20%20Final.pdf (accessed 22 January 2013).

Heward, S., Hutchins, C., & Keleher, H. (2007). Organisation change: key to capacity building and effective health promotion. *Health Promotion International, 22*(2), 170–178.

Kemp, L., & Harris, E. (2012). The challenges of establishing and researching a sustained nurse home visiting program within the universal child and family health service system. *Journal of Research in Nursing, 17*(2), 127–138.

Kickbusch, I., Wait, S., Maag, D. (2005). Navigating health: the role of health literacy. www.emhf.org

Lynch, J., Law, C., Brinkman, S., Chittleborough, C., & Sawyer, M. (2010). Inequalities in child health development: some challenges for effective implementation. *Social Science & Medicine, 71*(7), 1244–1248.

Mathena, K. (2002). Nursing manager leadership skills. *The Journal of Nursing Administration, 32*(3), 136–142.

Milio, N. (1987). Making healthy public policy: developing the science by learning the art: an ecological framework for policy studies. *Health Promotion, 2*(3), 263–274.

Ministry of Health. (2010). *Kōrero Mārama: Health literacy and Maori results from the 2006 Adult literacy and life skills survey*. Wellington: MOH NZ.

Ministry of Health New Zealand (MOH NZ). (1998). *Child Health Strategy*. Wellington: MOH NZ. Retrieved from http://www.health.govt.nz/publication/child-health-strategy (accessed 22 January 2013).

Ministry of Health New Zealand (MOH NZ). (2000a). *The New Zealand Public Health and Disability Act 2000*. Wellington: MOH NZ. Retrieved from http://www.legislation.govt.nz/act/public/2000/0091/latest/DLM80051.html (accessed 22 January 2013).

Ministry of Health New Zealand (MOH NZ). (2000b). *The New Zealand Health Strategy*. Wellington: MOH NZ. Retrieved from http://www.health.govt.nz/publication/new-zealand-health-strategy (accessed 29 January 2013).

Ministry of Health New Zealand (MOH NZ). (2001). *The Primary Health Care Strategy*. Wellington: MOH NZ. Retrieved from http://www.health.govt.nz/our-work/primary-health-care (accessed 22 January 2013).

Ministry of Health New Zealand (MOH NZ). (2002). *Breastfeeding: A guide to action*. Wellington: MOH NZ. Retrieved from http://www.health.govt.nz/publication/breastfeeding-guide-action (accessed 22 January 2013).

Ministry of Health New Zealand (MOH NZ). (2006). *A guide to developing public health programs: a generic program logic model*. Wellington: MOH NZ. Retrieved from http://www.moh.govt.nz/notebook/nbbooks.nsf/0/6C8C1C9F05649A94CC25717300087A91/$file/public-health-programme-v2-may07.pdf (accessed 22 January 2013).

Ministry of Health New Zealand (MOH NZ). (2008). *Early childhood oral health*. Wellington: MOH NZ.

National Breastfeeding Advisory Committee of New Zealand. (2009). *National strategic plan of action for breastfeeding 2008–2012: National Breastfeeding Advisory Committee of New Zealand's advice to the Director-General of Health*. Wellington: Ministry of Health New Zealand.

New Zealand Breastfeeding Authority. (n.d). Retrieved from www.babyfriendly.org.nz/ (accessed 22 January 2013).

Nutbeam, D., & Bauman, A. (2006). *Evaluation in a nutshell: A practical guide to the evaluation of health promotion programs*. Sydney: McGraw-Hill.

Peerson, A., & Saunders, M. (2009). Health literacy revisited: what do we mean and why does it matter? *Health Promotion International, 24*(3), 285–296.

Public Health Advisory Committee. (2005). *A guide to health impact assessment: A policy tool for New Zealand*. Wellington: Public Health Advisory Committee.

Queensland Health. (2010a). *Preventative health: Strategic directions 2010–2013*. Brisbane: Queensland Government. Retrieved from http://www.health.qld.gov.au/ph/documents/pdu/ph_stratdir2010_13.pdf (accessed 28 June 2012).

Queensland Health. (2010b). *Making tracks towards closing the gap in health outcomes for Indigenous Queenslanders by 2033 – implementation plan 2009–2010 to 2011–2012*. Brisbane: Queensland Health. Retrieved from http://www.health.qld.gov.au/atsihealth/documents/makingtracks/making_tracks_plan.pdf (accessed 28 June 2012).

Queensland Health. (2010c). *Making tracks towards closing the gap in health outcomes for Indigenous Queenslanders by 2033 – policy and accountability framework*. Brisbane: Queensland Health. Retrieved from http://www.health.qld.gov.au/atsihealth/close_gap.asp (accessed 28 June 2012).

Rohleder, M., & Apatu, A. (2009). *Health impact assessment: Implementation of Oral Health Strategy location of a community clinic in Flaxmere*. New Zealand: Hawke's Bay District Health Board, Hawke's Bay. Retrieved from http://www.health.govt.nz/our-work/health-impact-assessment/completed-nz-health-impact-assessments/implementation-oral-health-strategy-location-community-clinic-flaxmere-hia (accessed 22 January 2013).

Subhi, R., & Duke, T. (2011). Leadership for child health in the developing countries of the Western Pacific. *Journal of Global Health, 1*(1), 96–104.

The University of Adelaide. (2011). *Recent papers published by our mental health researchers*. The University of Adelaide. Retrieved from http://www.adelaide.edu.au/childrens_research/research/mental_health/publications/ (accessed 27 October 2012).

Tones, K., & Tilford, S. (2001). *Health promotion: Effectiveness, efficiency and equity* (3rd ed.). Cheltenham: Nelson Thornes.

UNICEF. (2012). *The State of the World's Children 2012*. UNICEF. Retrieved from http://www.unicef.org/sowc2012/pdfs/SOWC%202012-Executive%20Summary_EN_13Mar2012.pdf (accessed 27 October 2012).

United Nations. (1990). *United Nations Convention on the Rights of the Child*. United Nations. Retrieved from http://www2.ohchr.org/english/law/crc.htm (accessed 22 January 2013).

VicHealth. (2008). *The partnership analysis tool: For partners in health promotion*. Carlton, Victoria: Victorian Health Promotion Foundation. Retrieved from www.vichealth.vic.gov.au (accessed 28 June 2012).

Vogel, A., & Mitchell, E. (1998). The baby friendly hospital initiative: evidence and implementation. In A. Beasley & A. Trlin (Eds.), *Breastfeeding in New Zealand: Practice, problems and policy* (pp. 169–192). Palmerston North: Dunmore Press.

Waters, E., Armstrong, R., Swinburn, B., et al. (2011). An exploratory cluster randomized controlled trial of knowledge translation strategies to support evidence-informed decision-making in local governments (The KT4LG study). *BMC Public Health, 11*(34), 1–8.

Wilkinson, J., Carryer, J., Adams, J., & Chaning-Pearce, S. (2012). *Evaluation of the Diabetes Nurse Specialist Prescribing Project. Report prepared for the New Zealand Society for the Study of Diabetes.* New Zealand: Massey University. Retrieved from http://healthworkforce.govt.nz/sites/all/files/DNS%20Final%20evaluation%20report.pdf (accessed 22 January 2013).

Wood, D., McCaskill, Q., Winterbauer, N., et al. (2009). Multi-method assessment of satisfaction with services in the medical home by parents of children and youth with special health care needs. *Maternal and Child Health Journal, 13*(1), 5–17.

World Health Organization (WHO). (1984a). *Glossary of terms used in the 'Health for all' series, numbers 1–8.* Geneva: WHO.

World Health Organization (WHO). (1984b). *Health promotion: Concepts and principles.* Report of a Working Group, 9–13 July. Copenhagen: WHO Regional Office for Europe. Retrieved from http://whqlibdoc.who.int/euro/-1993/ICP_HSR_602__m01.pdf (accessed 23 January 2013).

World Health Organization (WHO). (1986). *Ottawa Charter for Health Promotion.* Geneva: WHO.

World Health Organization (WHO). (1988). Adelaide Recommendations on Healthy Public Policy. Second International Conference on Health Promotion, Adelaide, South Australia, 5-9 April 1988. Retrieved from http://www.who.int/healthpromotion/conferences/previous/adelaide/en/print.html (accessed 9 March 2013).

World Health Organization (WHO). (2001). *Evaluation in health promotion: Principles and perspectives.* Geneva: WHO. Retrieved from http://www.euro.who.int/__data/assets/pdf_file/0007/108934/E73455.pdf (accessed 22 January 2013).

World Health Organization (WHO). (2005). *The Bangkok Charter for Health Promotion in a Globalized World.* Geneva: WHO. Retrieved from http://www.who.int/healthpromotion/conferences/6gchp/hpr_050829_%20BCHP.pdf (accessed 22 January 2013).

World Health Organization. (2008). *Closing the gap in a generation: Health equity through action on the social determinants of health.* Geneva: WHO.

World Health Organization. (2010). *Adelaide Statement on Health in All Policies.* Geneva: WHO.

World Health Organization (WHO), UNICEF. (1989). *Protecting, promoting and supporting breast-feeding: The special role of maternity services.* Geneva: WHO.

World Health Organization (WHO), UNICEF. (1990). *The Innocenti Declaration: Breastfeeding in the 1990s – A global treatise.* Geneva: WHO.

World Health Organization (WHO), UNICEF. (2003). Global Strategy for Infant and Young Child Feeding. Geneva: WHO. Retrieved from http://whqlibdoc.who.int/publications/2003/9241562218.pdf (accessed 22 January 2013).

Chapter 3

TOWARDS PARTNERSHIP: INDIGENOUS HEALTH IN AUSTRALIA AND NEW ZEALAND

Evelyn Hikuroa, Vicki Holliday

LEARNING OUTCOMES

Reading this chapter will help you to:

» distinguish between Indigenous peoples and ethnic minorities

» discuss the impact of colonisation on the health of Indigenous peoples with specific reference to Australia and New Zealand

» identify social, economic and political processes that perpetuate inequalities in health between Indigenous and non-Indigenous peoples

» identify key health issues affecting Aboriginal and Torres Strait Islander peoples and Māori

» recognise the potential of nursing and midwifery to improve the health outcomes for Indigenous children, young people and their families.

Introduction

The health status of Indigenous children and their families in Australia and New Zealand contradicts the first-world ranking of these countries. In many instances the health statistics for Aboriginal and Torres Strait Islander peoples and Māori are more reflective of third-world countries, particularly in relation to child health. Ongoing documentation of inequalities in health outcomes between Indigenous people and their non-Indigenous compatriots has become a common feature in the literature, so common it's as if the disparities are somewhat ordinary and therefore acceptable (Reid, Robson & Jones, 2000). An essential starting point for action to address inequalities is to view them correctly as inequities and to acknowledge the gulf in health outcomes between Indigenous and non-Indigenous peoples as unjust and definitely unacceptable. This chapter, therefore, aims to assist students, practising nurses and midwives to recognise the role they can play, as members of their professions and the wider health system, in reducing health inequities and providing culturally safe, high-quality and evidence-based care to Indigenous families.

Although some health professionals, including nurses and midwives, do not see the relevance of colonisation, acknowledging the significance of history as a determinant of disparate patterns of health between Indigenous and non-Indigenous peoples is arguably a critical step in education for change. Exploration of the experiences of Aboriginal and Torres Strait Islander peoples and Māori will lead to an understanding that Indigenous health issues are not only rooted in historical events but that they are perpetuated in ongoing processes of colonisation that continue to marginalise them in their own countries. The reader is, therefore, invited to engage critically and thoughtfully with the insights in this chapter and to consider the implications for nursing and midwifery practice and health service delivery.

Defining Indigenous

The *Macquarie Dictionary* defines 'Indigenous' as 'originating in and characterising a particular region or country'. The term 'Indigenous' has been identified as problematic by some writers due to its general application to any country or land. This lack of specific acknowledgement of the Australian context diminishes their Aboriginality (New South Wales Health, 2004). Therefore, where possible, this chapter uses the term 'Aboriginal and Torres Strait Islander peoples' to refer to the diversity of languages, cultural practices and spiritual beliefs of the first inhabitants of Australia. Aboriginal peoples from different parts of Australia have their own names, such as Koori, Yamaji, Nunga, Murri and Yolngu. These names are specific to various regions and are only used when referring specifically to that region (New South Wales Health, 2004). Outside of Australia, the term 'aboriginal' is also used as a synonym for 'indigenous'.

Aboriginal and Torres Strait Islander culture is said to be one of the oldest continuing cultures in the world, dating back more than 40,000 years. There have been many debates regarding the number of Aboriginal and Torres Strait Islander peoples and the number of language groups prior to colonisation. The population estimate is dependent on the text source and varies from 300,000 to more than a million, with the number of language groups reported as between 200 and 250 (Aboriginal and Torres Strait Islander Commission [ATSIC], 1998).

As tribal people, the tangata whenua or Indigenous people of New Zealand identify themselves by the names of their hapu (sub-tribe) and iwi (tribe). Renaming was an early process of colonisation and the adjective Māori, meaning ordinary or normal, was used as a noun to 're-identify' them as one homogenous group (Smith, 1999). As the name is now universally known, the term Māori is used to refer to the Indigenous people of New Zealand.

Māori and Aboriginal and Torres Strait Islander peoples belong to an international network of Indigenous communities who are unified in a collective struggle for their rights as first peoples. These rights are derived from their status as descendants of the original occupants of the lands and territories they now inhabit with others. The others include the colonisers, who have become the majority, and migrant or ethnic minorities, who came later. In the fervour to promote 'multiculturalism', it is important to distinguish between Indigenous peoples and ethnic minorities (Maaka & Fleras, 2005). Indigenous peoples occupy a unique political space and should not be 'redefined' as ethnic minorities in their own countries. The differences lie in the historical relationship that exists between the Indigenous peoples and the colonising power (the Crown), and their status does not depend on numbers in the population (Jackson, cited in Robson & Reid, 2001).

Definition of health and wellbeing

For Aboriginal and Torres Strait Islander peoples and Māori, health is conceptualised differently from the descriptions in their governments' policies, which reflect the World Health Organization's principles for health and wellbeing (1986). The following statement from the National Aboriginal Health Working Party (1989) provides insight into the health concepts of Aboriginal and Torres Strait Islander peoples:

> Aboriginal health is not just the physical well being of an individual but is the social, emotional and cultural well being of the whole community in which each individual is to achieve their full potential thereby bringing about the total well being of their community. It is a whole-of-life view and includes the cyclical concept of life-death-life. (page ix).

See Box 3.1, which presents an example of the interrelatedness of the child, wellbeing and community.

These views are consistent with Māori health concepts. Mason Durie's Whare Tapa Wha model is a contemporary framework that draws key elements from Māori philosophy to depict health as four dimensional (Durie, 1998). Using the walls of a house to symbolise health, these dimensions are named wairua (spirituality), hinengaro (mental wellbeing), whanau (family) and tinana (physical wellbeing). Put simply, health is dependent on the harmony and stability between and within all four dimensions.

> **Box 3.1 Collectivism and Aboriginal childrearing**
>
> It is interesting to consider the traditional values of collectivism invested in childrearing practices among Aboriginal peoples, while at the same time being careful to neither stereotype nor homogenise. The literature available around contemporary childrearing practices in Aboriginal families is limited. However, traditional Aboriginal childrearing practices, which still influence Aboriginal families living in remote and many urban parts of Australia, provide some insight into collectivism in childrearing.
>
> The Aboriginal perspective on childrearing is based on a collectivist view of family and social life that sees responsibility for the rearing of children invested in many people. According to this view, children come to trust in the capacity and commitment of a multitude of people to care for them and nurture them through childhood and into adulthood (Howard, 2006). A collectivist society depends on their relationships and obligations to significant others. Collectivists describe themselves by referring to the groups they belong to, the land which they are from, and not their individual rewards or results (Howard, 2006).
>
> Traditionally, Aboriginal children are seen as self-reliant and are encouraged to regulate their own behaviour and development (Kearins, 1984, 2000). In traditional family function, children help care for younger children and assist with household tasks from an early age (Kearins, 2000). Independence in learning is highly regarded and developmental skills and behaviour are determined by the child (Kearins, 1984). Traditionally, Aboriginal children are raised in an environment that is not verbally directed, nor are they required to stay in close proximity to their carers; they are hence relatively free to explore their world. Observational or visual channels are thus important in the learning style.
>
> Aboriginal infants are viewed as autonomous individuals capable of indicating their own needs. It is the signals provided by the infant that will determine a response such as feeding and the need for comfort (Brown, 2000). These learning pathways are possible in a collective environment, and contrast with the individualised, regulated and isolated environment of some western childrearing models.

History of colonisation and its contemporary effects on Indigenous families

All over the world, colonisation has followed a pattern of cultural destruction, dispossession of people from their land and natural resources, political disempowerment and death (Durie, 2005; Maaka & Fleras, 2005). Following European settlement, Indigenous populations in both Australia and New Zealand rapidly declined as a direct result of conflict and the introduction of European diseases that they had no defences against. The social and cultural organisations of Indigenous groups were undermined and their spiritual belief systems challenged by western secular and religious ideas and organisations. Furthermore, the firmly held belief of the European settlers that Indigenous peoples were inferior led to laws that denied them citizenship (Eckermann, Dowd, Chong et al., 2006).

Australia

In Australia, the declaration of European settlers in 1778 that stated Australia was an empty land, or 'terra nullius', had far-reaching consequences that reside today in contemporary Australian society. In 1992, in the historic Mabo case, eastern Torres Strait Islanders (Meriam peoples of the Murray Islands) contested for native title to their lands. The High Court of Australia overturned the ruling of terra nullius, and this paved the way for more appropriate recognition of Aboriginal sovereignty (Bessarah, 2000). Aboriginal and Torres Strait Islander peoples traditionally had strong connections between family, culture and the land. The effects of colonisation with non-Indigenous policies have weakened those links, which in turn has had a major impact on the health of many of these people (Mathews, 1998, 2004).

Aboriginal and Torres Strait Islander peoples suffered under various state governments' so-called 'protectionist' policies, such as the *Aborigines Protection Act 1869* (Vic), the *Aboriginal Protection and Restriction of the Sale of Opium Act 1897* (Qld), the *Aborigines Act 1905* (WA) and the *Aborigines Protection Act 1909* (NSW). The protection (segregation) policy did not achieve its aims and was replaced by policies of assimilation (1950s–1960s). The consequence of both the 'protection' and 'assimilation' policies was that many thousands of Aboriginal children were removed from their parents (Broome, 2002); this practice did not stop in the 1960s. These children are known as the 'Stolen Generation' and a national inquiry into the separation of Aboriginal and Torres Strait Islander children is documented in the 'Bringing them home' report (Human Rights and Equal Opportunity Commission, 1997), which outlines the ongoing removal of children from their families in the decades following the protection and assimilation policies. On the tenth anniversary of the Royal Commissions, a report entitled 'Us taken-away kids: commemorating the "Bringing them home" report' (Australian Human Rights Commission, 2007) was released.

The next policy shift was integration (1967–1972), encouraging Aboriginal peoples to adopt European ways and abandon their culture (Human Rights and Equal Opportunity Commission, 1997). The people of Australia voted in a referendum in 1967 to remove two discriminatory clauses in the 1901 constitution. This resulted in governments being prohibited from passing special laws relating to Aboriginal peoples. Aboriginal peoples were also to be recognised as Australian citizens and be included in the census (Human Rights and Equal Opportunity Commission, 1997).

Many Aboriginal and Torres Strait Islander people use the term 'invasion' or refer to Australia Day on 26 January each year as 'Invasion Day' or 'Survival Day'. The term invasion is also commonly used interchangeably with colonisation in journals, texts and discussions. As students you might consider researching additional resources to further your knowledge and understanding.

New Zealand

At the time New Zealand was being colonised, Britain had started to acknowledge the harm being brought to Indigenous peoples in territories it had invaded. Unlike colonisation in Australia, however, Māori were offered a treaty, and in 1840 the Treaty of Waitangi was signed by Māori and the British Crown. Although it is described as the 'founding document' of New Zealand, laying the foundation has been fraught and the Treaty remains the subject of ongoing political and public dispute (Durie, 1998; Orange, 2004; Reid & Cram, 2005; Walker, 2004).

As an agreement between two parties, the Treaty articulates a relationship between Māori and the Crown. Explicit in the Treaty is the promise to Māori that they would be protected from the detrimental effects of colonisation. Importantly, Māori would retain their lands and natural resources and the right to exercise authority over them (self-determination or tino rangatiratanga) (Durie, 1998). Guarantees were also made to Māori in relation to equity and citizenship, ensuring they would enjoy with their Treaty partner equal access to the benefits of a new society (Reid & Cram, 2005).

Ongoing debate about the Treaty of Waitangi centres on questions of British intent and motivation for a Treaty and differing perceptions of whether Māori sovereignty was ceded or not. These questions are fuelled by inconsistencies between the Māori and English texts and disagreement about which text is the 'right' one. In reality, and regardless of which text is recognised, the promises in neither text have been fulfilled. Present-day inequalities between Māori and other New Zealanders in social, economic and health status do not reflect the achievement of equity or that access to the benefits of society has been equal. Needless to say, nor did Māori retain their land and natural resources, let alone the right to exercise authority over them.

Following the signing of the Treaty of Waitangi, the settler government was quickly established without Māori, their Treaty partner, and through mainly legislative processes Māori were effectively dispossessed of their land and their sovereignty (Durie, 1998; Orange, 2004; Walker, 2004). Like colonisation in Australia and elsewhere, assimilation was a key agenda item and, well into the 1960s, policies including urbanisation saw the loss of Māori language, culture, tribal unity and identity − all critical determinants in the health of Indigenous peoples.

Ongoing impact on contemporary families

The emergence of Indigenous peoples as a social movement has led to international acknowledgement of the historic and lingering impacts of colonisation on Indigenous communities throughout the world (Sissons, 2005; Smith, 1999). To appreciate the impact of land loss on the health of Indigenous peoples, it is necessary to understand their relationship with the natural environment. Apart from the universal value of land as an economic base and place to live, for Indigenous peoples the land is the foundation of social unity and cultural identity and the source of spiritual sustenance (Durie, 1998; National Aboriginal Health Working Party, 1989).

It should need no explanation, therefore, that when people are dispossessed of their land, their spiritual, social and economic wellbeing will suffer immediately and for generations after. Evidence of this can be seen in the measurement of deprivation (see Figure 3.1). In New Zealand the NZDep Index measures socioeconomic position by assigning a decile score from 1 (least deprived) to 10 (most deprived). Māori are overrepresented in very deprived areas with over half living in deciles 8, 9 and 10. Regardless of what measuring tools are used, poverty for Indigenous peoples in Australia and New Zealand was created in the past, and it continues in the present.

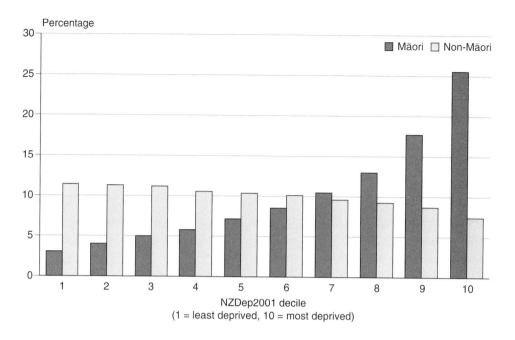

FIGURE 3.1 Deprivation by ethnicity in New Zealand
Robson B, Harris R (eds). *Hauora: Māori Standards of Health IV. A study of the years, 2000-2005*, p. 27. Wellington: Te Rōpū Rangahau Hauora a Eru Pōmare. Data: Ministry of Health 2002. *Reducing Inequalities in Health.* Wellington: Ministry of Health, New Zealand.

Racism

Prior to discussing specific health issues experienced by Aboriginal and Torres Strait Islander peoples and Māori it is imperative to define and discuss racism. Racism refers to the belief that groupings of people are based on genetic similarities rather than on social agreements between people. Racism, like sexism and classism, is about power. 'It is the approach by which one dominant racial group has and maintains power over another racial group and subordinates it' (Smith, 2004).

Most of us would declare ourselves 'non-racist' and would find it difficult to accept that racism continues to be a significant and widespread problem. However, although overt racism has become increasingly socially unacceptable, racism still exists. As Mellor, Bynon, Maller et al. (2001) contend, subtle or 'covert' racism occurs in the context of everyday living, such as shopping, using public transport and eating in restaurants and, importantly, accessing mainstream services, including health, welfare, education and the justice system.

Understanding our own actions and prejudices and taking responsibility for how these can affect service delivery is one of the most significant things we can do to improve services for individuals and groups who are marginalised by the system. Most of us do not intend to be racist in our attitudes, but every time we assign a negative feeling towards someone based on their culture, language, behaviour or beliefs, this is racism. It usually happens because we have a different cultural

> **Box 3.2** Critical questions and reflections: Challenging the stereotypes
>
> Flo, an Aboriginal Health Education Officer (AHEO or, in the community controlled sector, may be referred to as an Aboriginal Health Worker [AHW]) who is a registered nurse, has been asked to present a cultural awareness workshop to student midwives in a local hospital. To allow sufficient time to set up the room, Flo arrives 15 minutes prior to the scheduled starting time. Flo is quite nervous and apprehensive about the presentation; she sits and waits for the students to arrive. As the students arrive, several of them start a conversation making comments such as 'typical Aboriginal person, always late'; 'I don't know why we have to be here anyway'; 'If they didn't drink, smoke and take drugs so much they would be just the same as everyone else'. Flo (who has fair skin) then stands up and introduces herself as the person who will be presenting to them, also letting them know that she had arrived 15 minutes before the presentation time to ensure that she was organised and ready to start on time.
>
> 1. Would you consider this to be ignorance or racism? Why? Reflect on your answer.
> 2. What were the judgements made by the midwives regarding the AHW and Aboriginal people?
> 3. How do you think this situation may have been averted?
>
> *Note*: there are a number of Aboriginal or Torres Strait Islander Nurses who are employed as Aboriginal Health Workers, Aboriginal Health Education Officers or their equivalent in the public and community controlled sectors. It is often the role of the AHW/AHEO to provide cultural awareness/respect training.

viewpoint from the person to whom we are offering services. These different values and beliefs result in us making assumptions to predict behaviours in individuals or groups who are different from ourselves and can lead us to stereotype or generalise (Willis & Shandell, 2007).

A stereotype and a generalisation may appear similar, but they function very differently. A 'generalisation' is a beginning point. It indicates common trends, but further information is needed to ascertain whether the statement is appropriate to a particular individual (Galanti, 1991). A 'stereotype' is an endpoint. No attempt is made to learn whether the individual in question fits the statement (Galanti, 1991). Stereotyping does not allow for individual differences within cultures and commonly victimises groups by blaming their cultures for perceived and negatively valued practices. In Box 3.2, you will find a reflective exercise that encourages you to challenge the stereotypes.

An important contributory factor to the poor health status of Aboriginal and Torres Strait Islander peoples and Māori is institutional racism. Institutional racism has been defined as:

> ... the ways in which racist beliefs or values have been built into the operation of social institutions in such a way as to discriminate against, control and oppress various minority groups. (McConnachie, Hollingsworth & Pettman, 1988).

Henry, Houston & Mooney (2004) provide several examples of institutional racism for Aboriginal and Torres Strait Islander peoples, as below:

- *Funding inequity*: overall funding of Aboriginal and Torres Strait Islander health care is not commensurate with extra need.
- *Different performance criteria for black and white*: for example, in Perth, Derbarl Yerrigan Aboriginal Medical Service funding was cut when an 'overspend' arose because of success in attracting clients. At the same time, the teaching hospitals' overspend was 120 times greater than that at Derbarl Yerrigan. The teaching hospitals were given an extra $100 million to cover their overspend.
- *'Body part' funding*: separate streams of money are provided for conditions such as diabetes and heart disease for a health service that is intended to be holistic. For example, there are 26 funding streams (and hence 26 separate accounts and 26 demands for accountability) for the Danila Dilba Aboriginal Medical Service in Darwin.
- *Differences in treatment regimens*: Aboriginal peoples in Western Australia born in the 1940s received low-cost nursing care; in contrast, a white cohort of the same age received higher cost technological care.
- *Inequitable Medicare funding of primary health care (Medicare Benefits Schedule plus Pharmaceutical Benefits Scheme)*: in Katjungka (a remote Aboriginal community), it is $80 per head per year; in Double Bay (an affluent Sydney suburb), it is $900 per head per year.
- *Cultural barriers to Aboriginal use of healthcare services*: there is inadequate funding to reduce these barriers (such as language barriers and lack of recognition of different constructs of health) for Aboriginal peoples (Henry et al., 2004).

To counter overt and covert racism within the Australian health system, a number of principles have been prepared for the *Cultural respect framework for Aboriginal and Torres Strait Islander health 2004–2009* (Australian Health Ministers' Advisory Council, 2004, pp. 8–9). They include:

- a holistic approach
- health sector responsibility
- community control of primary healthcare services
- working together
- localised decision making
- promoting good health
- building the capacity of health services and communities
- accountability for health outcomes.

In addition to this strategy, in August 2012 the Australian Government launched the National Anti-Racism Strategy. The implementation of this strategy will play an important role in the Australian Government response to closing the gap in Indigenous disadvantage. The implementation of this strategy will be monitored by the Australian Human Rights Commission (2012), working in partnership with a number of government and non-government organisations. The overarching aim of the strategy is:

> to promote a clear understanding in the Australian community of what racism is, and how it can be prevented and reduced. (Australian Human Rights Commission, 2012).

Determinants of health and current health status

The relationships between health and social factors including housing, employment, poverty and education have been well documented (Marmot, 1998), and it is well established that the health and welfare indicators for Aboriginal and Torres Strait Islander peoples and Māori remain consistently worse than those of non-Indigenous groups. The relationship between disadvantage and poor health is complex, but the major influences include low educational achievement, low income, low employment rates, inadequate housing and transport, exposure to pollutants, poor access to health services and reduced access to healthy foods (Richardson & Prior, 2005). Conversely, the relationship between advantage and good health is relatively straightforward. The health and welfare of non-Indigenous Australians and New Zealanders remains consistently better than Indigenous groups. A shift in focus from explanations about the poor health status of Indigenous peoples to the good health of their fellow countrymen and women provides a different lens to view inequalities. Questions should be asked about what creates advantage rather than why some groups are disadvantaged. To be explicit, what has created the social, economic and health advantages enjoyed by the non-Indigenous?

For Indigenous peoples in Australia and New Zealand, the residual effects of land alienation, asset loss and social destruction explain not only why Māori, Aboriginal and Torres Strait Islander peoples are disproportionately represented in lower socioeconomic strata but also why non-Indigenous people are represented in the higher socioeconomic strata. See Chapter 1 for a discussion of social gradient and risks and protective factors for children's health. Table 3.1 offers a summary of the latest demographic data available.

Māori health

Data on Māori health status is easily accessed on Ministry of Health and Statistics New Zealand websites and from a substantial body of ongoing research. The *Hauora Standards of Māori Health* series is an important resource, which provides analysis from a Māori perspective. Of interest to nurses and midwives, the most recent edition (*Hauora Standards of Māori Health IV*) spotlights the issues of poor access to health and health care and unequal treatment in healthcare services as major factors contributing to poorer health outcomes for Māori.

A summary of Māori health issues highlights the following disparities: a greater number of low birthweight newborns and greater mortality in the first 5 years of life; the sudden infant death syndrome (SIDS) rate is four times higher than for non-Māori; children and adolescents have a higher risk of both accidental and non-accidental injury; and rates of youth suicide are increasing along with mental illness, drug and alcohol abuse and injury and death from road traffic accidents and violence.

Māori children and young people also have a higher incidence than non-Māori of a range of infectious illnesses, such as pneumonia, tuberculosis, rheumatic fever and, more recently, meningococcal disease. In adulthood, Māori have a higher risk of

TABLE 3.1 Demographic data on Indigenous peoples

INDICATOR	NEW ZEALAND	AUSTRALIA
Population	Total: 4,178,658	Total: 21,505,717 million
	Māori: 565,329 (14.6%)	Aboriginal and Torres Strait Islander: 548,369 (2.5%)
Post school qualifications	Total: 40%	Total: 61%
	Māori: 30%	Aboriginal and Torres Strait Islander: 40%
Unemployment	Total: 5.1%	Total: 3.5%
	Māori: 11%	Aboriginal and Torres Strait Islander: 15.1%*
Median income	Total: $24,000	Total: $38,480
	Māori: $20,900	Aboriginal and Torres Strait Islander: $23,920
Median age	Total: 35.5 years	Total: 37 years
	Māori: 22.7 years	Aboriginal and Torres Strait Islander: 21 years

*Excludes Community Development Employment Program (CDEP, which is Work for the Dole) participants.
Source: The Statistics New Zealand census (2006), Ministry of Health New Zealand (n.d.), Australian Institute of Health and Welfare (2011) and Australian Bureau of Statistics (2011).

cancers, cardiovascular disease and diabetes. Māori, therefore, bear a disproportionate burden of risk, morbidity, disability and mortality in every major disease category.

A review of government reports, research and statistical data (Ministry of Health New Zealand, 2003, 2005, 2006) illustrates 'systematic disparities in health outcomes, in the determinants of health, in health system responsiveness and in the health workforce' (Reid & Robson, 2006).

Aboriginal and Torres Strait Islander health

In Australia, Aboriginal and Torres Strait Islander men can expect to live 11.5 years less than non-Indigenous men and Aboriginal and Torres Strait Islander women 9.7 years less than non-Indigenous women (Australian Institute of Health and Welfare, 2011; see Figure 3.2).

The population graph by age, sex and Indigenous status (Figure 3.2) shows that the Aboriginal and Torres Strait Islander population is significantly younger than the non-Indigenous population in the 0–24 age group, which engenders many considerations when developing and implementing programs and services.

Morbidity data indicate that chronic disease (including respiratory disease, cardiovascular disease, renal disease and diabetes) remains the highest causative factor in the morbidity and mortality of Aboriginal and Torres Strait Islander peoples (Australian Institute of Health and Welfare, 2011).

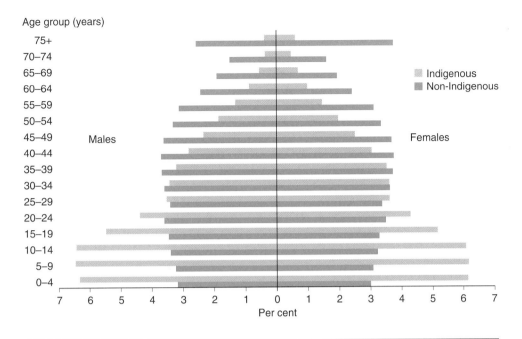

FIGURE 3.2 Age structure, by sex and Indigenous status, 2006
Australian Institute of Health and Welfare (AIHW) 2011 The health and welfare of
Australia's Aboriginal and Torres Strait Islander people, an over view 2011. Cat. No.
IHW 42. Canberra: AIHW.

Aboriginal and Torres Strait Islander women are more likely to have their babies at a
younger age than non-Indigenous women, with 19.7% aged less than 20, compared to
3.2% of non-Indigenous mothers (Li, Zeki, Hilder & Sullivan, 2012). These babies will
grow having a reduced life expectancy and increased morbidity and comorbidities
compared to non-Indigenous babies (Australian Institute of Health and Welfare, 2011).

Aboriginal and Torres Strait Islander babies have a higher death rate than non-
Indigenous babies with the most common causes being birth trauma, fetal disorders,
premature birth and reduced fetal growth. Although the incidence of SIDS has
improved and is now reported as being 7%, it remains higher than non-Indigenous
babies (Australian Institute of Health and Welfare, 2011).

Childhood mortality between the ages of 0 and 14 is twice the rate of
non-Indigenous children. Death due to respiratory disease occurs more than 4 times
more frequently than in non-Indigenous children and other external causes are
3 times more likely (Australian Institute of Health and Welfare, 2011). For children,
morbidity statistics indicate that, in 2003–2004, Aboriginal and Torres Strait Islander
infants were more likely to be hospitalised than other infants, whereas Indigenous
and other children aged 1–14 years were hospitalised at similar rates.

The Australian Institute of Health and Welfare (AIHW) report (2011) outlines some
improvements in health status but also notes that there is still a lot of work to be done.
The AIHW report highlights the following statistics for children and young adults:

- Asthma is the most common long-term condition (16%).
- Diabetes is less prevalent than in adults but type 1 diabetes is still around 9%.

- Hospitalisation is more likely for Aboriginal or Torres Strait Islander children or young people than non-Aboriginal children or young people.
- 33% of Aboriginal or Torres Strait Islander young people (aged 18–24 years) have been diagnosed with or reported a mental health illness.
- Vaccinations are less likely to be up-to-date.
- There is a higher exposure to violence both in the home and outside of the home.
- Aboriginal or Torres Strait Islander children have the highest rates of hearing impairment leading to total or partial hearing loss as a result of otitis media.
- Injury/poisoning is 1.7% higher for Aboriginal or Torres Strait Islander children and young adults than non-Aboriginal children and young adults.
- Smoking rates are higher, with 4 out of 10 young Aboriginal or Torres Strait Islander people aged 15–24 years smoking, and they were nearly 3 times more likely to live in a household that smoked.
- Harmful levels of alcohol for young Aboriginal or Torres Strait Islander people aged 19–24 years were reported as 23% compared to 14% for non-Aboriginal people of the same age.
- Young Aboriginal or Torres Strait Islander people are at higher risk of substance misuse than non-Aboriginal people of the same age.
- Aboriginal or Torres Strait Islander children and young people are less likely to consume the daily recommended dietary intake (Australian Institute of Health and Welfare, 2011, chapters 5 & 6, pp. 61–87).

Aboriginal children are at a higher risk of being diagnosed with both infectious and non-infectious diseases, often leading to long-term chronicity (Australian Institute of Health and Welfare, 2011). The report also identifies some concerning statistics that have resulted from the Northern Territory Emergency Response Child Health Check initiative. The health checks have revealed that 12% of children had suppurative otitis media, which is 3 times the rate which the WHO classes as a public health problem. It also states that the other countries that have been classified at this level include Tanzania, India and Guam (Australian Institute of Health and Welfare, 2011, p. 82). The Australian Institute of Health and Welfare report revealed: a significant increase in trachoma reported as over 5% in most areas, which is endemic (2011, p. 82); 62% of Aboriginal children in the top end of NT and Central Australia were diagnosed with rheumatic fever (2011, p. 82); and Aboriginal or Torres Strait Islander children were 3 times more likely to be hospitalised with a diagnosis of pneumonia in Central Australia, with 14% being reported in Western Australia (2011, p. 83).

The ongoing poor health status of Aboriginal and Torres Strait Islander peoples can be directly attributed to their low social gradient, an ongoing impact of colonisation. Ring and Brown (2002) argue that, although there have been strategies and programs to improve access to health services, more needs to be done. It could be argued that the development of additional strategies is wasting resources that should be spent on implementing strategies such as the National Aboriginal Health Strategy (National Aboriginal Health Working Party, 1989) that have never been totally implemented (Ring & Brown, 2002).

In the past there have been many policies, strategies, services and initiatives developed in an attempt to improve access to services for Aboriginal and Torres

Strait Islander people; however, many of these services worked in isolation. To gain the greatest benefit there must be collaboration at all levels (Australian and state governments, non-government organisations, Aboriginal community controlled organisations (ACCHO), local Aboriginal and Torres Strait Islander communities).

The Australian Government made a commitment to close the gap within a generation when the government, opposition, Human Rights Commission and peak Aboriginal and Torres Strait Islander health organisations signed a Statement of Intent in March 2008 (Human Rights and Equal Opportunity Commission, 2008). The signing of the Statement of Intent was timely as it happened just 5 weeks (13 February 2008) after the Prime Minister, The Hon. Kevin Rudd, gave a formal apology to the Aboriginal and Torres Strait Islander people who were forcibly removed from their families (Human Rights and Equal Opportunity Commission, 2008).

There was also a National Partnership Agreement signed off by the Australian Government, states and territories. Key priorities were set and funding was made available for some of the work needed to close the gap within a generation. All states and territories are required to report back to the Australian Government regularly on the outcomes and achievements (Australian Government, Council of Australian Governments, 2008).

The Close the Gap Committee and the Health Leadership Forum continue to monitor the progress of 'closing the gap' with collaboration and consultation, meeting regularly to lobby government and organise the Close the Gap Day celebration, which is held in March each year (to find out more about this you can look up Close the Gap on the Oxfam site, National Congress of Australia's First Peoples and Human Rights Commission, Aboriginal and Torres Strait Islander Social Justice – see 'Useful resources').

Even though there has been some improvement in the rates of morbidity and mortality for Aboriginal and Torres Strait Islander children and young people, as discussed in the previous paragraphs, there remain concerning statistical data indicating rates of disease or infection that are absent or minimal within the non-Indigenous communities. This paints a picture of a future of health inequity including disadvantage, poor health and shorter life expectancy.

To begin to arrive at a more positive picture, one of good health, increased levels of employment and a life expectancy equal to that of non-Indigenous people, it is important that we all work collaboratively to '*close the gap within a generation*' (Human Rights and Equal Opportunity Commission, 2005).

The role of nursing and midwifery in reducing inequalities

As a nurse or midwife, the extent of disparities in health, and individual capacity to address them, may be overwhelming. However, significant improvements in services can be achieved through recognition that:

- health inequities exist and why
- 'doing health business as usual' maintains or increases health inequalities

- individuals can contribute to change
- individuals can initiate change
- nursing and midwifery professional groups can participate in political process (e.g. submissions to government).

As they represent the largest group of health professionals in health settings, nurses and midwives form a powerful group. Improving access to health services and improving the quality of health care to Indigenous peoples is within the scope of nursing and midwifery practice and can be key in reducing inequalities. In New Zealand the theory and application of cultural safety in nursing and midwifery practice has been described as a means of improving health outcomes for Māori. In addition, nurses and midwives can play an important role in improving quality of care by recognising and challenging unequal or differential treatment identified earlier in the section on racism.

Cultural safety and Māori

Concepts related to cultural safety, such as cultural competence and cultural responsiveness, have emerged in recent times in other health disciplines. Although similar in regard to desired outcomes, cultural safety focuses on the power imbalance that exists between the health professional and the consumer of health care rather than efforts to behave in 'culturally appropriate' ways.

The idea of cultural safety was conceived by Māori nurses in relation to their concerns about Māori health status and their negative experiences of health services (Ramsden, 2002). The initial journey of cultural safety was fraught with public protest, government enquiry and initial concerns from within nursing education itself because it was considered to reflect an unnecessary emphasis on Māori (Ramsden, 2002). As a concept it was introduced into New Zealand nursing education in 1990 and has since gained international interest across a range of disciplines. It is often contrasted with the theory of transcultural nursing, which is similar to cultural competence as it advocates the need to study the cultural practices and ideas of population groups in order to provide appropriate nursing care. The significant difference between the two approaches is that cultural safety requires nurses to look at their own cultural practices and ideas, and the impact these may have on clients for whom they are providing care (Ramsden & O'Brien, 2000).

Cultural safety was initiated by Māori about Māori concerns but, under pressure from various quarters, it underwent a 'metamorphosis' to the point where the concept now relates to all persons. Although the theory is no longer specific to Māori, the Nursing Council of New Zealand states that nurses have a 'social mandate to improve health outcomes for Māori', and their expectations are made explicit in *Guidelines for cultural safety: the Treaty of Waitangi and Māori health in nursing practice and education* (Nursing Council of New Zealand, 2011). This document, as the title suggests, identifies principles related to cultural safety, the Treaty of Waitangi and Māori health, to guide nurses towards the delivery of better care in their interactions with Māori. (See Box 3.3 for application of the Treaty in practice.)

Box 3.3 Critical reflection: Application of the Treaty of Waitangi in nursing and midwifery practice

Among the New Zealand public, interest in the Treaty of Waitangi and understanding of it vary according to personal and political views. The same variation occurs in nursing despite the fact that, as a student or registered nurse, you are assessed regularly on your ability to apply the 'principles of the Treaty' in your practice (competency 1.2) (Nursing Council of New Zealand (NCNZ), 2012). What examples are you able to offer when you are undergoing a clinical assessment or appraisal on the application of the Treaty in your practice? Do you explain to your assessor that you apply 'the 3 P's' in your interactions with Māori and then name the principles of protection, participation and partnership or, worse still, do you say that you 'practise the famous 3 P's with all my patients'. If so, have you ever been challenged to elaborate or, on the other hand, did you feel the assessor was quite happy with your 'evidence' and quickly moved to competency 1.3?

There is a considerable lack of understanding of the evidence required to prove competence in this area. The following points may help nurses to clarify what is expected by the NCNZ in regard to competency 1.2 and the role of nurses to improve Māori health outcomes.

» A good starting point for nurses is to know that the NCNZ has derived four principles from the Treaty of Waitangi to guide nursing practice. These are outlined in the NCNZ publication *Guidelines for cultural safety, the Treaty of Waitangi and Māori health in nursing education and practice* (Nursing Council of New Zealand, 2011). So nurses should make reference to these four principles when they are being assessed, not the 3 P's, which were developed by the Royal Commission on Social Policy in 1988. Although they are similar, the NCNZ principles are specific to nursing practice.

» Application of the Treaty in practice relates to nurses' relationships with Māori, not to 'all people' or 'all patients'.

» Principles 1, 2 and 3 assist nurses to recognise the rights of Māori to self-determination and the role of nurses to work in partnership with Māori clients and their whanau as well as Māori community groups and agencies. Partnership in the context of a Treaty relationship is not just about nursing sick Māori people and 'involving them in all aspects of nursing assessment, planning, intervention and evaluation'. That form of partnership is the right of 'all patients' and is fundamental in the provision of nursing care. So nurses should reflect on how they interpret and enact partnership with Māori in the context of the Treaty. Principle 3 speaks of the opportunity to improve health outcomes for Māori through the provision of health care and the delivery of health service that reflects Māori values and belief systems.

» Principle 4 focuses on the role of the nurse to facilitate the same access and opportunities to health and health care for Māori as non-Māori. This can be achieved in a number of ways. Firstly, with a sound understanding of current health issues and government health targets nurses will recognise Māori health as a government priority and find opportunities to contribute to positive health gain for Māori, in their everyday practice.

» Using the prevention of rheumatic fever as an example, all nurses regardless of practice setting should know that the rates of rheumatic fever in New Zealand are considered to be 'third world' and Māori children, with their Pacific Island cousins, are most at risk. They should know that currently the New Zealand government has invested considerable funding into the prevention of rheumatic fever. Importantly, nurses can play a significant role in reducing rheumatic fever by staying abreast of current guidelines for the management of sore throats (Heart Foundation, 2012) and seizing every opportunity to ensure they are implemented. The recommended pathway for the

Box 3.3 Continued

screening and subsequent treatment of a child with a group A streptococcal infection is clearly defined and, if adhered to, can prevent the onset of acute rheumatic fever. A significant barrier in the implementation of these guidelines is a lack of knowledge by health professionals and failure to follow them. Nurses can intervene when these guidelines are not adhered to and question why, for example, screening did not take place or why the treatment prescribed was not for the recommended 10 days. Nurses can also work with whanau to enhance their understanding of sore throats: how to reduce the risk of throat infections, how to be assertive when they seek medical attention (to ensure appropriate treatment) and the importance of completing the 10-day course of antibiotics for the treatment of group A streptococcal infections.

These practice examples all illustrate how nurses and midwives can improve access to health for Māori and go some way to demonstrate application of the Treaty of Waitangi in practice. As a profession nursing can fulfil a wider role in Māori health advocacy by participating at the political level. Some recent examples of action taken by nursing organisations include: the presentation of submissions to the Parliamentary Māori Select Committee on the impact of tobacco on Māori (College of Nurses, 2010; New Zealand Nurses Organisation, 2010; Smokefree Nurses Aotearoa/New Zealand, 2010) to the Māori Select Committee enquiry into the determinants of health for Māori children (New Zealand Nurses Organisation, 2012a); and submissions to the NZ Government Green Paper on Vulnerable Children (New Zealand Nurses Organisation, 2012b).

With regard to Indigenous peoples, assumptions cannot be made about cultural identity. As an example, in a midwifery context the spiritual significance for Māori of the whenua (placenta) is recognised and it is common practice now, following the birth, to offer it to the whanau (family) for burial. This practice is a positive response to the needs of Māori in health service delivery and bodes well for the possibility of future changes. However, for those Māori who have been removed from their cultural information, being offered the whenua could be offensive and even disturbing. The complexity of culturally safe practice becomes abundantly clear in this example and the recent development of Tikanga Best Practice policies by District Health Boards aims to further enhance the provision of culturally safe health service to Māori. These policies take into account diversity among Māori, but reflect widely accepted Māori belief systems and practices related to health care.

Although it is difficult to measure the effect of cultural safety education and policy in improving Māori health, the success of Māori initiatives in improving access to health services and long-term health gain is more significant (Ministry of Health New Zealand, 2013). In the last two decades, the development of Māori health services has provided Māori peoples with more options in terms of health service delivery (see Box 3.4). These initiatives are still controlled by the Crown, but they reflect in varying degrees the right of Māori to determine their own health outcomes (self-determination).

Culturally safe practice, as a means of improving access to health service and of addressing health inequalities, is simply based on effective communication, analysis of one's own cultural biases and a willingness to neutralise the power imbalance that is inherent in nurse–client relationships.

Box 3.4 Practice highlight: Māori health providers

Turuki Health Care is a Māori health provider in South Auckland. It has a focus on women, children and whanau and provides a range of health and social services. Nurses, midwives, doctors, community health workers, social workers, breastfeeding advocates, lactation consultants and administration staff work collaboratively to promote their goals of wahine and whanau oranga (wellbeing of women and the whole whanau). Kaumatua (Māori elders) as well as traditional Māori health practitioners in the areas of Mirimiri (massage) and Rongoa (Māori medicine) provide additional support and kaupapa Māori approaches (Māori world view) in the delivery of services.

TAONGA has established facilities also in South Auckland that provide secondary school education for teenage mothers and childcare for their infants. The students are predominantly Māori and come from the local community. Based at this facility is a Māori nurse whose specialties include well child nursing and adolescent health. She collaborates with visiting Plunket nurses, midwives, youth health services, teachers and other community agencies to ensure continuity of care for the students and their babies. Her own role is comprehensive and includes a teaching component covering sexual health, parenting, growth and development, breastfeeding and child protection. She uses the HEADSS assessment tool to identify the needs of the young women, and home visiting enhances her ability to support them, their babies and their partners in the context of the wider whanau. The role of this nurse has been critical in the success of students completing their school qualifications and, therefore, enhancing their health potential in the future. TAONGA is currently undertaking research to evaluate the long-term benefits of its service to students.

Cultural safety/respect from an Aboriginal and Torres Strait Islander perspective

The *Cultural respect framework for Aboriginal and Torres Strait Islander health 2004–2009* (Australian Health Ministers' Advisory Council, 2004) defines cultural respect as 'recognition, protection and continued advancement of the inherent rights, cultures and traditions of Aboriginal and Torres Strait Islander cultures' (p. 7). The framework was developed after extensive consultation to address issues of inequity and cultural safety for Indigenous peoples with the goal being to 'uphold the rights of Aboriginal and Torres Strait Islander peoples to maintain, protect and develop their culture and achieve equitable health outcomes' (p. 7). Furthermore, the framework aims to ensure that cultural respect is embedded in the provision of health service, policies and strategies. It is the responsibility of health service administrators in states and territories to work collaboratively with Aboriginal and Torres Strait Islander peoples to implement the framework at the state and local levels.

The Congress of Aboriginal and Torres Strait Islander Nurses (CATSIN) was established in 1997 as a forum for Aboriginal and Torres Strait Islander nurses. The initial priorities for CATSIN were to improve recruitment and retention of Indigenous nurses and to ensure that CATSIN had input in decision making at all levels of government (Congress of Aboriginal and Torres Strait Islander Nurses, 2006). The *Getting em n keeping em* report (Indigenous Nursing Education Working Group, 2002, p. 50) of the Indigenous Nursing Education Working Group endorsed the

> **Box 3.5** Practice highlight: An Aboriginal maternal and infant health strategy
>
> The New South Wales Aboriginal maternal and infant health strategy (AMIHS) aims to improve the health of Aboriginal women during pregnancy and decrease perinatal morbidity and mortality. The aim is to commence patient-centred antenatal care prior to the 20th week of the pregnancy. This is achieved through the establishment of small teams consisting of a community midwife and an Aboriginal health worker (AHW) or health education officer (AHEO). These teams provide community-based, continuity-of-care services and education for Aboriginal women in collaboration with medical, midwifery, paediatric and child and family health staff.
>
> The team approach, where an AHW/AHEO and a midwife work together in a primary healthcare model to provide continuity of care, is a major strength of the AMIHS. A number of innovative community development projects have been undertaken as part of the AMIHS. These include art programs, peer education and partnerships with other organisations (New South Wales Health, 2005).

Aotearoa model of cultural safety (from the Nursing Council of New Zealand) in nursing and midwifery.

Cass, Lowell, Christie et al. (2002) promote the development of interpersonal relationships between health service providers and clients as a necessity to improve health outcomes. In their study, Cass et al. advocate the development of strategies for non–Indigenous health service providers to communicate effectively with Indigenous clients and families. Although the study was carried out with the Yolngu people (from East Arnhem Land), strategies can be developed and adapted with other Aboriginal and Torres Strait Islander communities. Strategies could include:

- Indigenous health service providers as cultural advisors
- Indigenous peoples as interpreters
- all staff to complete cultural respect/cultural safety programs
- Indigenous health service providers to be included as part of the multidisciplinary team
- consultation with Indigenous communities
- respect for cultural beliefs and practices (Cass et al., 2002).

Box 3.5 provides an example of a strategy and associated team-based service.

Working in partnership

As already identified, the provision of culturally safe care is reliant on the health provider recognising the social, cultural and environmental influences on the health of individuals and community groups. Communication in health provider and patient/family relationships was also highlighted above as a critical strategy in improving health outcomes.

Partnership models provide an effective and growing methodology, grounded in strengthening and enabling (see Chapter 1 for a discussion of strengths approaches). Partnership models provide an alternative to the long-dominant expert systems model (Giddens, 1990) that accompanied biomedical approaches to health care. Within this approach the practitioner, as the expert, determines the health needs of clients and offers advice, education and other strategies to address these needs. The expert model assumes domination and control of the health interaction by the professional (Elkan, Kendrick, Hewitt et al., 2000).

This model fails to recognise or respect the centrality of the clients' role in determining their own health. It also fails to address problems that relate to the cultural, social, historical and environmental influences of health and wellbeing. In an area as complex as Aboriginal, Torres Strait Islander and Māori health, the expert model fails to recognise the multiple layers of complexity that influence this population's health and wellbeing.

Working in partnership requires clinicians to transfer the focus of professional attention away from 'problems', 'deficits' and 'weaknesses', and towards the strengths or power of the client or community. This orientates the professional towards developing a collaborative and equal partnership with clients, focusing on building individual, family and community assets (De Jong & Miller, 1995). A major premise of the partnership model is that all clients have strengths and capabilities and are more likely to respond to interventions that build on these, rather than identify weaknesses and deficits (Darbyshire & Jackson, 2004; Dunst, Boyd, Trivette & Hanby, 2002). Partnership models that focus on strengths aim to increase participants' capabilities and feelings of self-worth (Darbyshire & Jackson, 2004).

Another important component of the partnership model is that there is an increasing emphasis on the expertise of the client (individual or collective). The assumption is that, with support, clients will discover their own way rather than learning to adopt some 'right way' defined by a clinician (Barnes & Freude-Lagevardi, 2003). Family-centred partnership involves professionals and family members working together in 'pursuit of a common goal' and is 'based on shared decision making, shared responsibility, mutual trust and mutual respect' (Dunst, 2000).

Developing a client's self-esteem is an important feature of partnership models. Working in a strengths-based or partnership model does not deny the expertise of the professional; it merely identifies the complementary expertise of the client (Davis, Day & Bidmead, 2002). A partnership model is particularly important when working with marginalised groups, such as Indigenous peoples who may be mistrustful of non-Indigenous 'experts' or authority figures. An important component of the principle of empowerment, embedded within partnership models, occurs when the professional believes in the client's ability to understand, learn and manage situations (Dunst & Trivette, 1996).

Partnership models for Aboriginal and Torres Strait Islander peoples will include existing service providers to enhance continuity of care, thus improving the patient journey. Many Aboriginal and Torres Strait Islander people source their health care from Aboriginal Medical Services (AMSs), which are also referred to as Aboriginal Community Controlled Health Organisations (ACCHOs). The first AMS was established in Redfern in the early 1970s. There are now over 140 AMSs throughout Australia. AMSs are predominantly funded by the Australian, state and territory governments to provide comprehensive primary healthcare services and programs to Aboriginal and Torres Strait Islander clients and communities (NACCHO). Each State and Territory has a peak Aboriginal Community Control Organisation.

The National Community Controlled Health Organisation (NACCHO) describes itself as the national peak organisation for Aboriginal health representing state and territory members and affiliates in the national arena (www.naccho.org.au).

As nurses and midwives you should familiarise yourselves with the Aboriginal Health Services in the vicinity of your workplace, including but not limited to Aboriginal and Torres Strait Islander health staff in the public health system or services and programs provided by the AMS or other government and non-government organisations.

Nurses often carry within themselves a heavy sense of their own responsibility that is incompatible with programs that respect clients as experts of their own lives. There may be a perceived justification for the views and kinds of programs being offered; however, it could be that the service has been offered historically without being reviewed or evaluated, and this model would more suitably be called 'nurse-centred care' rather than the preferred model of 'patient-centred care'. Shared decision making between professionals and clients is essential, particularly in the area of maternal, child and youth health services. All clinicians can examine their own communication style and biases, for our own prejudices and judgements impact greatly on our ability to work in partnership. This awareness is particularly important when working with Aboriginal and Torres Strait Islander families. If clinicians believe that their clients are unable or unwilling to take control of their own lives, long-term health gains will be difficult to achieve. Working in partnership requires clinicians to assist individuals to develop, secure and use their own resources that will promote or foster a sense of control and self-efficacy (Rodwell, 1996). Reflect on these concepts as you undertake the activity in Box 3.6.

Box 3.6 Critical questions and reflections: Assessment of an 18-year-old

You have been asked to do a home visit to assess Milly, an 18-year-old Aboriginal woman, who is approximately 20 weeks pregnant and has had no antenatal care to date.

Milly has a 15-month-old son, Tom, and they live with Milly's mother, Jane, aged 35, and her three siblings of whom Milly is the eldest.

When you arrive at the house with your colleague you find that Milly appears distracted and hesitant to answer questions as she is more concerned about her mother, who has been unwell for a number of days and unable to get out of bed. Jane has a history of diabetes and hypertension.

When you are able to begin obtaining information from Milly, she tells you that Tom was born at 32 weeks after starting premature labour. You observe that Tom is not walking, is underweight and has a runny nose and discharging ears.

Milly tells you that she had a negative experience during her first pregnancy, especially in the antenatal period. She felt that the midwives and doctors were judgemental when she was accused of smoking and misusing alcohol and drugs during her pregnancy, which led to her premature labour. Milly insists that she does not and never has smoked or misused drugs or alcohol.

Milly tells you that she has had intermittent vaginal bleeding and she has long periods of nausea and vomiting and generally feeling unwell. She has not made an appointment with the GP to review these issues.

1. Reflect on how you would begin to address the issues raised by Milly.
2. What steps would you take to engage with Milly to form a trusting relationship?
3. What are the top five priorities to address for Milly and her family?
4. How and why are these issues named top five priorities?

Conclusion

The issues for Aboriginal, Torres Strait Islander and Māori children, young people and their families are rooted in the past. However, the means to address them lie in the present. Recognising and accepting these historical influences is imperative for nurses and midwives if they are to develop a critical awareness of how the dominant Australian and New Zealand groups continue to marginalise Aboriginal and Torres Strait Islander families. Recognising the fundamental right of Indigenous peoples as first peoples to determine their own futures is the broad brushstroke that needs to shape current attitudes. The immediate need is effective health service delivery grounded in cultural safety and current and evidence-based practice, where nurses and midwives acknowledge the past and move forward by working in partnership that builds on family and community strengths.

KEY POINTS

» Indigenous peoples are distinct from ethnic minorities.

» Colonisation has had a dramatic and long-standing impact on the health of Indigenous peoples in Australia and New Zealand.

» Aboriginal, Torres Strait Islander and Māori conceptualisations of health are all-encompassing, inclusive of the individual and collective, physical and metaphysical and sustain links among people, history and land.

» Continuing social, economic and political processes exist today that contribute to inequalities in health between Indigenous and non-Indigenous peoples.

» Cultural safety and cultural respect are at the heart of reform.

» All nurses and midwives need to practise from a critically self-aware position in order to understand and enact principles of cultural safety.

» Strengths-based partnership models of practice are enabling and capacity building. They build respect, esteem and skills.

USEFUL RESOURCES

Australian Bureau of Statistics (ABS) 2005 *The health and welfare of Australia's Aboriginal and Torres Strait Islander peoples.* ABS [Cat. No. 4704.0]. ABS, Canberra.

Australian Government 2012 Closing the gap clearinghouse. Retrieved from http://www.indigenous.gov.au/closing-the-gap-clearinghouse-offers-new-evidence-for-policy-makers/ (accessed 26 February 2013)

Australian Government 2012 *Closing the gap: Indigenous chronic disease.* Retrieved from http://www.health.gov.au/tackling-chronic-disease (accessed 26 February 2013)

Australian Government 2012 *Closing the gap: Indigenous reform agenda.* Retrieved from http://www.fahcsia.gov.au/our-responsibilities/indigenous-australians/programs-services/closing-the-gap (accessed 26 February 2013)

Australian Government 2012 *Racism: it stops with me*. Retrieved from http://www.indigenous.gov.au/launch-of-the-national-anti-racism-strategy-racism-it-stops-with-me/ (accessed 26 February 2013)

Australian Government Office of Aboriginal and Torres Strait Islander Health (OATSIH) 2012 *Improving health in Aboriginal Torres Strait Islander mothers, babies and young people*. Retrieved from http://www.health.gov.au/internet/h4l/publishing.nsf/content/respack-litreview (accessed 14 January 2013)

Australian Human Rights Commission 2007 *Us taken-away kids: commemorating the 10th anniversary of the 'Bringing them home' report*. Retrieved from http://www.humanrights.gov.au/bth/taken/us_taken_away2007.pdf (accessed 26 February 2013)

Australian Human Rights Commission: Aboriginal and Torres Strait Islander social justice: http://humanrights.gov.au/social_justice/index.html

Australian Human Rights Commission 2012 *Racism: it stops with me*. Retrieved from http://itstopswithme.humanrights.gov.au/ (accessed 26 February 2013)

Australian Indigenous Health Infonet (a 'one-stop info-shop' for people interested in improving the health of Indigenous Australians): www.healthinfonet.ecu.edu.au/

Centre for Midwifery, Child and Family Health, University of Technology Sydney 2006 *NSW Aboriginal maternal and infant health strategy evaluation: final report*. NSW Health, Sydney

Congress of Aboriginal and Torres Strait Islander Nurses (CATSIN): www.catsin.org.au

Health Promotion Forum 2002 *TUHA-NZ: a treaty understanding of hauora in Aotearoa-New Zealand*. Retrieved from www.hpforum.org.nz (accessed 26 February 2013)

Human Rights and Equal Opportunity Commission, Aboriginal and Torres Strait Islander Social Justice Commissioner 2008 *Close the gap Indigenous health*. Retrieved from http://humanrights.gov.au/social_justice/health/statement_intent.html (accessed 15 January 2013)

Massey University Māori Studies (a range of publications on Māori interests are cited, including a bibliography of Mason Durie): http://www.massey.ac.nz/massey/research/centres-research/te-mata-o-te-tau/

Ministry of Health New Zealand (section devoted to Māori health information and publications): http://www.health.govt.nz/our-work/populations/maori-health

National Aboriginal Community Controlled Health Organisation (NACCHO) (representative body for Aboriginal Community Controlled Health Services): http://www.naccho.org.au/

National Congress of Australia's First People: http://nationalcongress.com.au

National strategic framework for Aboriginal and Torres Strait Islander peoples' mental health and social and emotional wellbeing 2004–2009, a 5-year plan: http://www.phcris.org.au/publications/infonet/2006/feb/framework.php

New South Wales Health 2000 *NSW Aboriginal maternal and infant health strategy evaluation.* NSW Health, North Sydney

Oxfam 2013 Close the gap campaign. Retrieved from https://www.oxfam.org.au/explore/indigenous-australia/close-the-gap/ (accessed 26 February 2013)

Secretariat of National Aboriginal and Islander Child Care Inc. *Footprints: a resource to where we are. A resource manual for Aboriginal and Torres Strait Islander children services.* Retrieved from http://www.snaicc.org.au/ (accessed 26 February 2013)

Statistics New Zealand: http://www.stats.govt.nz/

Statistics New Zealand census 2006 Quickstats about Māori (revised March 2007). Retrieved from http://www.stats.govt.nz/Census/2006CensusHomePage/QuickStats/quickstats-about-a-subject/maori/work-and-income-ko-nga-mahi-me-nga-whiwhinga-moni.aspx (accessed 26 February 2013)

Tikanga best practice policies. Retrievable internally from Auckland District Health Board and Counties Manukau District Health Board

Treaty of Waitangi (available on a number of sites). The following provides further historical background to events leading up to and following the Treaty: http://www.nzhistory.net.nz/taxonomy/term/133

References

Aboriginal and Torres Strait Islander Commission (ATSIC) (1998). *As a matter of fact: Answering the myths and misconceptions about Indigenous Australians.* Woden, ACT: Commonwealth of Australia.

Australian Bureau of Statistics (ABS) (2011). *Australian social trends March 2011: Education and wellbeing.* Canberra: Australian Government. Retrieved from http://www.ausstats.abs.gov.au/ausstats/subscriber.nsf/LookupAttach/4102.0Publication23.03.116/$File/41020_Indigenouseducation_Mar2011.pdf (accessed 11 January 2013).

Australian Government, Council of Australian Governments (COAG) (2008). *National partnership agreement on closing the gap in Indigenous health outcomes: Implementation plan.* Canberra: Australian Government. Retrieved from http://www.health.gov.au/internet/main/Publishing.nsf/Content/closinggap-tacklingchronicdisease/$File/commonwealth_implementation_plan.pdf (accessed 16 January 2013).

Australian Health Ministers' Advisory Council (2004). *Cultural respect framework for Aboriginal and Torres Strait Islander health 2004–2009.* Canberra: Australian Government.

Australian Human Rights Commission (2007). *Us taken-away kids: Commemorating the 10th anniversary of the 'Bringing them home' report.* Retrieved from http://www.humanrights.gov.au/bth/taken/us_taken_away2007.pdf (accessed 26 February 2013).

Australian Human Rights Commission (2012). *National anti-racism strategy.* Canberra: Australian Human Rights Commission.

Australian Institute of Health and Welfare (AIHW) (2011). *The health and welfare of Australia's Aboriginal and Torres Strait Islander people, an overview 2011* [Cat. No. IHW 42]. Canberra: AIHW.

Barnes, J., & Freude-Lagevardi, A. (2003). *From pregnancy to early childhood: Early interventions to enhance mental health in children and families.* London: Mental Health Foundation.

Bessarah, D. (2000). Working with Aboriginal families. In W. Weeks & M. Quinn (Eds.), *Issues facing Australian families* (3rd ed.). Sydney: Pearson Education Australia.

Broome, R. (2002). *Aboriginal Australians: Black responses to white dominance, 1788–2001.* Sydney: Allen & Unwin.

Brown, I. (2000). The socialisation of the Aboriginal child. In P. Dudgeon, D. Garvey, & H. Pickett (Eds.), *Working with Indigenous Australians: A handbook for psychologists* (pp. 293–305). Perth: Gunada Press, Curtin Indigenous Research Centre, Curtin University of Technology.

Cass, A., Lowell, A., Christie, M., et al. (2002). Sharing the true stories: improving communication between Aboriginal patients and healthcare workers. *Medical Journal of Australia, 176*(10), 466–470.

College of Nurses (2010). *Submission on the Maori Affairs Select Committee's Inquiry on the Tobacco Industry and the Consequences of Tobacco Use for Maori.* New Zealand: Palmerston North. Retrieved from http://www.nurse.org.nz/submissions-2010-1.html (accessed 27 February 2013).

Congress of Aboriginal and Torres Strait Islander Nurses (CATSIN) (2006). *Education statement.* Sydney: CATSIN. Retrieved from www.catsin.org.au (accessed 26 February 2013).

Darbyshire, P., & Jackson, D. (2004). Using a strengths approach to understanding resilience and build health capacity in families. *Contemporary Nurse, 18,* 211–212.

Davis, H., Day, C., & Bidmead, C. (2002). *Working in partnership with parents: The parent advisor model.* London: Psychological Corporation Limited.

De Jong, P., & Miller, S. (1995). How to interview for client strengths. *Social Work, 40,* 729–737.

Dunst, C. (2000). Revisiting 'Rethinking early intervention'. *Topics in Early Childhood Special Education, 20,* 95–104.

Dunst, C., Boyd, K., Trivette, C., & Hanby, D. (2002). Family-oriented program models and professional helpgiving practices. *Family Relations, 51,* 221–229.

Dunst, C., & Trivette, C. (1996). Empowerment, effective helpgiving practices and family-centered care. *Pediatric Nursing, 22,* 334–343.

Durie, M. (1998). *Whaiora: Māori health development* (2nd ed.). Auckland: Oxford University Press.

Durie, M. (2005). *Indigenous health reforms: best health outcomes for Māori in New Zealand.* Calgary: Paper presented at the Unleashing Innovation in Health, Care Alberta's Symposium on Health.

Eckermann, A., Dowd, T., Chong, E., et al. (2006). *Binan Goonj: Bridging cultures in Aboriginal health* (2nd ed.). Sydney: Elsevier.

Elkan, R., Kendrick, D., Hewitt, M., et al. (2000). The effectiveness of domiciliary health visiting: A systematic review of international studies and a selective review of the British literature. *Health Technology Assessment Programme*, *4*. Retrieved from http://www.hta.ac.uk/fullmono/mon413.pdf (accessed 26 February 2013).

Galanti, G. (1991). *Caring for patients from different cultures*. Philadelphia: University of Pennsylvania Press.

Giddens, A. (1990). *The consequences of modernity*. Cambridge: Polity Press.

Heart Foundation (2012). Algorithm 4: a guide for sore throat management. *The National Health Foundation of New Zealand and the Cardiac Society of Australia and New Zealand 2006*. Retrieved from http://www.heartfoundation.org.nz/order-resources/product_view/872/algorithm-4-a-guide-for-sore-throat-management (accessed 27 February 2013).

Henry, B., Houston, S., & Mooney, G. (2004). Institutional racism in Australian healthcare: a plea for decency. *Medical Journal of Australia*, *180*, 517–520.

Howard, D. (2006). *Mixed messages: Cross-cultural management in Aboriginal community controlled health services*. Darwin: Phoenix Consultancy.

Human Rights and Equal Opportunity Commission (HREOC) (eds) (1997). *Report of the national inquiry into the separation of Aboriginal and Torres Strait Islander children from their families*. Retrieved from http://www.humanrights.gov.au/pdf/social_justice/bringing_them_home_report.pdf (accessed 26 February 2013).

Human Rights and Equal Opportunity Commission (2005). *Social justice report 2005: Aboriginal and Torres Strait Islander Social Justice Commissioner. Report 3/2005*. Sydney: McMillan Printing. Retrieved from http://humanrights.gov.au/social_justice/sj_report/sjreport05/pdf/SocialJustice2005.pdf (accessed 15 January 2013).

Human Rights and Equal Opportunity Commission, Aboriginal and Torres Strait Islander Social Justice Commissioner (2008). Close the gap Indigenous health. Retrieved from http://humanrights.gov.au/social_justice/health/statement_intent.html (accessed 15 January 2013).

Indigenous Nursing Education Working Group (2002). *Getting em n keeping em*. Report to Commonwealth Department of Health and Ageing, Office for Aboriginal and Torres Strait Islander Health. Retrieved from http://catsin.org.au/wp-content/uploads/GettingEmAndKeepingEm.pdf (accessed 11 January 2013).

Kearins, J. (1984). *Child-rearing practices in Australia: Variation with lifestyle*. Perth: Education Department of Western Australia.

Kearins, J. (2000). Children and cultural difference. In P. Dudgeon, D. Garvey, & H. Pickett (Eds.), *Working with Indigenous Australians: A handbook for psychologists*. Curtin, Perth: Gunada Press, Curtin Indigenous Research Centre.

Li, Z., Zeki, R., Hilder, L., & Sullivan, E. (2012). *Australia's mothers and babies 2010. Perinatal statistics series no. 27* [Cat. No. PER 57]. Canberra: AIHW National Perinatal Epidemiology and Statistics Unit.

Maaka, R., & Fleras, A. (2005). *The politics of indigeneity: Challenging the state in Canada and Aotearoa New Zealand*. Dunedin: University of Otago Press.

Marmot, M. G. (1998). Improvement of social environment to improve health. *Lancet*, *351*, 57–61.

Mathews, C. (2004). *Healthy children: A guide for child care* (2nd ed.). Sydney: Elsevier.

Mathews, J. (1998). The Menzies School of Health Research offers a new paradigm of cooperative research. *Medical Journal of Australia*, *169*, 625–629.

McConnachie, K., Hollingsworth, D., & Pettman, J. (1988). *Race and racism in Australia.* Sydney: Social Science Press.

Mellor, D., Bynon, G., Maller, J., et al. (2001). The perception of racism in ambiguous scenarios. *Journal of Ethnic and Migration Studies, 27,* 473–488.

Ministry of Health New Zealand (MOH NZ) (n.d.). Retrieved from http://www.health.govt.nz/our-work/populations/maori-health (accessed 26 February 2013).

Ministry of Health New Zealand (MOH NZ) (2003). *Decades of disparity: Ethnic mortality trends in New Zealand 1980–1999.* MOH NZ, Public Health Intelligence Occasional Bulletin Series. Retrieved from http://www.moh.govt.nz/notebook/nbbooks.nsf/0/37A7ABB191191FB9CC256DDA00064211/$file/EthnicMortalityTrends.pdf (accessed 26 February 2013).

Ministry of Health New Zealand (MOH NZ) (2005). *Decades of disparity II: Socioeconomic mortality trends in New Zealand 1981–1999.* MOH NZ, Public Health Intelligence Occasional Bulletin Series. Retrieved from http://www.kaupapamaori.com/assets//decades_disparity/disparities_report2.pdf (accessed 26 February 2013).

Ministry of Health New Zealand (MOH NZ) (2006). *Decades of disparity III: Ethnic and socio-economic inequalities in mortality, New Zealand 1981–1999.* MOH NZ, Public Health Intelligence Occasional Bulletin Series. Retrieved from http://www.otago.ac.nz/wellington/otago024509.pdf (accessed 26 February 2013).

Ministry of Health New Zealand (MOH NZ) (2013). *Report on the performance of general practices in Whānau Ora collectives as at September 2012.* Wellington: MOH NZ.

National Aboriginal Health Working Party (1989). *A national Aboriginal health strategy.* Canberra: Department of Health and Ageing.

New South Wales Health (2004). *Communicating positively: A guide to appropriate Aboriginal terminology.* Sydney: NSW Department of Health. Retrieved from http://www.health.nsw.gov.au/pubs/2004/pdf/aboriginal_terms.pdf (accessed 26 February 2013).

New South Wales Health (2005). *NSW Aboriginal maternal and infant health strategy evaluation.* North Sydney: NSW Health.

New Zealand Nurses Organisation (2010). *Submission to the Maori Affairs Select Committee on the Inquiry into the tobacco industry in Aotearoa and the consequences of tobacco use for Maori.* New Zealand: Wellington. Retrieved from http://www.nzno.org.nz/Portals/0/Docs/Activities/Submissions/2010-01%20%20Inquiry%20into%20Tobacco%20Industry%20in%20Aotearoa%20NZNO.PDF (accessed 27 February 2013).

New Zealand Nurses Organisation (2012a). *Submission to the Maori Affairs Committee on the Inquiry into determinants of wellbeing for Maori children.* New Zealand: Wellington. Retrieved from http://www.nzno.org.nz/Portals/0/2012-03%20Inquiry%20into%20%20determinants%20of%20wellbeing%20for%20Maori%20children%20FINAL.pdf (accessed 27 February 2013).

New Zealand Nurses Organisation (2012b). *Submission to the Ministry of Social Development on the Green paper for vulnerable children.* New Zealand: Wellington. Retrieved from http://www.nzno.org.nz/Portals/0/Docs/Activities/Submissions/2012-02-28%20Green%20paper%20on%20vulnerable%20children%20NZNO%20submission%20final.pdf (accessed 27 February 2013).

Nursing Council of New Zealand (2011). *Guidelines for cultural safety: The Treaty of Waitangi and Māori health in nursing practice and education.* Wellington: Nursing Council of New Zealand. Retrieved from www.nursingcouncil.org.nz (accessed 26 February 2013).

Nursing Council of New Zealand (2012). *Competencies for registered nurses.* New Zealand: Wellington. Nursing Council of New Zealand. Retrieved from http://www.nursingcouncil.org.nz/download/98/rn-comp2012.pdf (accessed 27 February 2013).

Orange C (2004). *An illustrated history of the Treaty of Waitangi.* Wellington: Bridget Williams Books.

Ramsden, I. (2002). Cultural safety and nursing education in Aotearoa and Te Waipounamu. Unpublished doctoral thesis, Victoria University, Wellington.

Ramsden, I., & O'Brien, L. (2000). Defining cultural safety and transcultural nursing. Kai Tiaka. *Nursing New Zealand, 6*(8), 4–5.

Reid, P., & Cram, F. (2005). Connecting health, people, and country in Aotearoa New Zealand. In K. Dew & P. Davis (Eds.), *Health and society in Aotearoa New Zealand* (pp. 33–48). Melbourne: Oxford University Press.

Reid, P., & Robson, B. (2006). The state of Māori health. In M. Mulholland (Ed.), *State of the Māori nation: Twenty-first-century issues in Aotearoa* (pp. 17–32). Auckland: Reed Books.

Reid, P., Robson, B., & Jones, C. (2000). Disparities in health: common myths and uncommon truths. *Pacific Dialog, 7*(1), 38–46.

Richardson, S., & Prior, M. (2005). Childhood today. In S. Richardson & M. Prior (Eds.), *No time to lose: The wellbeing of Australia's children.* Melbourne: Melbourne University Press.

Ring, I., & Brown, N. (2002). Indigenous health: chronically inadequate responses to damning statistics [Crisis]. *Medical Journal of Australia, 177*(11), 629–631.

Robson, B., & Reid, P. (2001). *Ethnicity matters: Māori perspectives.* Wellington: Statistics New Zealand.

Rodwell, C. (1996). An analysis of the concept of empowerment. *Journal of Advanced Nursing, 23*, 305–313.

Sissons, J. (2005). *First peoples: Indigenous cultures and their futures.* London: Reaktion Books.

Smith, J. (2004). *Australia's rural and remote health: A social justice perspective.* Melbourne: Tertiary Press.

Smith, L. (1999). *Decolonising methodologies: Research and Indigenous peoples.* London: Zed Books.

Smokefree Nurses Aotearoa/New Zealand (SNANZ) (2010). Supplementary submission on the Maori Affairs Select Committee's Inquiry on the Tobacco Industry and Consequences of Tobacco Use for Maori. Retrieved from http://www.smokefreenurses.org.nz/Whats+Going+On/Submissions.html (accessed 26 February 2013).

Statistics New Zealand census (2006). Quickstats about Māori (revised March 2007). Retrieved from http://www.stats.govt.nz/Census/2006CensusHomePage/QuickStats/quickstats-about-a-subject/maori/work-and-income-ko-nga-mahi-me-nga-whiwhinga-moni.aspx (accessed 26 February 2013).

Walker, R. (2004). *Ka whawhai tonu matou, struggle without end*, revised edn. Auckland: Penguin Books.

Willis, K., & Shandell, E. (2007). *Society, culture and health: An introduction to sociology for nurses*. Melbourne: Oxford University Press.

World Health Organization (WHO) (1986). Ottawa charter for health promotion. Geneva: WHO. Retrieved from http://www.who.int/healthpromotion/conferences/previous/ottawa/en/ (accessed 26 February 2013).

Chapter 4

PRACTICE INTEGRITY: ADVOCACY, ETHICS AND LEGAL ISSUES

Jenny Fraser, Helen Stasa

LEARNING OUTCOMES

Reading this chapter will help you to:

» explore the role of advocacy in nursing children, young people and their families

» understand the obligation to advocate for children, young people and their families

» consider the relationship between advocacy, ethics and lawful practice

» analyse ethical frameworks for nursing practice

» recognise the relevance of the United Nation's *Declaration of the Rights of the Child* to nursing practice

» analyse contentious clinical cases to integrate knowledge of advocacy for children, young people and their families

» critically analyse the nursing responsibilities and priorities within practice relating to families at risk, children's rights and child protection legislation.

Introduction

Nurses working in paediatric, child and youth health settings operate within a framework informed by lawful scope of practice and ethical standards. One of the features that distinguishes practice for nurses who work in such settings is that they may sometimes be required to act as an advocate for clients. This chapter presents a review of the nurse's role as advocate for children, young people and families, and examines this role across the landscape of children and youth health services. The chapter also presents a number of practical examples, which are designed to assist you in thinking through the important factors governing advocacy in the nursing context.

Nursing shares the role of patient advocate with a number of other health professions (such as medicine and psychology) (Davis-Alldritt, 2012) and, since the mid-1990s, nursing has included advocacy as one of the fundamental roles in its scope of practice (Mallik & Rafferty, 2000). For instance, the International Council of Nurses (ICN), (2006b) lists advocacy as a 'key nursing role', and this commitment is expressed through professional codes of conduct set at the domestic level (Australian Nursing and Midwifery Council, 2002; New Zealand Nurses Association, 1995). More precisely, the ICN code of ethics, which is relevant to nursing practice in both Australia and New Zealand, explicitly stipulates that nurses are responsible for acting as advocates for the needs and welfare of patients, for the profession of nursing and for the interests of colleagues in nursing (2006a). Nevertheless, ambiguous interpretations of the concept of patient advocacy continue to pose a number of problems for nurses in practice. Hence, an overview of what advocacy means in general, and for nurses working with children, young people and their families in particular, is necessary.

Advocacy: What is it?

At the broadest level, an advocate is someone who pleads for, or speaks on behalf of, another person or entity who is unable or unwilling to speak for themselves (Oxford English Dictionary, 2012). The concept of advocacy in nursing has developed over the past three decades from two distinct sources:

1. theoretical writings
2. research studies.

Theoretical work and model development was begun in the late 1970s and early 1980s by American writers such as Curtin (1979) and Gadow (1980), and was later expanded by Gates (1994) and Mallik (1997a, 1997b, 1998) in the United Kingdom.

Models developed from these writings essentially focused on the role of nurses in promoting patient rights and supporting self-care (see O'Connor and Kelly [2005] for a detailed review and critique of these models). This meant that, in assisting patients to exercise their rights to self-determination, nurses were obligated to provide information and support decision making led by patients. In other words, this perspective conceives of nurse advocates as playing an enabling role, whereby they provide information to clients, with the client making the decision.

However, the difficulty for nurses was to disentangle dimensions of paternalism (the practice of restricting the freedoms and responsibilities of subordinates or dependants in what is considered to be their best interests [Oxford English Dictionary, 2012]) and advocacy. As O'Connor and Kelly (2005) contend, this approach led to definitions that simply interpreted patient advocacy as information-giving by nurses and receiving by patients. Follow-up support by nurses was not incorporated into this conception of advocacy.

Research studies have since been conducted to expand upon the earlier theoretical work, and to empirically test the main theoretical assumptions (Mallik, 1997a, 1997b, 1998; Mallik & Rafferty, 2000; O'Connor & Kelly, 2005). This body of research has helped to conceptualise advocacy in nursing in terms of nurses' actual, lived experiences, rather than from a purely theoretical basis. Importantly, these studies have suggested that some consensus is beginning to emerge (Jezewski, 1993; Mallik & Rafferty, 2000; O'Connor & Kelly, 2005).

In their study of Irish nurses, O'Connor and Kelly (2005) were able to identify two important elements fundamental to understanding patient advocacy:

1. clinical advocacy
2. organisational advocacy.

Specifically, *clinical advocacy* occurs at a proximal level to the nurse–patient relationship, with nurses acting on behalf of patients regarding healthcare or treatment options. In other words, clinical advocacy is typically conceived of as a relationship between individual nurses advocating on behalf of individual patients (Mahlin, 2010). However, as Mahlin (2010) suggests, although such individual advocacy is a worthy goal, it does not address systematic issues.

In contrast, *organisational advocacy* takes a broader, more distal approach, and involves nurses acting on behalf of patients at a systems level. Thus, organisational advocacy extends the nurse–patient relationship by situating this relationship within the broader healthcare system. A nurse's role is to mediate or interpret the system as required while attempting to facilitate patient autonomy.

Advocacy in the child, youth and family health context

Although it may not be possible to offer a precise definition of patient advocacy as it applies to child and youth health nursing practice, it is important to examine key elements of the concept, including:

*   children's rights and healthcare
*   decision-making frameworks
*   ethical decision making and informed consent.

This chapter highlights implications for clinical nursing practice throughout, and then provides more specific reference to child protection legislation influencing nursing practice. Advocacy in the context of therapeutic relationships with children, young people and their families is then considered, with a number of case studies presented.

Human rights, child rights and advocacy

The United Nations *Declaration of the Rights of the Child* (United Nations, 1989) sets international standards for protecting the interests and rights of children. The Convention was adopted by the United Nations in 1989 and has been ratified in all but two countries (Somalia and the United States) to date (The World Organisation for Cross-border Co-operation in Civil and Commercial Matters, 2012). Australia ratified the convention in 1991, followed by New Zealand in 1993 (United Nations Treaty Collection, 1989). In regards to health care, the *Declaration* explicitly states that the child 'shall be entitled to grow and develop in health … (and) shall have the right to adequate nutrition, housing, recreation and medical services' (United Nations Treaty Collection, 1989).

Other relevant international human rights laws applicable to children and young people include the child's right to medical treatment located in Article 3 of the *Universal Declaration of Human Rights*, which provides that 'everyone has a right to life' (and the treatment required to sustain life), and Article 12(1) of the United Nation's International Covenant on Economic, Social and Cultural Rights, which recognises 'the right of everyone to the enjoyment of the highest attainable standard of physical and mental health' (cited in Breen, 2006, p. 48). Article 19 of the Convention (United Nations, 1989) goes further and obligates state parties to intervene to 'protect the child from all forms of physical and mental violence, injury or abuse, neglect or negligent treatment' (cited in Breen, 2006, p. 49).

Of particular importance in relation to nursing children and young people is that we accept that individuals have the right to make informed choices about the care they receive. Article 13(1) provides that:

> The child shall have the right to freedom of expression; this right shall include the freedom to seek, receive and impart information and ideas of all kinds, regardless of frontiers … (United Nations, 1989).

At the same time, advocacy usually means supporting children and young people in the context of their parents' rights and obligations to protect the child. In more recent times, the importance of parental autonomy in child healthcare delivery and decision making has posed the problem of advocacy versus paternalism for nurses practising within a family-centred framework. A common experience for nurses working with children, young people and their families is negotiating parent–child conflict in treatment preference, particularly for children with a chronic illness. Advocacy is made more complex when we accept children's rights as paramount. The child's degree of autonomy and capacity to consent to treatment determines their ability to exercise their rights (Breen, 2006). As children grow older and develop decision-making skills, their right to consent to treatment and research participation must be respected (Breen, 2006).

Nonetheless, it is possible that situations may arise in which the preferences of parents may conflict with what is thought to be in the healthcare interests of the child. In such circumstances, nursing staff have an important role to play in advocating to ensure the child's rights are protected, while also acknowledging the rights of the parents (Woolley, 2005). An example helps to make this issue clear. One of the fundamental doctrines of the Jehovah's Witness Society (a Christian religious organisation) is a prohibition against receiving whole blood transfusions (Elder, 2008; Harrison, 2008; Woolley, 2005). This ban was introduced in 1945 and, since then, Jehovah's Witness parents have fought for their rights to refuse blood products on behalf of their children even if, without such products, survival is unlikely (Elder, 2008; Woolley, 2005). However, as Woolley suggests, although courts in the western world recognise parents' rights to raise their children in a way in which they see fit, these rights may not be absolute (Guichon & Mitchell, 2006; Woolley, 2005). In Australia, for example, the child's rights are seen as paramount, and every Australian jurisdiction has legislation that permits certain medical procedures (including whole blood transfusions) to be performed in the absence of parental consent (Woolley, 2005). This is a clear example where child, paediatric and family health nurses may be called upon to play an advocacy role to help reach an agreement.

Practice implications

There is growing support for models of nursing care that are patient-centred (Dancet, D'Hooghe, Sermeus et al., 2012; Murphy, 2012; Stewart, Ryan & Bodea, 2011). Within paediatric, child and youth health nursing settings, the term *family-centred care* is used to describe a model of care that focuses on issues such as the involvement of parents in the care of their child, consideration of the children's perspectives and increasing children's involvement in their treatment and treatment decisions (Scarfe, Redshaw, Wilson & Dengler, 2012). MacKean, Thurston and Scott (2005) argue that family-centred care emerged as best practice in children's health settings from the widespread interest in patient advocacy, citing hospital visiting rights for parents as one outcome of the advocacy movement.

The child (and the nurse) must rely on parents making such treatment and other healthcare decisions based on the child's best interests, as they are recognised as having the authority to act on behalf of the child (Breen, 2006). However, as was shown in the previously presented example of Jehovah's Witnesses and whole blood transfusions, attempting to balance the interests of the child and the parents often can be a complex procedure (Elder, 2008; Harrison, 2008; Woolley, 2005). It is therefore important to review models of family-centred care that emphasise training of parents to assume responsibility for care and decision making and move towards truly collaborative relationships between families and nurses.

Advocacy for children, young people and their families extends beyond shifting care responsibility back to families, and requires strategies for the development and maintenance of ongoing collaborative engagements. This is particularly important as the relationships between parents, young people and nursing staff may change over time, particularly when the child reaches an age at which they may be able to generate their own autonomous preferences regarding treatment. A key feature of this collaboration is the ability of nurses to help facilitate plans for care and treatment.

To illustrate the principles of advocacy in the context of family-centred care, consider a young child admitted to a paediatric ward setting for ongoing surgical treatment to correct congenital talipes. On admission, her mother reveals that she has left her three other children with a babysitter and needs to get back to them, leaving the child in hospital with only the staff to care for her.

The qualities and skills required to advocate for this family, the child, her mother and siblings at home waiting for their mother to come home are complex. The advocacy role in relation to the child, the parent and family must be managed within the context of a busy paediatric setting. There may be an expectation that parents will be available to provide children's care in hospital.

In this example, the nurse advocate is required to balance the competing needs of the child, parent and the family as a whole. This will involve considering the child's need for support and assistance in making decisions about her care (particularly given that the condition is ongoing), her mother's ability to provide care for all four of her children and the other children's needs. In this situation, it may be in the best interests of the child, parent and family if the mother returns home to care for her other children, while remaining in close contact with the nursing staff about the child's progress.

Decision-making frameworks

As Kelly and colleagues note in their recent work, 'it is generally accepted that families have the best interests of their children at heart and that it is within the family unit that children's rights are maintained' (Kelly, Jones, Wilson & Lewis, 2012, p. 198). Where children cannot consent to participate in treatment or research that will benefit them, they rely on adults (typically their parents or guardians) to protect them and to act in their best interests. Children's welfare, meaningful informed consent and respect for patients must therefore be upheld in both treatment and research activities (Diekema & Stapleton, 2006). Issues surrounding children and young people's consent to medical treatment will now be examined, followed by those related to research.

Using a developmental approach, increasing responsibility is afforded to children in healthcare decisions as they mature. This view is strongly supported by writers such as Dickey and colleagues, who argue that minors who possess the capacity and capability to make reasoned decisions about their health care should be involved in such decisions, irrespective of their age (Dickey, Kiefner & Beidler, 2002). However, the normative moral issue of whether children ought to have a role in healthcare decision making is separate from the empirical question of whether the law presently allows for such involvement. Children in Australia, for example, may assent (voluntarily agree) to treatment or to participate in research before legal autonomy, but it is their parents who must give consent. Box 4.1 provides the guidelines for age-of-majority legislation across Australian jurisdictions.

Box 4.1 Guidelines for age-of-majority legislation in Australia

In most jurisdictions, pursuant to age-of-majority legislation, the age of majority is 18. Beyond that age, people can make their own medical decisions in the same ways as any other adult. In New South Wales and South Australia, the age for making medical decisions is 14 and 16, respectively (*Minors (Property and Contracts) Act 1970* (NSW), section 49). A person who gives medical or dental treatment to a person under the age of 16 is protected from liability if a parent or guardian has consented; a practitioner who performs medical or dental treatment on a person 14 years or older with the consent of that person is similarly protected from liability. In South Australia, under the *Consent to Medical Treatment and Palliative Care Act 1995* (SA), section 6, a person 16 years of age or older may make decisions about their own medical treatment as validly and effectively as an adult.

Adolescence is a particularly challenging developmental stage as young people move towards the autonomy of adulthood. Parental duty to protect the child gives way to the young person's ability to make independent decisions competently (Larcher, 2005). Consent for clinical treatment must be adequately informed and freely given by a competent individual (the definition of 'competence' will be discussed in more depth later). Parents thus have legal power to consent on behalf of the young person if the young person is deemed not competent (for example, in cases of severe cognitive impairment).

However, difficulty arises when the young person is competent and either refuses treatment or seeks treatment against the wishes of the parents (Woolley, 2005). This is a difficult issue, and one in which laws vary widely internationally (Woolley, 2005). The NSW Law Reform Commission states that 'to give young people and their parents coexisting rights to consent to medical treatment means that unresolved conflicts between the wishes of a competent young person and those of his or her parents in relation to proposed medical treatment are generally resolvable ultimately by litigation, in which the best interests of the child will be the primary consideration' (Law Reform Commission New South Wales, 2004). The points being made here are that the child's welfare has ultimate importance and that, when treatment preference decisions conflict, the resolution should favour the best interests of the child.

Interestingly, Breen (2006) argues that, during the past decade, New Zealand's government and judiciary have succeeded in placing children's rights before those of parents. Breen cites a number of cases related to that country's obligations as a State Party to the Convention on the Rights of the Child to uphold Article 6, for example, recognising that 'every child has an inherent right to life in stating that parties should ensure to the maximum extent the survival and development of the child' [1996] NZFLR 670, 671, and using provisions pertaining to 'the right to life in Article 6(1) of the International Covenant on Civil and Political Rights' [198] NZFLR 998, 1000–01, 1003 (cited in Breen, 2006, p. 46).

Another fundamental principle in relation to consent to medical treatment is termed *Gillick competence*, which is based on the House of Lords ruling in *Gillick v West Norfolk Area Health Authority* 1985 (Law Reform Commission New South Wales, 2004; Woolley, 2005) cited in Breen (2006, p. 54). The Gillick principle holds that some children are legally competent to consent to medical treatment. More precisely, the ruling states that 'if a child under 16 could demonstrate sufficient understanding and intelligence to understand fully the treatment proposed they could give their consent to treatment', rather than medical professionals having to seek the advice of the child's parents (Woolley, 2005, p. 717). This ruling only applies to medical treatment that has clear potential for direct benefit to the health of the child. It is also important to remember that the Gillick principle applies only to a decision to receive treatment – it does not apply in cases of refusing treatment. An example of this is an adolescent managing cystic fibrosis who refuses a heart–lung transplant against the parents' wishes.

In Australia, the law is clear that a child can give legally informed and effective consent to medical treatment using a Gillick assessment, although it is not obligatory. Indeed, it is still argued that Australian law is inadequate in upholding children's rights to medical treatment without parental consent.

Decision making about the healthcare treatment of children and young people is influenced by the values, beliefs and attitudes of the individuals involved. It is important that nurses:

- recognise power inequity in the relationship between parents and the healthcare agency or institution
- recognise that inequity also exists in the relationship between parents and children
- enact their role as advocate
- facilitate children's and parents' decision making
- advocate for the child
- assist parents in identifying options consistent with their values
- clarify their own values, beliefs and attitudes, and thereby recognise their own biases and potential for influencing parents.

The study in Box 4.2 examined factors influencing nurses' ethical beliefs.

Nevertheless, problems of terminology leave the child at risk, as they are open to interpretation. For example, the concepts of 'best interests' and 'informed consent' are problematic. It is often difficult to determine what is in a person's 'best interests' at a particular time, as this requires detailed knowledge of the relevant circumstances, and this knowledge is often hard to gain. Similarly, questions arise about how much information the subject requires in order for their consent to be said to be properly 'informed'. Given the important role that these concepts play in discussions of advocacy, it is clearly a priority to accurately define what is meant by such terms. Moreover, the definitions of child and young person are subject to the various laws in each relevant jurisdiction, and an individual who is defined as a 'child' in one jurisdiction may be deemed to be a 'young person' in another (Law Reform Commission New South Wales, 2004). As advocate, the nurse can assist children, young people and families in forming an understanding of the relevant laws, and play a pivotal role in making sure that risks are reduced and child rights are upheld. An example helps to illustrate advocacy in practice. Consider when parents will not give consent for full and complete immunisation for their children as recommended. According to Diekema (2005), there are three important considerations for the healthcare professional:

1. Does this constitute medical neglect and thus reportable neglect?
2. How high is the risk of harm to others?
3. What is the best response?

Diekema (2005, p. 1429) suggests that, in attempting to answer these questions, the health professional will need to:

- assess the decision-making framework of the parents
- address any misinformation or miscalculation of risk versus benefit

---

Box 4.2 Research highlight

Read the article by Davis, Schrader and Belcheir: Influencers of ethical beliefs and the impact on moral distress and conscientious objection. *Nursing Ethics* 2012; 19(6), 738.

This article provides insight into the relationship between ethical beliefs, moral distress and conscientious objection in clinical practice. You are encouraged to consider this research when reflecting on practice integrity in nursing children and young people.

- acknowledge risk and the potential for harm, placing it in the context of harm versus benefit
- respect the decision eventually reached (with exception).

Returning to the Jehovah's Witness example helps to make this process clear. Suppose an 8-year-old child from an orthodox Jehovah's Witness family is admitted to hospital suffering from a condition that requires him to undergo a surgical procedure that typically involves the use of transfused whole blood – some examples of such procedures are outlined elsewhere (Chau, Wu, Ansermino, Tredwell & Purdy, 2008; Digieri, Pistelli & de Carvalho, 2006; Effa-Heap, 2009; Guichon & Mitchell, 2006; Huebler, Boettcher, Koster et al., 2007; Kacka, Kacki, Merak & Bleka, 2010).

Following Diekema's (2005) outline, in this case the nurse advocate would need to be mindful of the parents' religious beliefs and how these may impact on their healthcare decision making. The nurse would also need to inform the parents of the child's chances of survival in the event that a blood transfusion is not used, as well as considering whether there are any suitable alternatives available (as some Jehovah's Witnesses allow for the use of blood components in surgery) (Elder, 2008; Harrison, 2008). Having provided the parents with this information, the nurse advocate will allow them to make a decision about whether the surgery is performed, and what products are used in the process. However, if it is believed that the welfare of the child will not be optimised by the parents' decision, this may constitute an exceptional case in which judicial interference may be required.

Practice implications

Another challenging situation is one commonly experienced by school health and other nurses working with young people. Consider 15-year-old Angela. Angela is already sexually active and not yet using any form of contraception. Her young boyfriend, 15-year-old Simon, is willing to use condoms but they are not always prepared and do not always use them. Angela implores the nurse not to tell anyone and wants information about how to avoid pregnancy.

Such a case provides a number of challenges for the nurse advocate, who needs to balance the interests of the client with those of the clients' parents. On the one hand, the nurse has a responsibility to respect the rights of this child and provide the necessary information and health advice, particularly as young people have a right to access such information (Cohen, 1994; Gabzdyl, 2010; Schmiedl, 2004). Yet, on the other hand, there is also a duty to uphold the parents' responsibility to protect their child. Conflicts between the health system and child and family perspectives on appropriate intervention and treatment may have to be resolved by legal means if other measures prove ineffective. This is more clearly understood when the influence of social and cultural context is considered in addition to the cognitive development of children and young people (Hallstrom & Elander, 2005). Judgement and decision-making skills develop throughout the early years and are moderated by emotional, cultural and social influences (Jacobs & Klaczynski, 2005).

Thus, children and young people's decision-making ability varies within and between communities according to their position within contemporary society. For example, in communities where children are viewed as possessions, the property of their parents and other adults, they may be viewed as dependent on adults and unable to make their own decisions. At the other end of the spectrum, in some communities children may be viewed as citizens with full rights to express their own opinions and make decisions on their own behalf (Hallstrom & Elander, 2005). Think again about 15-year-old Angela and the school health nurse. The nurse must make clinical decisions based on the child's community and the cognitive and emotional development of the child, as well as social and cultural considerations. National and international legislation and conventions designed to protect the rights and interests of children and young people outlined in the previous section must also be taken into account.

Ethical decision making and informed consent in research

As with consent for clinical treatment, the age at which a child can give informed consent to participate in research and under what conditions they may legally do so rely on individual characteristics, although national regulations exist to protect children in this domain. In Australia, a series of guidelines is available through the National Health and Medical Research Council (2007), which detail what steps should be taken to ensure that research does not pose a risk to child participants. Human Research Ethics Committees are charged with the responsibility to ensure that research that does not meet a child or young person's interests does not proceed. The guidelines stress four requisite conditions for the conduct of research with children and young people, namely:

1. the importance of the question(s)
2. that the need for the participation of children/young people is indispensable, as no other source is available to provide answers to the question(s)
3. the appropriateness of the methodology
4. the research is conducted in such a way as to protect their physical, emotional and psychological safety.

The parameters for gaining consent are also stipulated in these guidelines, which state that consent must be gained from:

the child or young person whenever he or she has the capacity to make this decision; and

(b) either (i) one parent, except when, in the opinion of the review body, the risks involved in a child's participation require the consent of both parents; or where applicable

(ii) the guardian or other primary care giver, or any organisation or person required by law. (NHMRC, 2007, p. 55).

The guidelines also stipulate the need for respect for the child and young person's right to refuse to participate.

All the same, the relationship between a child's consent and the consent of parents in social research remains ambiguous in this document. For instance, what if a situation arises where the child agrees to participate, and the parents do not give consent? And when is it considered necessary to obtain both parents' consent, rather than just a single parent's consent? These are difficult issues, which require further elucidation. Until 1964, the only international code of research ethical standards was the International Military Tribunal's Nuremberg Code, which was created in the aftermath of the Second World War (Annas & Grodin, 1995). In 1964, the *Declaration of Helsinki* (1964, revised 1974, 1983, 1989, 1996, 2000, 2002, 2004) was established following a powerful history of children's rights abuses in research participation (see Diekema, 2006), and has resulted in the adoption of a set of child-specific principles (World Medical Association, 2005). The declaration states explicitly that 'permission from the responsible relative replaces that of the subject' (World Medical Association, 2005). However, at the same time the *Declaration* stipulates that children must also assent to participate. Indeed the policy (World Medical Association, 2004) states:

> When a subject deemed legally incompetent, such as a minor child, is able to give assent to decisions about participation in research, the investigator *must obtain* that assent in addition to the consent of the legally authorized representative. (emphasis added).

The requirement for informed consent and provision of an appropriate (usually written) explanation of the study is a critical element. This is where the nurse can act in the role of patient advocate. In explaining the nature of the study, everyday plain language must be used without losing the essence of the study's intention and risks (Green, Duncan, Barnes & Oberklaid, 2003). In particular, consideration must be given to parent's literacy capacity. The Australian Bureau of Statistics' report on Australian population literacy levels provides strong evidence for the need to ensure that parents are well informed if written explanations for consent are relied on (Australian Bureau of Statistics, 2006). The report found that approximately 7 million (46%) Australians aged 15 to 74 years had poor or very poor prose literacy skills, with only 2.5 million (16%) having good or very good skills. The remaining 5.6 million (37%) held minimum proficiency, being able to just cope with everyday life needs for literacy. Therefore, information provided to parents for gaining consent must be targeted to the ability of simple or minimum levels of literacy competency (Green et al., 2003). This is to ensure that the parents or guardians fully understand the nature of the research prior to giving or withholding consent. The nurse advocate may be required to assist parents and guardians in understanding the terminology used in the information sheets.

Useful guidelines and considerations for nurses planning to do research with children are:

- the child must assent to participation according to the World Medical Association (2004) principles
- the child's assent is given in addition to the consent of the legally authorised representative (usually the parent)
- parental consent provides consent to approach the child to participate and does not override the child's right to refuse to participate
- children as young as 5 years are capable of giving voluntary assent
- informed assent means that the child agrees to the conditions of participation
- all information about the research must be provided in developmentally appropriate terms
- the child's participation is voluntary and assent is sought away from parental influence.

Child protection and legislation

Within Australian and New Zealand societies, the dynamics of the family have changed considerably over recent decades. One such change has been the rising numbers of blended families with step-parents and single-parent families raising children with little and sometimes no extended family support (Australian Bureau of Statistics, 2012). The rising incidence and changing patterns of illicit drug use are other recent social changes, and they extend into the population of women of childbearing age (Australian Institute of Health and Welfare, 2007). Escalating use of psychostimulants, in particular, for which we have few treatment options, challenges delivery of health services (Australian Institute of Health and Welfare, 2005). Nurses can find they are in a unique position to support and advocate for children, young people and their families living under conditions of such adversity. However, with that role comes a legal, moral and ethical responsibility that must be clear to the nurse.

These responsibilities are particularly important in the prevention of child abuse and neglect (CAN), which is a complicated issue involving a multifaceted response from health providers and other relevant services. CAN are concepts that are defined by communities with much variation. Similarly, the response of these communities to CAN also varies considerably (Mathews, Walsh & Fraser, 2006).

The legal duty of nurses to report suspected CAN varies across Australian and New Zealand jurisdictions (see Mathews et al., 2006). There are differences in the extent of the duty, the extent of the harm caused to the child that qualifies as reportable and the types of abuse that are reportable. Differences occur between jurisdictions on whether it applies to cases of past CAN, perceived likely future CAN or both (Australian Institute of Family Studies, 2012). Due to these variations, nurses need to be familiar with the legislation that exists in the particular state or territory in which they work.

For example, Queensland and Victoria impose a condition on the consequences of sexual abuse to make it reportable, while five other jurisdictions do not (Mathews et al., 2006). The broad definition of reportable neglect in New South Wales relies on sound assessment if high rates of unsubstantiated reports are to be avoided. Abuse may be one or a combination of the four major types: physical abuse, sexual abuse, psychological/emotional abuse or child neglect. In some jurisdictions, such as Victoria and WA, nurses are not required to report suspected emotional or psychological abuse. In considering whether to report suspected CAN, the nurse advocate will need to weigh up the likely consequences of such a report and the probable effects on both the child and the family, which may be difficult to foresee.

Clearly, the opportunity to act as patient advocate for children, young people and their families is a privilege. Not only must the nurse be aware of the community standards and legal obligations for reporting, but as an advocate they must inform and support families to be aware of what is acceptable and what is not. However, it is important to remember that advocacy can, and often does, lead to conflict. When confronted by conflicting commitments and responsibilities, the nurse must make an assessment of risk and act legally and ethically (Mallik, 1997a). At the same time, commitment to supporting a family in their actions or decisions for their child may need to be compromised. This is a moral choice, but one that is constrained by legal mandates (e.g. to report suspected child abuse or neglect) and institutional power. The decision to advocate for children, young people and their families can have damaging emotional effects on nurses if risks are taken and, in certain cases, legal penalties may be applied. Consider the legal implications of findings from a South Australian study, where nurses reported that they had not, in some cases, reported suspected cases of child abuse and neglect despite a legal mandate to do so (Nayda, 2002, 2004). Nayda's (2004) research showed that reluctance to report was motivated by concerns for poor outcomes for both the nurse and the family. She also found differences between reporting by paediatric and emergency department nurses: emergency department nurses were more likely to shift responsibility to medical staff; paediatric nurses were more confident in their ability to assess and report suspected cases.

It is important to contextualise these judgements within lawful scope of practice and ethical standards. Consider a relationship that is truly collaborative. Parents do not wish to expose their children to harm. At the same time, the nurse practises within a framework that is principled, moral, ethical and legal. Respect for each of these positions within the collaborative and therapeutic relationship assists in taking actions in the best interests of the child and family.

Therapeutic relationships, advocacy and the context of child protection

Therapeutic relationships are a feature of nurse/child/family relationships in both acute care settings for sick children and young people and community healthcare settings for well children and young people. Specific characteristics of these relationships and how they differ are detailed in Chapter 5 but, for the purposes of this chapter, they are referred to more broadly. Nurses are responsible for structuring the relationship so that boundaries remain intact, the advocacy and caring roles are preserved and positive outcomes can be achieved for both children/young people and their families.

Families with particular characteristics face increased challenges in raising their children. The contemporary emphasis on early intervention and prevention programs for such families reflects wider concern that CAN are more about parenting capacity, or parental competence and emotional regulation, than individual psychopathology (Holzer, Bromfield, Richardson & Higgins, 2006).

The focus is on the parent–child relationship and the way in which the parent responds to behavioural and emotional development of the child. Nurses in clinical practice across the range of healthcare settings play a significant role in this effort.

In order to assist in fostering supportive parent–child relationships, it is important that the nurse has high levels of knowledge and is alert to and conscious of any emotional reactions, discomfort or feelings that may influence their ability to remain objective and interact in a non-judgemental manner. An awareness of biases, projected opinions and feelings is also important, as it is these subtle cues that a child or parent may pick up on that impact negatively on the therapeutic relationship (Davis et al., 2002). The nurse's counselling and interpersonal skills are essential to the initiation and maintenance of these relationships (Davis et al., 2002; Heffernan, Quinn Griffin, McNulty & Fitzpatrick, 2010; O'Connell, 2008). These skills should not be underestimated because neglect and abuse have significant detrimental effects on a child's physical or emotional health, development and wellbeing, and an appropriately skilled professional may be able to have a decisive influence in helping to eliminate, or at the very least reduce, incidences of CAN (Gould, Clarke, Heim et al., 2012; Widom, White, Czaja & Marmorstein, 2007).

Whether or not the nurse is required by law to report a case of suspected CAN, there is an ethical and moral obligation to protect children from further harm. This would require an extended and ongoing relationship between the nurse and the family. The action to report abuse to the appropriate authority should not impose on this relationship, but enhance its influence by providing valuable assistance and support not previously available. On the other hand, the results of Nayda's (2004) research indicate that many nurses do not believe that this is a possible outcome and that the family is more likely to be alienated from mainstream services.

Nurses in a position to develop and maintain productive relationships with families of vulnerable children are often also in a position to make regular home visitations. Opportunities to work closely with families in a sustained way, such as through a home visitation service, are crucial to assisting families struggling with the demands of parenting (Cramer, Crumley & Klassen, 2003; Kemp, Harris, McMahon et al., 2011; Kitzman, Olds, Cole et al., 2010; Norr, 2011; O'Brien, Moritz, Luckey et al., 2012; Olds, Kitzman, Cole et al., 2010; Stubbs & Achat, 2012). However, it is vital to ensure that nurses who are undertaking home visits to vulnerable families are adequately prepared for this work. A recent study of home visitation in the USA found that home-visiting nurses reported that they had been drawn to working in a home-visiting service for the opportunity to work intensively with vulnerable and high-risk families (Zeanah, Larrieu & Boris, 2006). However, they were initially unprepared for the intensity and chronicity of their caseloads, citing intimate–partner violence, child abuse, incest and psychopathology as:

- characteristics that interfered with the success of their home-visiting work, and
- requiring mental health nursing skills beyond the base training of home-visiting nurses (Zeanah et al., 2006).

Current initiatives in the suite of home-visiting strategies thus include those targeting specific high-risk family factors such as domestic violence and parental psychopathology (Boris, Larrieu, Zeanah et al., 2006).

If a constructive effort is to be made to assist and support families to establish effective parenting, it is crucial that nurses avoid critical, judgemental or aggressive attitudes towards possible perpetrators (Humphreys & Campbell,, 2011). Specific training is required and, if the research summarised above continues to demonstrate effective outcomes for children, nurses will be increasingly engaging in more specific home-visiting treatments. Although most parents easily engage in the therapeutic relationship, the most vulnerable families tend to be those least likely to access services. Remember that healthcare professionals, and the services they represent, may be perceived as the 'wolf in sheep's clothing', with the single intention to report suspected CAN. This can occur especially in families who already feel alienated by mainstream services (Fraser et al., 2000).

Conclusion

This chapter explored the role of advocacy within the scope of nursing children, young people and their families. The tensions between advocacy, ethics and lawful practice were considered within the framework of therapeutic relationships with families and the overall issue of children's and young people's safety. Clinical cases were highlighted to integrate an understanding of advocacy within healthcare practices and nursing responsibilities and priorities relating to families at risk, children's rights and child protection legislation.

KEY POINTS

» Advocacy is a key role in nursing children, young people and their families.
» Moral, ethical and legal obligations impact on advocacy for children, young people and their families.

CRITICAL QUESTIONS AND REFLECTIONS: LEGAL POSITION, ADVOCACY AND SKILLS

Troy is a quiet and shy 10-year-old boy. He confides to the school nurse that he is very sad because he accidentally broke his dad's favourite mug. He says his dad told him he is worthless, should never have been born and is nothing but trouble. When you ask, Troy says that this is how his father always talks to both him and his mother, and that it is okay because his father never really does anything to hurt them.

Legal position

1. In your opinion, do you think that this is a case of child abuse? Why or why not?
2. Is it reportable by law in your jurisdiction? If yes, is it reportable by a registered nurse and to whom does the nurse report?
3. How much harm to the child does there need to be for a report to be made?
4. Do you fear reprisals from reporting suspected or known child abuse? If so, why?
5. Do you fear reprisals from not reporting suspected or known child abuse? If so, why?

Advocacy role

1. Do you think it is in the child's best interests to report child abuse? Why or why not?
2. Do you think it is in the family's best interests to report child abuse? Why or why not?

Skills and competencies

1. What would be your personal strengths as a nurse in this case?
2. What would be your personal limitations as a nurse in this case?

Elisha is a 4-year-old girl frequently admitted to the paediatric hospital for review of eczema treatments. Elisha's parents have given consent in writing for her to participate in a research study that will examine the relationship between child behaviour problems, parent management of child behaviour and eczema treatments. The parents have spent a long time participating in the study by completing questionnaires and being interviewed. An important component of the study is observation data of parent/child interactions. When the nurse researcher sets up for the observation, Elisha says she doesn't want to be observed and wants the nurse to go away and not come back.

1. How can the nurse respond to act in the best interests of the child?
2. How can the nurse respond to act in the best interests of the family?

Isaiah is a 7-year-old boy admitted to the paediatric surgical unit for major abdominal surgery related to a congenital malformation of his left kidney. His parents are Jehovah's Witnesses and the paediatric surgeon will request that the family is prepared for the possibility of him having to receive a blood transfusion intraoperatively.

1. How can the nurse respond to act in the best interests of the child?
2. How can the nurse respond to act in the best interests of the family?

USEFUL RESOURCES

An Bord Altranais (Irish Nursing Board): www.aba.ie

Australian Human Rights Commission: www.hreoc.gov.au/

Australian Institute of Family Studies: www.aifs.gov.au

Australian Nursing and Midwifery Council: www.anmc.org.au

International Council of Nurses: www.icn.ch

National Council of State Boards of Nursing (United States): www.ncsbn.org

Nursing and Midwifery Council (United Kingdom): www.nmc-uk.org

United Nations *Convention on the Rights of the Child* (2001): http://treaties.un.org/Pages/ViewDetails.aspx?src=TREATY&mtdsg_no=IV-11&chapter=4&lang=en (a full list of countries that have ratified the convention is provided)

References

Annas, G. J., & Grodin, M. A. (1995). *The Nazi doctors and the Nuremberg Code: Human rights in human experimentation.* New York: Oxford University Press.

Australian Bureau of Statistics (ABS). (2006). *Adult literacy and life skills survey, summary results, Australia* [Cat. No. 4228.0]. ABS, Canberra.

Australian Bureau of Statistics (ABS). (2012). *Australian social trends, March quarter* [Cat. No. 4102.0]. ABS, Canberra.

Australian Institute of Family Studies. (2012). *Mandatory reporting of child abuse and neglect.* Melbourne: Australian Institute of Family Studies.

Australian Institute of Health and Welfare (AIHW). (2005). *National drug strategy household survey – detailed findings* [Cat. No. PHE 66]. Canberra: AIHW. Retrieved from http://www.aihw.gov.au/publication-detail/?id=6442467781 (accessed 22 January 2013).

Australian Institute of Health and Welfare (AIHW). (2007). *Statistics on drug use in Australia 2006.* Drug Statistics Series No. 18. Canberra: AIHW.

Australian Nursing and Midwifery Council (ANMC). (2002). *Code of ethics for nurses in Australia.* Canberra: ANMC.

Boris, N., Larrieu, J., Zeanah, P., et al. (2006). The process and promise of mental health augmentation of nurse home-visiting programs: data from the Louisiana nurse–family partnership. *Infant Mental Health Journal, 27*(1), 26–40.

Breen, C. (2006). *Age discrimination and children's rights: Ensuring equality and acknowledging difference.* Boston: Martinus Nijhoff Publishers.

Chau, A., Wu, J., Ansermino, M., Tredwell, S., & Purdy, R. (2008). A Jehovah's Witness child with hemophilia B and factor IX inhibitors undergoing scoliosis surgery. *Canadian Journal of Anesthesia, 55*(1), 47–51.

Cohen, P. (1994). The role of the school nurse in providing sex education. *Nursing Times, 90*(23), 36–38.

Cramer, K., Crumley, E., & Klassen, T. (2003). Are home visiting programs more effective than the standard of care at preventing injury in children who are at risk for injury? Part A. *Paediatrics & Child Health, 8*(4), 227–228.

Curtin, L. (1979). The nurse as advocate: a philosophical foundation for nursing. *Advances in Nursing Science, 1*(3), 1–10.

Dancet, E., D'Hooghe, T., Sermeus, W., et al. (2012). Patients from across Europe have similar views on patient-centred care: an international multilingual qualitative study in infertility care. *Human Reproduction, 27*(6), 1702–1711.

Davis, H., Day, C., & Bidmead, C. (2002). *Working in partnership with parents: The parent adviser model.* London: Psychological Corporation.

Davis, S., Schrader, V., & Belcheir, M. J. (2012). Influencers of ethical beliefs and the impact on moral distress and conscientious objection. *Nursing Ethics, 19*(6), 738–749.

Davis-Alldritt, L. (2012). All about advocacy. *NASN School Nurse, 27*(2), 62–63.

Dickey, S., Kiefner, J., & Beidler, S. (2002). Consent and confidentiality issues among school-age children and adolescents. *Journal of School Nursing, 18*(3), 179–186.

Diekema, D. (2005). Responding to parental refusals of immunization of children. *Pediatrics, 115*(5), 1428–1431.

Diekema, D. (2006). Conducting ethical research in pediatrics: a brief historical overview and review of pediatric regulations. *Journal of Pediatrics, 149*, 3–11.

Diekema, D., & Stapleton, F. B. (2006). Current controversies in pediatric research ethics: proceedings introduction. *Journal of Pediatrics, 149*, 1–2.

Digieri, L., Pistelli, I., & de Carvalho, C. (2006). The care of a child with multiple trauma and severe anemia who was a Jehovah's Witness. *Hematology, 11*(3), 187–191.

Effa-Heap, G. (2009). Blood transfusion: implications of treating a Jehovah's Witness patient. *British Journal of Nursing, 18*(3), 174–177.

Elder, L. (2008). Re: Faith held by Jehovah's Witnesses does not always forbid blood transfusions. *Paediatrics & Child Health, 13*(4), 334–341.

Fraser, J. A., Armstrong, K. L., Morris, J., et al. (2000). Home visiting intervention for vulnerable families with newborns: follow-up results of a randomised controlled trial. *Child Abuse and Neglect, 24*(11), 1399–1429.

Gabzdyl, E. (2010). Contraceptive care of adolescents: overview, tips, strategies, and implications for school nurses. *Journal of School Nursing, 26*(4), 267–277.

Gadow, S. (1980). Existential advocacy: philosophical foundation in nursing. In S. F. Spicker & S. Gadow (Eds.), *Nursing images of reality* (pp. 79–101). New York: Springer.

Gates, B. (1994). *Advocacy: A nurses' guide.* London: Scutari Press.

Gould, F., Clarke, J., Heim, C., et al. (2012). The effects of child abuse and neglect on cognitive functioning in adulthood. *Journal of Psychiatric Research, 46*(4), 500–506.

Green, J. B., Duncan, R. E., Barnes, G. L., & Oberklaid, F. (2003). Putting the 'informed' into 'consent': a matter of plain language. *Journal of Paediatrics and Child Health, 39*, 700–703.

Guichon, J., & Mitchell, I. (2006). Medical emergencies in children of orthodox Jehovah's Witness families: three recent legal cases, ethical issues and proposals for management. *Paediatrics & Child Health, 11*(10), 655–658.

Hallstrom, I., & Elander, G. (2005). Decision making in paediatric care: an overview with reference to nursing care. *Nursing Ethics, 12*(3), 223–238.

Harrison, C. (2008). Re: Faith held by Jehovah's Witnesses does not always forbid blood transfusions. *Paediatrics & Child Health, 13*(4), 341.

Heffernan, M., Quinn Griffin, M., McNulty, R., & Fitzpatrick, J. (2010). Self-compassion and emotional intelligence in nurses. *International Journal of Nursing Practice, 16*(4), 366–373.

Holzer, P., Bromfield, L., Richardson, N., & Higgins, D. (2006). *Child abuse prevention: What works? The effectiveness of parent education programs for preventing child maltreatment.* Retrieved from http://www.aifs.gov.au/nch/pubs/brief/rb1/rb1.html (accessed 4 July 2012).

Huebler, M., Boettcher, W., Koster, A., et al. (2007). Transfusion-free cardiac reoperation in an 11-kg Jehovah's Witness child by use of a minimized cardiopulmonary bypass circuit. *Texas Heart Institute Journal, 34*(1), 108–111.

Humphreys, J., & Campbell, J. (Eds.), (2011). *Family violence and nursing practice* (2nd ed.). New York: Spring Publishing.

International Council of Nurses (ICN). (2006a). *The ICN Code of ethics for nurses.* Retrieved from www.icn.ch/icncode.pdf (accessed 22 January 2013).

International Council of Nurses (ICN). (2006b). *The ICN Definition of nursing.* Retrieved from www.icn.ch/definition.htm (accessed 22 January 2013).

Jacobs, J. E., & Klaczynski, P. A. (2005). *The development of judgement and decision making during childhood and adolescence.* New Jersey: Lawrence Erlbaum Associates.

Jezewski, M. A. (1993). Culture brokering as a model for advocacy. *Nursing in Health Care, 14*, 78–85.

Kacka, K., Kacki, W., Merak, J., & Bleka, A. (2010). Use of recombinant activated factor VII for reduction of perioperative blood loss during elective surgical correction of spine deformity in a Jehovah's Witness. *Ortopedia Traumatologia Rehabilitacja, 12*(5), 448–458.

Kelly, M., Jones, S., Wilson, V., & Lewis, P. (2012). How children's rights are constructed in family-centred care: a review of the literature. *Journal of Child Health Care, 16*(2), 190–205.

Kemp, L., Harris, E., McMahon, C., et al. (2011). Child and family outcomes of a long-term nurse home visitation programme: a randomised controlled trial. *Archives of Disease in Childhood, 96*(6), 533–540.

Kitzman, H., Olds, D., Cole, R., et al. (2010). Enduring effects of prenatal and infancy home visiting by nurses on children: follow-up of a randomized trial among children at age 12 years. Prenatal and infancy home visiting by nurses. *Archives of Pediatrics & Adolescent Medicine, 164*(5), 412–418.

Larcher, V. (2005). Consent, competence, and confidentiality. In R. Viner (Ed.), *ABC of adolescence* (pp. 5–8). Oxford: Blackwell.

Law Reform Commission New South Wales. (2004). *Issues Paper 24 – Minors' consent to medical treatment*. Retrieved from http://www.lawlink.nsw.gov.au/lrc.nsf/pages/ip24chp01 (accessed 22 June 2012).

MacKean, G. L., Thurston, W. E., & Scott, C. M. (2005). Bridging the divide between families and health professionals' perspectives on family-centred care. *Health Experiences, 8*(1), 74–85.

Mahlin, M. (2010). Individual patient advocacy, collective responsibility and activism within professional nursing associations. *Nursing Ethics, 17*(2), 247–254.

Mallik, M. (1997a). Advocacy in nursing – a review of the literature. *Journal of Advanced Nursing, 25*, 130–138.

Mallik, M. (1997b). Advocacy in nursing – perceptions of practising nurses. *Journal of Clinical Nursing, 6*, 303–313.

Mallik, M. (1998). Advocacy in nursing: perceptions and attitudes of the nursing elite in the United Kingdom. *Journal of Advanced Nursing, 28*, 1001–1011.

Mallik, M., & Rafferty, A. M. (2000). Diffusion of the concept of patient advocacy. *Journal of Nursing Scholarship, 32*(4), 399–404.

Mathews, B., Walsh, K., & Fraser, J. A. (2006). Mandatory reporting by nurses of child abuse and neglect. *Journal of Law and Medicine, 13*(4), 505–517.

Murphy, B. (2012). Regarding 'National Health and Hospital Reform Commission final report and patient-centred suggestions for reform' by T. Jowsey, L. Yen, R. Wells and S. Leeder. *Australian Journal of Primary Health, 18*(1), 2–3.

National Health and Medical Research Council (NHMRC). (2007). *National statement on ethical conduct in human research*. Canberra: NHMRC.

Nayda, R. (2002). Influences on registered nurses' decision making in cases of suspected child abuse and neglect. *Child Abuse Review, 11*(3), 168–178.

Nayda, R. (2004). Registered nurses' communication about abused children: rules, responsibilities and resistance. *Child Abuse Review, 13*(3), 188–199.

New Zealand Nurses Association (NZNA). (1995). *Code of ethics*. Wellington: NZNA.

Norr, K. (2011). Children benefit up to the age of 12 years old from prenatal and infancy home visiting by nurses; with reduced substance use, improved academic performance and reduced mental health problems. *Evidence-Based Nursing*, *14*(1), 6–7.

O'Brien, R., Moritz, P., Luckey, D., et al. (2012). Mixed methods analysis of participant attrition in the nurse–family partnership. *Prevention Science*, *13*(3), 219–228.

O'Connell, E. (2008). Therapeutic relationships in critical care nursing: a reflection on practice. *Nursing in Critical Care*, *13*(3), 138–143.

O'Connor, T., & Kelly, B. (2005). Bridging the gap: a study of general nurses' perceptions of patient advocacy in Ireland. *Nursing Ethics*, *12*(5), 453–467.

Olds, D., Kitzman, H., Cole, R., et al. (2010). Enduring effects of prenatal and infancy home visiting by nurses on maternal life course and government spending: follow-up of a randomized trial among children at age 12 years. Prenatal and infancy home visiting by nurses. *Archives of Pediatrics & Adolescent Medicine*, *164*(5), 419–424.

Oxford English Dictionary. (2012). *Oxford English dictionary* (3rd ed.). Oxford: Oxford University Press.

Scarfe, G., Redshaw, S., Wilson, V., & Dengler, L. (2012). Heart to heart: a programme for children on a cardiac ward. *British Journal of Nursing*, *21*(2), 98–102.

Schmiedl, R. (2004). School-based condom availability programs. *Journal of School Nursing*, *20*(1), 16–21.

Stewart, M., Ryan, B., & Bodea, C. (2011). Is patient-centred care associated with lower diagnostic costs? *Healthcare Policy = Politiques de sante*, *6*(4), 27–31.

Stubbs, J., & Achat, H. (2012). Health home visiting for vulnerable families: what has occurred and what is yet to arrive? *Australian Journal of Primary Health*, *18*(1), 23–30.

The World Organisation for Cross-border Co-operation in Civil and Commercial Matters. (2012). *What is the difference between signing, ratifying and acceding to a Hague Convention?* Retrieved from http://www.hcch.net/index_en.php?act=faq.details&fid=38 (accessed 19 June 2012).

United Nations Treaty Collection. (1989). Chapter IV: Human rights 11. *Convention on the Rights of the Child*. Retrieved from http://treaties.un.org/Pages/ViewDetails.aspx?src=TREATY&mtdsg_no=IV-11&chapter=4&lang=en (19 June 2012).

Widom, C., White, H., Czaja, S., & Marmorstein, N. (2007). Long-term effects of child abuse and neglect on alcohol use and excessive drinking in middle adulthood. *Journal of Studies on Alcohol & Drugs*, *68*(3), 317–326.

Woolley, S. (2005). Children of Jehovah's Witnesses and adolescent Jehovah's Witnesses: what are their rights? *Archives of Disease in Childhood*, *90*, 715–719.

World Medical Association (WMA). (2004). *Ethical principles for medical research involving human subjects*. Helsinki: 18th World Assembly, 1964. Revised 54th WMA World General Assembly, Tokyo.

World Medical Association (WMA). (2005). *Recommendations guiding medical doctors in biomedical research involving human subjects*. Helsinki: 18th World Assembly, 1964. Revised 52nd WMA World General Assembly, Edinburgh.

Zeanah, P., Larrieu, J., & Boris, N. (2006). Nurse home visiting: perspectives from nurses. *Infant Mental Health Journal*, *27*(1), 41–54.

Chapter 5

COMMUNICATION WITH CHILDREN, YOUNG PEOPLE AND FAMILIES - A FAMILY STRENGTHS-BASED APPROACH

Lindsay Smith, Karen Ford

LEARNING OUTCOMES

Reading this chapter will help you to:

» understand how the historical position of children in health care has influenced contemporary standards of communicating with children, young people and families

» describe a child-centred approach to communication with children and families

» respect the views of children and young people by assisting them to participate in decision making related to their health care

» assess family strengths and incorporate family strengths into healthcare practice with children, young people and families

» apply positive communication skills to clinical practice with children, young people and families.

Introduction

Communication is defined as the giving and receiving of messages or, perhaps more appropriately, the exchange of meaning producing mutual understanding (O'Toole, 2012). The mutual exchange of information is inherent to effective communication and involves reciprocity and a two-way process of sharing information. This requires a common language that is more than just words, and includes emotions, behaviour, symbols and signs. Further, information that is shared needs to be both accurate and authentic to move towards shared understanding (Lucock, Lefevre, Orr et al., 2006, p. 3). Communicating with children and young people offers unique challenges in achieving shared understanding. Differences in age, gender, socio-cultural experiences and personal assumptions can impact on the development of shared understanding. For example, ineffective communication with a child could result from the nurse using language the child does not yet understand. Fear and mistrust can also prevent shared understanding so it is essential that the child's fears are acknowledged and alleviated.

It is important that communication with children, young people and families is based on fundamental skills of good communication technique, developing mutual understanding and a therapeutic relationship. Stein-Parbury (2009, pp. 52–53) outlines how communication competence is based on a therapeutic use of self and a balance between responsiveness (being able to listen to and understand others) and assertiveness (being able to express yourself). The reader is referred to both the O'Toole (2012) and Stein-Parbury (2009) texts for further details on developing fundamental communication skills and a therapeutic relationship. This chapter will help build your skills in forming therapeutic relationships with children, young people and their families through developing:

1. a style of communication – positive communication for health professionals – that is strengths-based, promotes a solution focus and can help strengthen nurse–child–family relationships
2. family assessment skills.

Historical position of the child in health care and its influence on communication

Traditionally, communication with children has been based on the assumption that the healthcare practitioner is the expert and this has promoted communication styles that tend to be one-way and authoritarian. Carlsson (2010) identified 'many professional relationships are often paternalistic and not empowering, for example when a health educator identifies risk behaviour and suggests changing that behaviour' (p. 28). An authoritarian/paternalistic style of communication has no place in contemporary paediatrics and child health care that recognises the rights of children and young people as active participants in their health care. Poor communication is counterproductive to efficient health care whereas positive and effective communication leads to improved health outcomes, saves time and benefits all involved.

Changes in society's view of children and childhood over time have also influenced communication with children. Nurse–child–family relationships have undergone changes since children were first admitted to hospitals and these relationships continue to undergo change. Sick and injured children were largely excluded from admission to the early hospitals, and were cared for in their homes with minimal assistance. During the 19th century, when children were beginning to be admitted to healthcare facilities, parents were soon excluded from being with their child in hospital except for a very short visiting time during the weekend, a situation that remained unchanged until the 1950s (Great Ormond Street Hospital, 2012; Telfer, 2008). The silencing of children and family exclusion were outcomes supported by the understandings of the time. Children in health care were expected to be quiet and compliant. The following quote from a children's nurse illustrates past (although not distant) nursing practices:

> I recall at one time children were well behaved, they were tied into their beds, so that busy nurses could keep track of them. There was order in the wards. Parents gave their child to the hospital to be treated. (Anonymous senior nurse, 1995, cited in Wood, 2008, pp. 119–120).

One of the most significant changes in children's and young people's health care in recent times has been the recognition that children have inherent rights and must be part of decision-making and communication processes (see the section 'Respecting the views of children'). It was only in the latter part of the 20th century that the concept of family participation and communicating with children became a feature of children's health care, particularly in hospital. In Australian hospitals, daily visiting for children was adopted in the 1950s and 1960s and mothers with young children were admitted in the late 1970s (Wood, 2008, p. 123). It is important to understand these past attitudes to nursing care of children, as current practice still struggles at times to totally break itself free from the restrictive attitudes recently prevalent in children's nursing. The ecology of child health care, which includes the physical space and the institutional policies, may still reflect past attitudes of silencing children. The ecology of child health care influences the nurse–child relationship and impacts on positive communication, sharing of decision making with children, the emotional response to the experience and implementation of family-centred care (Bishop, 2012).

Studies of separation and attachment have had a profound influence on the way infants and children are cared for in hospitals. The development of hospital policies and practices that support the care of children in the context of the family is in part a direct result of this influence. The effects of separation or the breaking of the attachment bond on the psychological wellbeing of the child were described by Robertson and Bowlby (1965), who identified three stages of grieving as protest, despair and detachment. Protest is characterised by crying and acute distress when the mother is lost to the child and the child tries to recapture her. Despair is characterised by increasing hopelessness, withdrawal and fewer efforts to be reunited with the mother. Detachment describes the child's behaviour of 'settling down' in the 'separation environment', where the child displays marked loss of attachment behaviours to the mother on her return (Bowlby, 1965, p. 214). Detachment, or 'settling down', was previously seen as a positive outcome although we now understand that children were communicating their deep distress of being separated from their parents through their behaviours of crying or withdrawal. Children's communications were *mis*-heard and misinterpreted by healthcare professionals based on their understandings of children and childhood of the time.

During health care children have been viewed as vulnerable and lacking capabilities, and this has resulted in a tendency to silence children and to limit communication with them. However, with our changing views of children as social actors in their own right – as social beings rather than 'becomings' – the traditional positioning of children is also subject to change (Hendrick, 2008, p. 42). When children are viewed as capable and intentional, the extent of their involvement and consultation in their care can be increased (Lucock et al., 2006, p. 14).

Respecting the views of children

The UN *Convention on the Rights of the Child* sets out the basic rights of children, and these include: the right to survival; to develop to the fullest; to protection from harmful influences, abuse and exploitation; and to participate fully in family, cultural and social life. A number of the articles in the *Convention on the Rights of the Child* relate to children's health care, and one of the core principles of the Convention is respect for the views of the child. Articles 12 and 13 are specifically relevant to communication with children. Article 12 relates to respect for the views of children and Article 13 to freedom of expression (UN, 1989).

> Article 12 encourages adults to listen to the opinions of children and involve them in decision-making. When healthcare decisions are being made that affect children, children have the right to say what they think should happen and have their opinions taken into account.

> Article 13 states that children have the right to get and share information, as long as the information is not damaging to them or others. The freedom of expression includes the right to share information in any way they choose, including by talking, drawing or writing.

The charters for children's and young people's rights in health care in Australia and in New Zealand were launched in 2010 (Children's Hospitals Australasia, 2010a, 2010b). Both charters refer specifically to: children's and young people's right to express their views, to be heard and taken seriously; their right to information in a form understandable to them; and their right to participate in decision making, and as appropriate to their capabilities, to make decisions about their care (Children's Hospitals Australasia, 2010a, 2010b). These charters are consistent with the rights expressed in the UN *Convention on the Rights of the Child* and also clearly articulate the rights of children and young people in terms of communication and participation. To facilitate their participation in decision making, health carers need to create an environment that is based on trust, the capacity to listen, information-sharing and sound guidance (Children's Hospitals Australasia, 2010a, 2010b; also see Box 5.1).

Box 5.1 Research highlight

Listening to children and young people and considering their views on their health care is a mark of respect, and can influence services that centre around their needs and choices. A qualitative study using appreciative enquiry by Carter, Coad, Bray et al. (2012) explored nursing services for children and young people in the family home. Their care needs ranged from relatively simple to highly technological interventions. In this UK study, children and young people were members of advisory groups who contributed to the study design and implementation. Focus group and interview participants included children and young people ($n = 27$), families ($n = 82$) and healthcare professionals ($n = 105$). Important enablers for care to be sustained at home were found to include effective communication, leadership and partnerships based on trust. The study findings have directly influenced government policy and practice. This work highlights the potential for children and young people to actively participate in research, even as researchers, and that when children and young people are listened to, care provision can move closer to best practice that meets their needs.

Positive communication - a style of communication to guide practice with children, young people and their families

Positive communication can be defined as a purposeful style of communication that recognises and builds on the strengths of the participants with the intent of enhancing developmental health outcomes and respecting human rights. Recent research in developmental health outcomes (see the bioecological theory of human development in Chapter 10) has indicated the importance of communication in developing optimal health outcomes. Positive communication enhances the efforts of healthcare professionals to support optimal health outcomes in children and families. Positive communication is a style of communication that: creates shared meanings at the level appropriate for the age of the child; has purposeful intent; is centred on the benefit of the other; incorporates a willingness to be bidirectional; is open to discovery and growth; is respectful of rights and autonomy; and seeks to identify and encourage strengths.

Kolucki and Lemish (2011) identified four principles for communicating with children through media and materials that support holistic development. These four principles of communication apply to all forms of communication with children. Following these four principles of communication will help achieve a positive communication style:

- Principle 1: communication should be age-appropriate and child-friendly.
- Principle 2: communication for children should address the child holistically.
- Principle 3: Communication should be positive and strengths-based.
- Principle 4: Communication should address the needs of all, including those who are most disadvantaged (pp ix–x).

The communication needs of children and young people are very different to those of adults. Health professionals caring for children are required to have a good understanding of children's communication skills as well as their physiological, psychological, intellectual and emotional development (Kennedy, 2001, p. 429). The special considerations that are required in relation to children's developmental needs mean that adult approaches are not suitable:

> They (children) experience and see the world differently. Children are in a constant state of growth and development which creates particular needs and demands which are of a different order from those affecting adult patients ... Children communicate their thoughts and feelings in a very different way from adults. (Kennedy, 2001, p. 419).

In addition, children are not one homogeneous group, and each child and young person needs to be considered as an individual with unique perspectives, experiences, needs and communication styles. Achieving positive communication with an infant is uniquely different to positive communication with a young person; however, all children at all ages communicate and must be listened to so that a shared understanding can be achieved. A 6-year-old child who has a chronic disease and has had multiple healthcare encounters will have different understandings and experiences and different communication needs compared to a 10-year-old child experiencing a first time admission to hospital for an acute illness. Infants, children and young people with language or speech difficulties, and those with developmental delay, present groups with their own special communication needs.

Effective communication with children displays several important elements: the ability to build trust, empathy and child centredness; the ability to listen and use creative communication techniques; and an understanding that communication is facilitated by enabling children's participation though empowerment and advocacy (Lucock et al., 2006). Carlsson, Bramhagen, Jansson and Dykes (2011, p. 472) recommend:

> when promoting empowerment the professional must not approach the subject from a paternalistic, controlling or decision-influencing standpoint but rather attempt to increasing the power of the individual they are supporting. To promote the individual's self-empowerment requires that the individual describes the problem, finds the solution themself, and acts to solve the problem.

This provides a challenge to child health nurses and allied health professionals to finds ways to empower children through helping them firstly describe their 'problem', then find a suitable solution and lastly enable children and families to take action fitting to their healthcare need.

Developing trust and sharing decision making through positive communication

Developing trust is one of the keys to achieving positive communication outcomes with children and young people. Nurses' use of age-appropriate language and play activities, providing explanations, enabling participation in decision making and goal setting, encouragement and adequate preparation for procedures all help build trust in the relationship. A child will be more trusting of nurses who communicate on their terms and in ways they can fully understand.

Children and young people also have a role and a right to determine the level of decision making and participation and this can vary in the same child in different circumstances. In general, there are no guidelines that regulate nurses delegating self-care tasks and enabling children and young people to participate in the decision-making process; however, the charters on children and young people's rights in health care are an excellent starting point. There are times, nevertheless, when nurses are required to implement care that challenges the connection that has developed in the relationship with the child or young person. Painful or distressing procedures and treatments are examples of this. At such times decisions need to be made about how much control lies with the child and the young person experiencing health care; however, at all times, what is in their best interests must inform the course of action. Issues of informed consent (see Chapter 4) and working within the scope of practice (see Chapter 4) should be articulated within the employer's policy and procedures manual and may determine appropriate actions in some situations.

Being held

According to the seminal work of Donald Winnicott (1965), the child's general physical and emotional growth is dependent upon a facilitating, holding environment. The holding environment describes the requirements for infants (and children) to grow and develop. A facilitating and supportive environment is necessary for children during their experience of illness (Ford, 2011) – a time that is recognised as a crisis for the child (Winnicott, 1965, p. 149).

Initially, holding consists of the mother's behaviour of making the totally dependent infant safe where the mother is able to meet the needs of her infant (Winnicott, 1965, p. 57). It is from the experience of being held that the infant develops an identity – the developing child is 'held', first of all, literally by the mother and later by the quality of its participation with the environment. According to Winnicott (1965), the term 'holding' represents 'not only the actual physical holding of the infant, but also the total environmental provision … in other words, it refers to a three-dimensional or space relationship with time gradually added' (p. 43). The holding environment is the necessary environment for the child to develop true personhood. The infant's experience of a protective space allows them to safely examine and interact with the things their world presents, even when they are frightened or alarmed and temporarily need to retreat to a safe place (Kahn, 2001, p. 262).

Although based in infancy, Winnicott's theories of development and holding also continue to be integral to the growing child and adolescent and the adult. The dependable meeting of the infant's physical needs and, later, the meeting of the child's psychological needs provides them with a way to develop and to meet the challenges they are presented with. At every stage, the child's growth is affected by the quality of the environment that supports their development (Van Buskirk & McGrath, 1999).

During health care, a facilitating, supportive, holding environment is essential for children to build understandings of their healthcare experience. The enabling environment includes both social and physical aspects and is experienced through positive communication and trusted connectedness between the nurse and the child. Holding environments encompass the nature of effective caregiving relationships considered to be intrinsic to human development, for it is 'within holding environments, [that] people demonstrate their care and concern for others in particularly skilful ways' (Van Buskirk & McGrath, 1999, p. 808). Being held during healthcare experiences is necessary for the child's safety and wellbeing. Parents and families are the primary ones who hold their child. Nurses enter into this holding environment through trust and positive communication, listening to both the verbal and the non-verbal communication of the child.

Family-centred care is a philosophical approach that has underpinned children's nursing for some time (Ahmann, 1994; Casey, 1988). The approach recognises the central role of the family in the child's life and essentially places the family at the heart of the child's care (Smith, Coleman & Bradshaw, 2006). One of the critiques of family-centred care is the passive role children are allocated within this model as the focus lies essentially with the adult participants – the parent, carer or health professional (Lambert, Glacken & McCarron, 2011). The risk is that the child may remain unseen and, we would argue, unheard when family-centred care does not recognise the child as a member of this partnership. If the child however, is recognised as a unique person and as an active participant within the partnership, their potential to participate in communication and their own decision making is realised and their rights are thereby also realised. This view then acknowledges the child as being 'in family', rather than the child 'and family'.

Family strengths

When the child is the centre of positive communication, nurses and healthcare professionals engage in positive communication with the whole family when caring for children and young people. There is a growing trend to understand families from a 'family strengths framework', to identify what families are doing well and what they can do to optimise positive outcomes. The family strengths framework is a positive approach to health care, looking at how families succeed and promote resilience. It proposes that all families have strengths, these strengths develop over time and strengths can be encouraged within all families (DeFrain & Asay, 2007). The family strengths framework is a solution-focused approach to health care (McAllister, 2007).

At the core of the family strengths framework is the concept that families function best through operational strengths that afford benefits. Although there is no commonly accepted definition for family strengths, Moore, Whitney and Kinukawa (2009) identify family strengths as 'the set of relationships and processes that inherently satisfy, support and protect families and family members, especially during times of adversity and change' (p. 1). Strengths are vital for optimising outcomes through challenging times, stressful periods and illness. The International Family Strengths Model has identified six common family strengths that appear to be universal in their importance to families (DeFrain & Asay, 2007). These are:

1. appreciation and affection
2. commitment to the family
3. positive communication
4. enjoyable time together
5. spiritual wellbeing
6. successful management of stress and crisis.

Not all families demonstrate similar strengths and how each family demonstrates strengths may differ from one family to another. Uniting families is a positive emotional connectedness towards one another, causing people in strong families to sacrifice for each other's wellbeing (Olson, DeFrain & Skogrand, 2010). All families have strengths that nurses can help the family draw on throughout health care. Positive communication is a strength that healthcare professionals share with families.

There is strong evidence around the importance of helping families develop family strengths to promote health outcomes and increase resilience to major life stressors (Moore et al., 2009; Olson et al., 2010; Smith, 2011). Children with positive social orientation, strong families and external community support have been identified as being able to cope more effectively with life changes than children without these protective factors (AIHW, 2012). Overwhelmingly, research and health advocates conclude that family strengths assist families to develop resilience, help overcome life challenges and crises and provide significant health and wellbeing benefits.

The strengths-based approach focuses on the client or family competencies, resources and capacities, and actively seeks to identify strengths within individuals and families creating a context for change (Wright & Leahey, 2009). As well, this approach leads to the development of clinician and client relationships based on partnership. (The important role of partnership in child, youth and family work is expanded across the chapters in this text.) Consequently, it is appropriate for nurses working with children and families to adopt aspects of the family strengths perspective and develop new roles such as family health nursing (see, for example, www.euro.who.int/en/what-we-do/health-topics/health-systems/nursing-and-midwifery/activities/education/family-health-nurse) into their clinical practice. Nurses caring for children should endeavour to develop a strong nurse–family relationship through positive communication and family strengths assessment.

Family strengths assessment: working with children, young people and families

To care effectively, nurses need to be equipped with a range of competencies and attributes. Among these competencies is the ability to undertake a comprehensive family assessment and to recognise the interplay of family, community and environment on children and young people's health. Assessing families is an important aspect of working with children and young people, as it recognises and values the child as being 'in family'. However, it is important to be aware also of situations when care for children and young people is provided 'outside of their natural family'. A specific example is that of homeless youth, who may be living in circumstances outside of their natural family and have particular health, social and financial concerns. In this situation, the family is whoever the young person identifies as their family and may include close social group members.

Wright and Bell (2009) justify the importance of nurses and midwives conducting comprehensive family assessments so that they better understand the family's experience of health or an illness event. Undertaking a thorough family assessment enables the development of an understanding of the family unit and what the health or illness event means to the family members, and identifies what they need during that time. A range of family assessment tools is available, each with different aims and scope. It is important to evaluate such tools as being fit for purpose. One family assessment tool available is the Australian Family Strengths Nursing Assessment Guide (AFS Nursing Assessment Guide – see below).

The Australian Family Strengths Research Project (Geggie, DeFrain, Hitchcock & Silberberg, 2000), the first Australian research to identify the language Australians use when talking about their strengths, identified eight qualities of strong Australian families, seven of which are family strengths. The eighth quality, resilience, captures the family's ability to withstand and rebound from crisis and adversity. The eight qualities are:

1. communication
2. togetherness
3. sharing activities
4. affection
5. support
6. acceptance
7. commitment
8. resilience.

These qualities of family strengths were identified by Australians as being important to them in the Australian Family Strengths Research Project and utilised to develop the AFS Nursing Assessment Guide.

The Australian Family Strengths Nursing Assessment Guide

Helping families identify and develop their strengths can instigate change in family functioning and increase family resilience (Patterson, 2002). Nurses can easily recognise strengths while listening to the family tell their story. Nurses can also observe strengths in the family's behaviour in response to the healthcare needs and challenges facing them. The AFS Nursing Assessment Guide (Table 5.1) is an assessment tool designed to provide nurses with a range of questions across the qualities of Australian family strengths (Geggie et al., 2000). In developing the assessment questions the language that Australians used to describe their family and how they interact together has been faithfully used. The AFS Nursing Assessment Guide can be used to initiate conversations with any family member that look for, support and encourage family strengths. This is a solution-focused strength of the tool.

The AFS Nursing Assessment Guide can help you encourage conversations with a family across the eight qualities of family strengths. The questions are asked as if concerning the family as a whole. For example, 'Tell me about when you talk openly with each other' refers to when the members of the family talk openly together. These questions, however, can be adapted to suit particular family and individual circumstances.

TABLE 5.1 Australian Family Strengths Nursing Assessment Guide v2

FAMILY STRENGTH	STRENGTH (S) OR GROWTH (G) AREA & COMMENTS
Togetherness • In your family, what shared beliefs really matter to you? • Do you share beliefs that really matter that you would like to follow during this admission/time of health care? • What are some of the things that cause you to celebrate together? • Can you tell me about some of your family's shared memories?	
Sharing activities • When does the family spend time together? • How often would you play together as a family? • Can you tell me about when you have good times together in your family?	
Affection • How do you show your love for each other? • How would others know you care about each other? • If I were to ask your best friend about how you care about each other, what would they say? • What sorts of things do you do for each other?	
Support • Can you tell me of times when you as a family 'share the load' and help each other? • What does it mean in your family to be 'there for each other'? • What new things have others in your family been encouraged to try?	
Communication • What helps your family to listen to each other? • Tell me about when you talk openly with each other. • Can you tell me about some of the times when you laugh together?	
Acceptance • In what ways does your family accept your individual differences? • When are you most likely to give each other space? • How do you show the members of your family that you respect each other's point of view? • What does 'forgiveness of each other' look like in your family? • What different responsibilities do each of you have?	

TABLE 5.1 Continued

FAMILY STRENGTH	STRENGTH (S) OR GROWTH (G) AREA & COMMENTS
Commitment • What helps you feel safe and secure with each other? • Can you list some of the things your family does for your community? • What rules do you have in your family and how should these be followed during this admission?	
Resilience • In what ways has this admission changed your plans? • What helps keep each other hopeful? • Can you tell me about when your family pulled together in a crisis? • When you have a problem, what helps you discuss your problems? • What do other people say they admire in your family?	
Spiritual wellbeing It is recommended that, with families who share beliefs that really matter to them, these further question/s are asked: • Is spiritual wellbeing an important strength for your family? • What do you do as a family to maintain your spiritual wellbeing? • Would you like help to maintain any of your spiritual activities during this admission/time of health care?	

The AFS Nursing Assessment Guide was developed by L Smith (2008) with permission from *Our scrapbook of strengths* (Family Action Centre and St Luke's Innovative Resources, 2003), using the language that Australian families use when talking about their own family and updated in 2013. The spiritual wellbeing section was added following evaluation of v1 and recent research evidence highlighting the positive impact of spiritual wellbeing on healthy outcomes (see Chapter 10).

The AFS Nursing Assessment Guide is not designed as a diagnostic tool that can classify or rank families according to their level of functioning. You cannot generate any type of score that is meaningful. Even a family that does not relate to any of the qualities of family strengths in the guide cannot be 'labelled' as having no strengths. Rather, only that the strengths included in the AFS Nursing Assessment Guide are not the ones that they currently include in their everyday activities. You may need to explore other strengths that the family value. The AFS Nursing Assessment Guide contains questions that can be asked of a child, young person or their family that assist in generating conversations. From conversations with families you can begin to walk more closely with the family in their effort to promote optimal developmental health and wellbeing for each other (see Box 5.2).

Box 5.2 Practice highlight

Here are some comments received from Registered Nurses in Australia about the AFS Nursing Assessment Guide and its clinical use:

'Using the AFS Nursing Assessment Guide was refreshing; it was nice to look at the positives in a person or family as opposed to the negative attributes. Nurses using this tool can identify strengths and then feed back to the family members, allowing families to develop goals and strengths to solve problems. Listening to families helped to build trust with them, improving our relationship in which the family felt they could share their feelings. This is a great step forward in client–nurse relationships as we are better able to include their strengths in our care plans.'

'The tool has enabled this family to have a better perception of the nurse engagement in the care of Mrs S. Ultimately this resulted in better acceptance of the nurse's role, more prompt acceptance of advice in the care and a better involvement by some family members. Some family members mentioned how using the AFS Nursing Assessment Guide has effectively helped them in realising how strong their family was and that together they will be able to manage even a challenging and distressing situation as their mother's illness.'

'I found using this tool with the family very easy – they felt comfortable answering the questions. I think they actually enjoyed discussing their strengths. The time-consuming aspect of using this guide is far outweighed by its benefits in terms of family and community development.'

Conducting a family strengths assessment

Here is a suggested approach to conducting a family strengths assessment using the AFS Nursing Assessment Guide. You may adapt this to suit your needs and the family's capacity.

Invite all the family to participate in this activity and work out when it would suit everyone for you to visit them. Let them decide who is in their family and who should be there. Don't be worried if other people are included; rather ask how everyone fits together (both the genogram and the ecomap are good for this – see McMurray & Clendon, 2011). Be careful, however, that some members of the family don't feel excluded, especially children and teenagers. This is an 'all in' activity! It may be necessary to just meet with those family members who are readily available; however, let them know that you are willing to work around their schedule. Let the family decide who, when and where within professional parameters that maintain safety.

Initially, identify for the family that you would like to have a conversation with them about how they relate to each other and that you want to learn what is important to them. You may like to mention that the focus of your discussion is on family strengths and, if necessary, you will redirect the conversations towards strengths. (There is an important place for deficit assessments; however, this is not the focus for this activity.)

Commence the conversation by asking the first or a relevant question in one of the qualities of Australian family strengths. Try to identify a quality for which you have noticed particular strength being displayed and make a statement reflecting what you see happening. For example, if the family members are enjoying spending time together, perhaps the father and children are playing together while things are getting organised, say 'I am really enjoying seeing how easy it is for you to play together' and ask 'How often would you play together as a family?' Ask participants if they believe that this is a quality that the family has, then place an 'S' (for strength) beside the question if they agree or 'G' (for growth) beside the question if this is an area where they want to grow further. From their answers encourage further conversation, such as what game is a family favourite? (If it is a board game, despite the temptation to get it out and have a game, please finish the assessment first.)

Where a family identifies that a question or quality is not relevant to them, just note 'not applicable'. There is no need to explore further at this stage. You may consider exploring other strength areas further as you walk beside the family at a later date.

From the family strengths nursing assessment you can build a picture for both yourself and the family of the strengths they embrace and the qualities that they want to further adopt or grow. Depending on your relationship and scope of nursing practice with the family, the insights that you gain about the family strengths can be incorporated into your nursing care. Subsequently, you can incorporate their strengths into your nursing care or you can discuss strategies to grow in different areas. Perhaps family communication was identified as an area for growth. The community health service may use this finding to identify a local need and offer a family communication workshop in the near future.

The first and perhaps most important outcome from the family strengths nursing assessment is the strengthening of the nurse–child–family relationship and the development of trust that is based on shared understanding and respect. Nursing is seen to value what is most important to the child and their family over other priorities.

Through identifying the strengths that a family uses, nurses may highlight for the first time that each family member offers something of value to each other, thus increasing the family's sense of purpose and unity. Recognising and encouraging family strengths helps demonstrate an understanding of the whole family's needs and hopes. Walking with the family in this way creates a connectedness that is unique to the nurse–child–family relationship. See Chapter 10 for application of the family strengths assessment to the young person.

Practical tips and techniques for developing a positive communication style with children and families

Children and young people express their views in many ways (Children's Hospitals Australasia, 2010a, b). Skills to enhance positive communication with children can be developed and the techniques embedded into clinical practice. In caring for children, nurses must attend closely to ways children communicate when words do not provide the means for them to be heard or when other methods are preferred by the child or young person. Here are a few tips that you may find useful.

1. *Gain the child's attention before talking.* This is best achieved if you are on the same level as the child and you have good eye contact (Harrelson, 2009). Get on the floor if you need to. If it is clean enough for them, it is clean enough

for you. Do, however, consider infection control issues when getting on the same level as the child. Sitting on one bed and then the next in a hospital setting can contribute to cross-infection. Rather than demanding that the child stop what they are doing, help the child to finish up with their activity before bringing their attention to the healthcare matter you want to talk with them about.

2. *Provide opportunities for children and young people to express themselves through play and art during their healthcare experience.* Children and young people have a natural ease expressing themselves though play and arts-based activities. Such methods can promote dialogue, enrich understandings of the child's experiences and enhance communication. The Association for the Wellbeing of Children in Healthcare (AWCH) identified that 'children have a basic need for play and it is a critical communication tool which can help the child understand their treatment and assist in recovery' (2008, p. 9). Providing opportunities for children and young people to express themselves through play and art during their healthcare experience presents another important method for enabling their rights to be heard. Engaging with children experiencing health care through play is a form of positive communication (Ford, 2011).

3. *Speak kindly and positively and be a good listener.* Encourage children and offer praise and thanks and use age appropriate words that the child recognises such as 'please' or 'ta' (Harrelson, 2009). Remember to be a good listener across every form of communication the child may be using, including crying or being quiet. Talk with children and not at them. Use positive directions when necessary; however, don't make demands and threats that are coercive and manipulative. Provide children and young people with the time and opportunity to ask questions (Lambert et al., 2011).

4. *Respect children's privacy.* Every effort should be made to respect a child's privacy; be courteous, provide explanations and ask permission. There are instances when a child or young person may request that an aspect of care is provided by a health professional of their own sex. It might be that some procedures will be planned for when their parent is present, or with the presence of a trusted member of staff (Department of Health, 2003, p. 15).

5. *Be truthful.* If a procedure is painful or unpleasant, provide a truthful explanation. Insertion of a cannula can be painful and saying it will not hurt is not respectful to the child. Acknowledge the child's fears and consider coping strategies that might assist, so the child has confidence and some level of control.

6. *Listen for and to children's communication of pain.* The FLACC pain assessment tool (Merkel, Voepel-Lewis, Shayevitz & Malviya, 1997), for example, is a validated tool that provides a useful guide for the assessment of pain in infants and preverbal children. FLACC stands for face, legs, activity, cry and consolability. The tool requires the nurse to assess a range of non-verbal communications such as the facial expression of the infant, their posture and activity, the nature of their cry and the degree to which they can be comforted. Previously, it was understood that infants do not feel pain as adults do, because the ways they communicated their pain were not understood. The result was that they did not receive adequate pain relief. When we understand and make sense of all the ways children communicate,

we are better able to respond effectively and meet their care needs. In this example, understanding how infants communicate their pain acknowledges their right to be heard but also their right to be protected from harm.

7. *Promote equality through communication with all children.* Children with language or speech difficulties present a group who may not be able to communicate through words. They may communicate through gesture, gaze or signing. Or they may use communication assistive devices such as a communication board that includes photos, pictures, words or symbols that they can indicate through gaze, finger or pointer stick. Increasingly, technological devices such as computers and tablets are being used to assist communication. Understanding the different ways that children communicate allows their rights to be heard and met. This might require that parents interpret for their child and teach nurses how to use these 'alternative' ways of communication effectively.

8. *Display caring attributes.* Children have identified qualities that they want in nurses and these include being 'friendly' and 'nice', 'kind' and 'helpful' (Pelander & Leino-Kilpi, 2004). These attributes are important features of positive communication because a friendly, positive and respectful stance provides a means for opening and maintaining positive communication with children and young people. Humour is described as a nursing intervention that nurses utilise through tone of voice, facial expressions and laughter (Sheldon, 1996, p. 1181) and provides an avenue for communication between the nurse and the child. Humour can provide a way for nurses to build rapport and a relationship with children. Communication by nurses using humour indicates their caring and humanness and that they are in tune with the child. Appropriate use of humour helps to break down barriers and establish the nurse–child relationship (Ford, 2011, p. 224).

9. *Spaces and physical environments also communicate messages to children and young people.* For example, art works by children for children displayed on the walls provide a very different message to long, white, 'sterile' corridors. Art work by children communicates a child friendly, safe environment compared to hospitals or clinics as scary, alien places and presents a recognisable children's space and place, where other children have been and had fun. The Tiles Project at the Mater Children's Hospital is a wonderful example of this (Creagh Sutton, 2005).

10. *Be approachable.* Wearing child friendly uniforms and bright print name tags, using the name of the child and your own name are all forms of positive communication that express that you are approachable and friendly.

All 10 positive communication tips are valuable and applicable in a broad range of healthcare settings including paediatric units and in community child health centres.

Conclusion

With shorter hospital admission times or limited time for health visits, there is a risk that the opportunities for communication with children and parents can be limited. Health professionals may make assumptions about what is being communicated or the level of understanding the child or family have about their health issue. The challenges nurses face include getting to know the individual child, their stories and their fears and anxieties (Ford, 2011). However, the importance of being able to listen to children and their families and to empower them with the information they need to make decisions remains. Nurses and midwives are well placed to lead and champion a new direction in health care of positive communication with children and families.

KEY POINTS

» Positive communication with children is built on trust and understanding the psychosocial, cognitive and emotional stages and challenges through infancy, childhood and into youth.

» Children's rights encourage adults to listen to the opinions of children and involve them in decision making.

» Family-centred care practices in nursing can be a means of promoting children's rights or can be a means of silencing children.

» An emphasis on the strengths and resources of families helps families develop positive attitudes towards their capabilities and helps to build trust in the nurse–child–family relationship.

CRITICAL QUESTIONS AND REFLECTIONS

1. Consider your own everyday communications with children – how you approach them and the language you use. How do you include children as active participants in discussions about care choices and planning?

2. After reading this chapter you are ready to undertake a family strengths assessment to apply the principles described to practice. Utilising the AFS Nursing Assessment Guide, engage in a conversation with a family as a group about their strengths and how their family functions across the eight qualities. Explore what goals the family are currently striving towards. Remember, not every strength needs to be explored with every family. What benefits do you think a family strengths assessment can have for clinical practice and promoting family health? What were the challenges to conducting your family strengths assessment?

USEFUL RESOURCES

Children's Hospitals Australasia (CHA) (2010a) *Charter on the rights of children and young people in healthcare services in Australia.* CHA/AWCH, Deakin, ACT.

Children's Hospitals Australasia (CHA) (2010b) *Charter on the rights of Tamariki children and Rangatahi young people in healthcare services in Aotearoa New Zealand.* CHA/Paediatric Society, New Zealand.

Stein-Parbury J, 2009 *Patient and person: Interpersonal skills in nursing*, 4th edn. Churchill Livingstone, Sydney.

UNICEF *Communicating with children. Principles and practices to nurture, inspire, educate and heal*. Retrieved from http://www.unicef.org/cwc/ (accessed 17 August 2012).

References

Ahmann, E. (1994). Family-centered care: shifting orientation. *Pediatric Nursing, 20*(2), 113–117.

Association for the Wellbeing of Children in Healthcare (AWCH). (2008). *Standards for the care of children and adolescents in health services*. Retrieved from http://www.awch.org.au/pdfs/Standards_Care_Of_Children_And_Adolescents.pdf (accessed 1 February 2013).

Australian Institute of Health and Welfare (AIHW). (2012). *Social and emotional wellbeing: Development of a Children's Headline Indicator* [Cat. No. PHE158]. Canberra: AIHW.

Bishop, K. (2012). The role of art in a paediatric healthcare environment from children's and young people's perspectives. *Procedia – Social and Behavioral Sciences, 38*, 81–88.

Bowlby, J. (1965). *Childcare and the growth of love*. Harmondsworth: Penguin Books.

Carlsson, A. (2010). *Child injuries at home. Prevention, precautions and interventions with focus on scalds*. Doctoral dissertation 2010. Sweden: Faculty of Health and Society, Malmö University.

Carlsson, A., Bramhagen, A.-C., Jansson, A., & Dykes, A. K. (2011). Precautions taken by mothers to prevent burn and scald injuries to young children at home: an intervention study. *Scandinavian Journal of Public Health, 39*, 471–478.

Carter, B., Coad, J., Bray, L., et al. (2012). Homebased care for special healthcare needs: community children's nursing services. *Nursing Research, 61*(4), 260–268.

Casey, A. (1988). A partnership with child and family. *Senior Nurse, 8*(4), 8–9.

Children's Hospitals Australasia (CHA). (2010a). *Charter on the rights of children and young people in healthcare services in Australia*. Deakin, ACT: CHA/AWCH.

Children's Hospitals Australasia. (2010b). *Charter on the rights of Tamariki children and Rangatahi young people in healthcare services in Aotearoa New Zealand*. New Zealand: CHA/Paediatric Society.

Creagh Sutton, K. (2005). *A study of the Mater Children's Hospital tile project. Unpublished Masters Thesis*. Australian Catholic University. Retrieved from http://dlibrary.acu.edu.au/digitaltheses/public/adt-acuvp105.11092006/02whole.pdf (accessed 12 May 2012).

DeFrain, J., & Asay, S. (2007). *Strong families around the world. Strengths-based research and perspectives*. New York: The Haworth Press.

Department of Health. (2003). *Getting the right start: National Service Framework for Children. Standard for hospital services*. Retrieved from http://www.dh.gov.uk/en/Publicationsandstatistics/Publications/PublicationsPolicyAndGuidance/DH_4006182 (accessed February 2013).

Ford, K. (2011). 'I didn't really like it, but it sounded exciting': admission to hospital for surgery from the perspectives of children. *Journal of Child Health Care*, 15(4), 250–260.

Family Action Centre and St Luke's Innovative Resources. (2003). *Our scrapbook of strengths*. Maryborough: Pyrenees Press.

Geggie, J., DeFrain, J., Hitchcock, S., & Silberberg, S. (2000). *The family strengths research report*. Newcastle: Family Action Centre, University of Newcastle.

Great Ormond Street Hospital. (2012). *Complete history of GOSH*. Retrieved from http://www.gosh.nhs.uk/about-us/our-history/complete-history-of-gosh/ (accessed 17 August 2012).

Harrelson, P. (2009). *Communicating with young children*. Virginia Cooperative Extension Publication 350–022. Virginia State University.

Hendrick, H. (2008). The child as a social actor in historical sources: problems of identification and interpretation. In P. Christensen & A. James (Eds.), *Research with children: Perspectives and practices* (pp. 40–65). New York: Routledge.

Kahn, W. (2001). Holding environments at work. *The Journal of Applied Behavioural Science*, 37(3), 260–279.

Kennedy, I. (2001). *The report of the public enquiry into children's heart surgery at the Bristol Royal Infirmary 1984–1995: Learning from Bristol*. London: The Stationery Office.

Kolucki, B., & Lemish, D. (2011). *Communicating with children. Principles and practices to nurture, inspire, excite, educate and heal*. New York: UNICEF.

Lambert, V., Glacken, M., & McCarron, M. (2011). Communication between children and health professionals in a child hospital setting: a Child Transitional Communication Model. *Journal of Advanced Nursing*, 67(3), 569–582.

Lucock, B., Lefevre, M., Orr, D., et al. (2006). *Teaching, learning and assessing communication skills with children and young people in social work education*. Social Care Institute for Excellence, University of Sussex. Retrieved from http://www.scie.org.uk/Index.aspx (accessed 6 February 2013).

McAllister, M. (2007). An introduction to solution-focused nursing. In M. McAllister (Ed.), *Solution-focused nursing. Rethinking practice* (pp. 49–62). Houndmills, UK: Palgrave.

McMurray, A., & Clendon, J. (2011). *Community health and wellness* (4th ed.). Sydney: Churchill Livingstone.

Merkel, S., Voepel-Lewis, T., Shayevitz, J., & Malviya, S. (1997). The FLACC: a behavioural scale for scoring postoperative pain in young children. *Pediatric Nursing*, 23(3), 293–297.

Moore, K. A., Whitney, C. W., & Kinukawa, A. K. (2009). *Exploring the links between family strengths and adolescent outcomes*. Research Brief Publication No. 2009–2020. Washington: Child Trends.

Olson, D., DeFrain, J., & Skogrand, L. (2010). *Marriages and families: Intimacy, diversity, and strengths* (7th ed.). USA: McGraw Hill.

O'Toole, G. (2012). *Communication. Core interpersonal skills for health professionals* (2nd ed.). Sydney: Elsevier.

Patterson, J. (2002). Understanding family resilience. *Journal of Clinical Psychology*, 58(3), 233–246.

Pelander, T., & Leino–Kilpi, H. (2004). Quality in pediatric nursing care: children's expectations. *Issues in Comprehensive Pediatric Nursing, 27*, 139–151.

Sheldon, M. (1996). An analysis of the concept of humour and its application to one aspect of children's nursing. *Journal of Advanced Nursing, 24*(6), 1175–1183.

Smith, L. (2008). Family assessment and the Australian Family Strengths Nursing Assessment Guide. In M. Barnes & J. Rowe (Eds.), *Child, youth and family health. Strengthening communities* (pp. 11–14). Sydney: Churchill Livingstone.

Smith, L. (2011). *Spiritual wellbeing and adolescent resilience. A case study of Australian youth attending one local church.* PhD dissertation, Australian Catholic University, Melbourne.

Smith, L., Coleman, V., & Bradshaw, M. (2006). Family-centred care. In A. Glasper & J. Richardson (Eds.), *A textbook of children's and young people's nursing* (pp. 77–88). Edinburgh: Churchill Livingstone.

Stein-Parbury, J. (2009). *Patient and person: Interpersonal skills in nursing* (4th ed.). Sydney: Churchill Livingstone.

Telfer, K. (2008). *The remarkable story of Great Ormond Street Hospital.* London: Simon & Schuster.

United Nations. (1989). *Convention on the Rights of the Child.* New York: United Nations General Assembly.

Van Buskirk, W., & McGrath, D. (1999). Organizational cultures as holding environments: a psychodynamic look at organizational symbolism. *Human Relations, 52*(6), 805–832.

Winnicott, D. W. (1965). *The maturational processes and the facilitating environment.* London: The Hogarth Press.

Wood, J. (2008). Bowlby's children: the forgotten revolution of Australian children's nursing. *Contemporary Nurse, 30*(2), 119–132.

Wright, L., & Bell, J. (2009). *Beliefs and illness. A model for healing.* Canada: Fourth Floor Press.

Wright, L., & Leahey, M. (2009). *Nurses and families: A guide to family assessment and intervention* (5th ed.). Philadelphia: FA Davis.

PART B

PRACTICE CONTEXTS IN CHILD,
YOUTH AND FAMILY HEALTH

Chapter 6

PREGNANCY AND BIRTH: HEALTH AND WELLBEING FOR THE WOMAN AND FAMILY

Rachel Reed, Margaret Barnes

LEARNING OUTCOMES

Reading this chapter will help you to:

» describe the maternity care systems in Australia and New Zealand and define concepts of continuity of care and partnership in maternity care

» describe how maternal health before and during pregnancy can influence the long-term health of the infant

» define the concept 'health literacy' and apply the concept to antenatal preparation of parents for pregnancy, birth and early parenting

» define attachment and describe the ways that attachment can be promoted in the early postnatal period

» describe the key factors that can influence breastfeeding in the early postnatal period.

Introduction

The decision to have a child or the discovery of pregnancy is an exciting time for most couples. It may also be challenging, depending on personal and social circumstances. It initiates a complex set of changes and transitions, which impact on the woman, her partner and her extended family in dramatic and sometimes unexpected ways. The challenges are biophysical, emotional and psychosocial and include the changing dynamics of the couple's relationship. A healthy pregnancy and good preparation for the important parenting transitions and family adjustments ahead are critical to ensure the best health and wellbeing of the woman, her child, her partner and other family members. The birth experience can have short-term and long-term implications for both the woman and her child. In this chapter, health in pregnancy, maternity services, options for antenatal care and birth, as well as parenting preparation, are discussed.

Clinical scenario 6.1
Setting the scene

This scenario introduces us to a woman early in her first pregnancy. It shows some of the challenges pregnant women and their families encounter, and the numerous pathways they follow towards the birth of a child.

Kay, aged 23, and her partner Richard, aged 25, live in Melbourne. They recently moved in together, and have discovered that they are expecting a baby.

Kay and Richard had not intended to start a family yet and, despite initially being shocked, they are now excited about becoming parents. Once Kay discovered she was pregnant she took steps to ensure her diet and lifestyle were healthy. However, by the time pregnancy was confirmed at 10 weeks, the fetus had already undergone significant development.

Preconception health

Ideally, women and their partners will consider their health and lifestyle prior to pregnancy. Cullum (2003) suggests that preconception refers to that time when a woman is fertile, but not pregnant, widening the potential for health care and health promotion among women prior to pregnancy. The aim of preconception health care is to identify and, if possible, modify biomedical, behavioural and social risks to a woman's health and prospective pregnancy (Centers for Disease Control, 2006). The focus of preconception care is to screen for risks, engage in health promotion and education and intervene when risks are identified (Centers for Disease Control, 2006). Preconception care aims to ensure that the woman entering pregnancy is in good health with as few risk factors as possible, which will optimise maternal and perinatal outcomes (Moos, Dunlop, Jack et al., 2008). However, most women receive fragmented care throughout the childbearing period and often only attend for care when there are signs of a pregnancy. Moos et al. (2008) suggest a continuum model of integrated care for women, where health providers build on what is learned about a woman's health and integrate health promotion opportunistically, prior to pregnancy. In this model, all women who are of reproductive age benefit from care and information that will influence their health at the time of a pregnancy.

The context of maternity care in Australia and New Zealand

Kay had her pregnancy confirmed at her local medical centre. Her general practitioner asked her what kind of maternity care she would like. Having no experience of the maternity system Kay decided she wanted to talk with Richard and explore their options before making a decision.

The provision of maternity care is influenced by the society and culture in which it takes place; therefore, maternity services vary considerably throughout the world. Although Australia and New Zealand are geographically close, the organisation of maternity services within these countries is very different. In New Zealand, women choose a lead maternity carer, and this person may be a midwife, a general practitioner or an obstetrician. Around 80% of women in New Zealand choose a midwife as their lead maternity carer (Ministry of Health New Zealand, 2011). In Australia, private and public maternity service options are available. In the public maternity system, women access maternity care with their general practitioner or with midwives and obstetricians at a local hospital, birth centre or clinic (Commonwealth of Australia, 2009). Within the private maternity system, women may choose an obstetrician or a privately practising midwife. Unlike private midwifery care, private obstetric care is covered by health insurance and subsidised by government. However, recently privately practising midwives have been able to register with Medicare, enabling women to claim rebates for antenatal and postnatal care (Nursing and Midwifery Board of Australia, n.d.).

New Zealand and Australia have distinct maternity systems, but the principles underpinning both systems are similar. These principles are: a commitment to community-based health care; continuity of care; and access to additional support via secondary and tertiary services where required (Commonwealth of Australia, 2009; MidCentral Health District Health Board, 2005; Ministry of Health New Zealand, 2000). Access to options within the maternity system varies considerably depending upon location. Women living in regional and remote areas often have limited access to services and care providers. In addition, in Australia personal circumstances such as health insurance can further limit options.

In New Zealand and Australia most women give birth in a hospital or a birth centre (Australian Institute of Health and Welfare, 2011; New Zealand College of Midwives and Midwifery and Maternity Providers Organisation, 2010). However, increasing numbers of women are choosing to give birth at home. This shift has been supported by the development of publicly funded homebirth services in response to consumer demand and a growing body of international research demonstrating that homebirth is a safe option for low-risk women. A small number of women choose to birth at home with an unregistered care provider or to 'freebirth' without a care provider (Dahlen, Jackson & Stevens, 2011).

Concepts of continuity and partnership in maternity care

Kay and Richard live in an Australian city with a range of maternity care options available. However, they found it difficult to decide which option was best for them and spent a few weeks researching their choices. Eventually, they both felt that it was important to have the same person providing care throughout the transition into parenthood. In addition, Kay wanted to birth at home and avoid intervention unless it was required. They interviewed a few independent midwives and chose one that they both felt comfortable with. Their midwife was Medicare eligible, which enabled them to claim back most of the cost of her services.

Maternity service strategies in both New Zealand and Australia maintain that continuity of care should be a fundamental aspect of all maternity service models (Commonwealth of Australia, 2011; MidCentral District Health Board, 2005). However, there is debate regarding what is meant by 'continuity of care'; for further exploration of this issue, see Box 6.1. There is also a commitment to increasing access

---

Box 6.1 Practice highlight: Continuity of care

The terms 'continuity of care' and 'continuity of caregiver' have been regarded by some practitioners as being equally acceptable or meaning the same thing. However, an examination of the extant literature reveals some subtle differences. Continuity of care is the care provided by different caregivers, but with a good overview of the woman's history and pregnancy to date through the use of clinical records (Medical Records Institute, 2006), whereas continuity of caregiver is defined as care provided by one person or a small group of caregivers throughout the maternity experience (Haggerty, Reid, Freeman et al., 2003).

Other terms used to describe this relationship were found by Haggerty et al., who were commissioned by the Canadian health services and policy research bodies to develop a common understanding of the concept of continuity. The additional terms include 'longitudinality', 'relational' or 'personal continuity' (p. 1219). Buetow (2004) borrowed the terms 'informational continuity' and 'relational or interpersonal continuity' from Haggerty et al. (2003), but challenged the fact that continuity of caregiver is focused on the *one* carer, who is usually a health professional, rather than on *all* those involved in care, such as family members, who will ask questions on behalf of the woman, listen to information provided and provide ongoing supportive care in the absence of the health professional.

The discussion paper *Primary maternity services in Australia: A framework for implementation* (Australian Health Minister's Conference, 2009) outlines research evidence supporting continuity of the midwifery carer during pregnancy, birth and the early postnatal period. This model is associated with a reduction in healthcare costs and the levels of intervention during labour, caesarean sections rates and the need for neonatal resuscitation at birth. In addition, this model of care results in enhanced experiences and satisfaction with care, greater preparedness for birth and early parenting and increased participation in decision making and has a positive influence on women's sense of self-confidence and self-esteem in the early postnatal period.

Critical question: barriers and restraints

As continuity of carer is considered to have positive impacts on the health and wellbeing of women and their families, what are the barriers and constraints to implementing such care in mainstream maternity services?

to midwifery-led care for women in Australia (Commonwealth of Australia, 2011). Midwifery care is underpinned by the concept of partnership whereby the woman makes decisions about her care, supported by her midwife (International Confederation of Midwives, 2010, 2011). The mother–midwife relationship is founded on the acknowledgement and respect of the woman's individual needs and circumstances. Midwives must provide women with adequate information in order to assist their decision making regarding available care options. Continuity of care assists with the development of the mother–midwife relationship.

Pregnancy: promoting health and preparation for parenthood

The health of the mother has a direct and long-term effect on the health of her baby. The importance of maternal health during pregnancy is becoming increasingly understood, in particular in relation to epigenetics (Godfrey, Gluck & Hanson, 2010; Hoyo, Murtha, Schildkraut et al., 2011; Martino & Prescott, 2011; Napoli, Infante & Casamassimi, 2011; Power, 2012; Suter, Ma, Harris et al., 2011). Berger, Kouzarides, Shiekhattar and Shilatifard (2009, p. 781) define an epigenetic trait as 'a stably heritable phenotype resulting from changes in a chromosome without alterations in the DNA sequence'. In terms of pregnancy, the study of epigenetics focuses on how particular factors, such as nutrition, 'switch on' expressions of particular genes. For example, babies who are born with a low birthweight have an increased risk of cardiovascular disease in later life (Eriksson, Forsén, Tuomilehto, Osmond & Barker, 2001). Epigenetic studies aim to identify the mechanism by which this genetic predisposition is initiated.

The connection between maternal health and infant health is not a new concept. The development of antenatal care occurred after World War II in an attempt to improve the health of the population by increasing surveillance of women's pregnancies (Arney, 1982). Today, antenatal care involves the regular performance of numerous tests and assessments aimed at determining the health of the mother and her developing baby (Sullivan, Kean & Cryer, 2006). The World Health Organization (2005) recommends that effective and appropriate antenatal care should be offered to all women. However, it questions some of the practices and interventions involved. Some interventions offered to women with a low-risk pregnancy are not effective, and many others have not been evaluated (Hofmeyr, Neilson, Alfirevic et al., 2008).

For Kay and Richard, antenatal care was focused on building a relationship with their midwife and information sharing. Their midwife also checked Kay's blood pressure and palpated her abdomen. Richard enjoyed being shown how the baby was lying in the uterus and hearing its heartbeat.

Kay and Richard were able to discuss the various screening tests and assessments available during their midwife visits. They decided to have only one ultrasound test during the pregnancy at 20 weeks gestation to check for any major congenital abnormalities, and to find out where the placenta was located.

Technological advances have also impacted on pregnancy and maternity care. The development of, and increased access to, artificial reproductive technologies (ART) has expanded the options available to the growing numbers of women experiencing infertility (Wang, Chambers & Sullivan, 2011). Although only 17.2% of treatment cycles result in a liveborn baby, success rates are improving, and in Australia and New

Zealand around 3% and 2%, respectively, of babies are conceived following some form of ART (Wang et al., 2011). Women who undergo ART are at increased risk of complications during pregnancy and birth; and their babies are more likely to be of low birthweight or have a congenital abnormality (Barnes, Roiko, Reed, Williams & Willcocks, 2012). Technological developments have also contributed to the ability to screen unborn babies for abnormalities. For example, there is now widespread routine use of ultrasound during pregnancy, despite unresolved concerns regarding the safety of this technology (Beech, 2008).

Social factors

Social and physical health factors are inter-related, and the health of a woman, her pregnancy and her baby are influenced by her social circumstances. In order to improve maternal health, social determinants of health such as housing, employment, environment etc. need to be addressed (Commonwealth of Australia, 2008). For example, a woman who is exposed to air pollution during pregnancy may increase the chance of her child developing asthma and allergies later in life (Baïz, Slama, Béne et al., 2011). Psychological stress during pregnancy increases the chance of the baby developing emotional, cognitive and mental health problems in childhood (Malaspina, Corcoran, Kleinhaus et al., 2008; Talge, Neal & Glover, 2007). Babies born following fetal growth restriction and, therefore, of low birthweight are at increased risk for developing cardiovascular and diabetic disease later in life (Barker, 2003). In addition to biophysical factors, there are many social determinants of low birthweight.

Spencer (2000, p. 194) suggests:

> … the birth weight of an infant reflects quality of the fetal environment and the length of gestation, which are influenced by intergenerational, genetic, constitutional, dietary and lifestyle factors. It is a pivotal point in the life-course continuum reflecting maternal health and predicting future health in childhood and adulthood.

Such interconnected factors influence the fetal and early childhood environment and may provide protection or place the child at risk.

Health behaviours are also influenced by social factors. For example, Indigenous women have higher rates of unhealthy behaviours such as smoking and alcohol use during pregnancy, and experience higher rates of ill health and poor outcomes compared to non-Indigenous women (Kildea, Kruske & Sherwood, 2010). However, such health behaviours must be considered within a social and cultural context. For example, a study by Passey, Gale and Sanson-Fisher (2011) explored Indigenous Australian women's reflections on smoking. They found that smoking provided the women with a way of 'belonging' and of asserting their group membership. Therefore, any attempts to reduce smoking rates amongst this group of women must address the social context of the behaviour.

Antenatal education

Pregnancy is a time when opportunities for health promotion present themselves, not only for the woman and family during this pregnancy and birth, but also for long-term health. One strategy used to frame this health promotion has been antenatal education.

Antenatal education programs are usually organised and delivered by the institutions providing birth services. A Cochrane review found insufficient evidence that antenatal education programs are beneficial or influence the outcomes or the experience of birth (Gagnon & Sandall, 2011). The review also suggests that the aim of programs run by institutions may be the explanation and justification of policies to encourage compliance. Another criticism directed towards antenatal education is that classes have traditionally focused on preparing for birth. New parents are increasingly voicing concerns about the lack of preparation for actual parenting (Barnes, Pratt, Finlayson et al., 2008; Ho & Holroyd, 2002; Renkert & Nutbeam, 2001).

An alternative approach to antenatal education is to focus on health literacy. The World Health Organization suggests that 'by improving people's access to health information and their capacity to use it effectively, health literacy is critical to empowerment' (Nutbeam, 1998, p. 357). Low health literacy will impact on a woman's own health knowledge and her ability to understand the care options available to her (Endres, Sharp, Haney & Dooley, 2004). Therefore, Shieh and Halstead (2009) argue that antenatal education should aim to increase a woman's health knowledge, self-efficacy and self-advocacy skills.

Kay and Richard chose not to attend the antenatal classes at the local hospital. Instead, they discussed topics with their midwife, read books, watched films and researched using the internet. Kay also attended a local mother's group and was able to gain information by talking with new mothers about birth and babies.

Traditionally, listening to the reflections of those who had already 'been there' prepared women for their own birth and mothering experience (Davis, 2004). Today, mothers continue to share birth stories, verbally, in writing and more recently via the Internet (Coates, 2007). Women not only learn practical information about pregnancy, birth and mothering through exchanging stories, they also gain ongoing emotional and social support (Carolan, 2005; Fabian, Rådestad & Waldenström, 2005; Farley & Widman, 2001; Savage, 2001).

Birth

In recent years childbirth has become increasingly medicalised. According to an Australian Institute of Health and Welfare report (2011) more than 80% of Australian women experience medical intervention to induce or speed up their labour; and more than 40% have their baby delivered by caesarean section or with the assistance of medical instruments. These statistics comprise data from all women giving birth, and the rates of intervention are likely to be even higher in the subset of first-time mothers. Unlike the Australian report, New Zealand's Maternity Clinical Indicator report focuses on the outcomes for first-time mothers only (Ministry of Health, 2011). Despite both countries having similar perinatal and maternal mortality statistics (World Health Organization, 2006, 2012), the intervention rates are significantly different. For example, the caesarean section rate in New Zealand is 16% compared to 30% in Australia.

The model of care and place of birth also influence the chance of a woman experiencing medical intervention. Intervention rates are highest in the Australian private sector, with around 50% of women undergoing a caesarean in some states (Australian Institute of Health and Welfare, 2011). Low-risk women birthing in a hospital setting are much more likely to undergo medical intervention than women giving birth at home or in a birth centre (Birthplace in England Collaborative Group, 2011; Davis, Baddock, Pairman et al., 2011; Kennare, Keirse, Tucker & Chan, 2010). A recent Australian study demonstrated that continuity of care by a primary midwife reduced the rates of intervention and improved outcomes for both women and their babies (McLachlan, Forster, Davey et al., 2012).

Medical intervention during birth can influence the short-term and long-term health of the mother, her baby and future pregnancies. For example, an infant born by caesarean has an increased risk of respiratory infections, asthma, digestive disorders, obesity and food allergies (Huh, Rifas-Shiman, Zera et al., 2012; Koplin, Allen, Gurrin et al., 2008; Laubereau, Filipiak-Pittroff, von Berg et al., 2004; Nunes & Ladeira, 2007; Thavagnanam, Fleming, Bromley, Shields & Cardwell, 2008). A woman who has a caesarean is at risk of complications such as haemorrhage and wound infection (Souza, Gülmezoglu, Lumbiganon et al., 2010), and she is also more likely to encounter complications during future pregnancies (Kennare, Tucker, Heard & Chan, 2007). Furthermore, a physiological vaginal birth prepares the mother and baby for early attachment and breastfeeding (Buckley, 2004). Hormones are released in response to uterine contractions and pain that initiate bonding behaviour following birth.

Kay gave birth to a healthy, 4.1-kg baby boy at home after a long and challenging labour, almost two weeks after her due date. Richard was thankful for the support of the midwife because he found it difficult to watch Kay experiencing pain. Kay felt deeply empowered by her birth experience.

Birth is not just a physical experience, and how a woman gives birth can have a long-lasting effect on her, emotionally and psychologically. The empowering nature of the birth experience has been identified in a number of studies (Callister, 2004; Cheyney, 2011; Halldórsdótti & Karlsdóttir, 1996; Kennedy et al., 2004). Women incorporate their birth experience into their sense of self, and this can result in increased self-confidence and self-esteem (Lundgren, 2005; Simpkin, 1991), which may assist with the subsequent challenges of motherhood. However, a negative experience of birth can also have long-term implications for a woman's psychological wellbeing. Women who give birth via caesarean section or assisted delivery (forceps or ventouse) are more likely to suffer emotional and psychological trauma (Soet, Brack & Dilorio, 2003). However, it is the sense of control and a lack of support from care givers that seem more important than the type of birth (Cigoli, Gilli & Saita, 2006; Czarnocka & Slade, 2000; Soet et al., 2003).

The transition following birth

Birth is a significant life event that initiates a sequence of changes and transitions, perhaps like no other during the life course. This transition is a major change for the woman, her partner and family. During this time, the woman as primary carer, but also her partner and other family members, has to get to know the baby, how the baby behaves and what these behaviours might mean, as well as giving basic care that provides for the baby's needs, warmth, comfort and contact and food. Basic skills in caring for a baby, such as hygiene, changing nappies, feeding and preventing distress and crying, are learned in the early weeks after birth. Learning to determine whether a baby is healthy or sick is another challenge for new parents, who may be afraid of over-reacting and seeking help too early or, even more so, of under-reacting and seeking help only when it is too late.

The importance of attachment

Attachment is the development of the strong relationship between a mother or a caregiver and a baby that leads to emotional security in the child. Bowlby (1969) observed infant–caregiver relationships and interactions, and theorised that the initial relationship is based on a set of innate signals that call the caregiver to the infant's side and that, during the first year of life, a true affectionate bond develops.

The importance of attachment was first signalled through the work of Bowlby (1969) and Ainsworth (1962), and more current thinking is highlighted in the World Health Organization document on the importance of caregiver–child interactions (2004). Bowlby, in his early work, emphasised the importance and the primacy of interpersonal relationships for young children and suggested that the formation of such relationships was as important to child survival as food, stimulation and physical care (World Health Organization, 2004).

Evidence suggests that it is not only social and psychological wellbeing that is influenced by secure attachment, but that children's neurological development occurs in response to social and interpersonal processes (Nelson & Bloom, 1997; Schore, 2001). The infant's brain has been described as being experience-dependent and experience-expectant in that new synaptic connections occur in response to experiences. Therefore, an infant's development is dependent upon sensory and motor stimulation (experiences) from caregivers, a kind of stimulation that occurs during affective interactions with responsive caregivers (World Health Organization, 2004). In Chapter 7 you will give further consideration to sensitive, responsive parenting during infancy. Here, we examine important initial interactions for the infant and mother (see Box 6.2).

Attachment and skin-to-skin contact

While the interaction between the infant and caregiver needs to be consistent and long-term, the experience around birth and the early postnatal period provides an opportunity to establish this relationship early. A mother's responsiveness to the signals from her baby is strongly influenced by the birth process and immediate post-birth period and the opportunities she is afforded to hold and get to know her baby undisturbed. It is therefore important to establish a birthing environment that encourages immediate and close contact.

One way in which attachment in the immediate post-birth period can be encouraged is via skin-to-skin contact, when the newborn baby is placed naked on the mother's chest with warm wraps across the baby's back. Skin-to-skin contact has been shown to positively influence breastfeeding outcomes and early mother–infant attachment as well as increasing the infant's cardiorespiratory stability (Moore, Anderson & Bergman, 2007).

Box 6.2 Research highlight

Schore and Schore (2008) build on the work of Bowlby and Ainsworth to describe a 'Modern Theory of Attachment', with an emphasis on the need for the mother to be psychobiologically attuned to the baby, so that the infant's arousal is appropriately responded to. To explore research further, see www.allanschore.com.

When Kieran was born, Kay held him to her chest. The midwife ensured he was dry and warm and that skin-to-skin contact was not disturbed so Kay and Richard could get to know their new baby. It wasn't long before Kieran began to search for the breast, and Kay was able to breastfeed uninterrupted. During pregnancy Kay read widely about the benefits of breastfeeding and would frequently discuss infant care and feeding with her midwife.

Supporting breastfeeding

Skin-to-skin contact and early breastfeeding are important to attachment and to the health and wellbeing of an infant in both the short and the longer term. Supporting breastfeeding is a key health promotion activity as the benefits of breastfeeding for infant, mother, family and community are well-recognised.

Breastfeeding is recognised as the optimal method of infant feeding and confers a number of health benefits for the infant, including reduced incidence of gastrointestinal illness (Kramer & Kakuma, 2012), respiratory illness, asthma and allergies (Oddy, 2004). Breastfeeding may also protect against the development of obesity (Arenz, Rückerl, Koletzko & von Kries, 2004) and type 2 diabetes (Owen, Martin, Whincup, Smith & Cook, 2006) in later life.

Exclusive breastfeeding for the first 6 months followed by breastfeeding and appropriate complementary food is recommended by the World Health Organization (WHO, 2003). In Australia and New Zealand the breastfeeding initiation rates are high, but this is followed by a sharp decline in exclusive breastfeeding over the first 6 months. For example in Australia, following a 92% initiation rate only 71% of infants were fully breastfed at 1 month, 56% at 3 months and only 14% at 6 months (Australian Health Ministers' Conference, 2009a, 2009b).

Improving breastfeeding rates, therefore, is a priority for both New Zealand and Australia. The Australian National Breastfeeding Strategy (2010–2015) aims to increase the percentage of babies fully breastfed from birth to 6 months with continued breastfeeding and complementary foods to 12 months and beyond. This strategy is an essential public health measure that has the potential to reduce the burden of acute and chronic disease for both women and infants. Similarly, the National Strategic Plan of Action for Breastfeeding 2008–2012 in New Zealand sets out strategies to protect, promote and support breastfeeding (National Breastfeeding Advisory Committee of New Zealand, 2009).

Factors that facilitate breastfeeding initiation, and are modifiable within practice settings, include implementation of the 'Ten steps to successful breastfeeding' at a service level, avoiding the use of narcotic analgesia in the first stage of labour and ensuring that skin-to-skin contact is routine and that mothers and infants are not separated (Forster & McLachlan, 2007). Factors that positively influence breastfeeding duration to 6 months (as recommended by WHO) include the woman's breastfeeding intention, breastfeeding self-efficacy and social support (Meedya, Fahy & Kable, 2010).

Supporting women and providing practical assistance and information for women during pregnancy and in the postnatal period is important to subsequent breastfeeding success. Practices in health facilities that facilitate and support breastfeeding are outlined in the 'Ten steps to successful breastfeeding' (UNICEF/World Health Organization, 2009), which are listed in Box 6.3. Implementation of these practices as routine ensures that maternity service environments promote, support and protect breastfeeding, and consider breastfeeding as the 'norm'.

The Baby Friendly Hospital Initiative (BFHI) was established by the World Health Organization and UNICEF in 1991, as a strategy to improve breastfeeding rates worldwide. The 10 Steps to Successful Breastfeeding are set out by UNICEF and the World Health Organization (UNICEF/World Health Organization 2009) and focus on practices that protect, support and promote breastfeeding.

There are now 152 countries worldwide that have implemented the BFHI. The Initiative is organised differently from country to country. To explore further how the initiative has been implemented and the impact of the initiative on breastfeeding, visit:

Australia: http://www.babyfriendly.org.au/

New Zealand: http://www.babyfriendly.org.nz/

United Kingdom: http://www.unicef.org.uk/babyfriendly/

United States of America: http://www.babyfriendlyusa.org/about-us/baby-friendly-hospital-initiative

For a global perspective visit: http://www.who.int/nutrition/topics/bfhi/en/

From these resources identify the 10 Steps to Successful Breastfeeding and consider the extent to which these have been implemented in your local services.

Much needs to be done, however, to provide ongoing support for women to maintain breastfeeding as recommended. Community groups play a vital role in this task. The Australian Breastfeeding Association (https://www.breastfeeding.asn.au/) provides a 24-hour breastfeeding helpline as well as online forums and face-to-face local meetings. The La Leche League in New Zealand (http://www.lalecheleague.org.nz/) provides support through local groups, online resources and a peer counselling program.

Conclusion

In this chapter, the focus was on the health services available to support a pregnant woman and significant others during pregnancy and into the immediate postnatal period. The importance of health promotion and the role of the midwife and nurse were explored as key in providing parents with information and skills that will enable them to make informed decisions about pregnancy care, birth and postnatal care.

KEY POINTS

» Continuity of care is recognised as an important principle in the provision of maternity care.

» The effectiveness of traditional antenatal education classes is not clear; however, parents may appreciate the support provided in the group situation.

» Secure attachment is important to short-term and long-term infant health.

» Breastfeeding affords numerous health benefits for both mother and infant.

CRITICAL QUESTIONS AND REFLECTION

1. What key information should be available for parents to consider when choosing their care provider and place of birth?

2. How can a woman improve her future infant's health before and during pregnancy?

3. What strategies may best meet the needs of parents attending antenatal education?

4. Given the importance of the experience of birth, how can care providers value this aspect of birth and implement best practice to support emotional/psychosocial health?

USEFUL RESOURCES

Australian Institute of Health and Welfare (AIHW), *Australia's mothers and babies 2009*: http://www.aihw.gov.au/publication-detail/?id=10737420870

Ministry of Health, New Zealand Maternity Clinical Indicators 2009: http://www.health.govt.nz/publication/new-zealand-maternity-clinical-indicators-2009-revised-june-2012

References

Ainsworth, M. (1962). The effects of maternal deprivation: a review of findings and controversy in the context of research strategy. In M. S. D. Ainsworth, R. G. Andry, R. G. Harlow, et al. (Eds.), *Deprivation of maternal care: A reassessment of its effects*. Geneva: World Health Organization.

Arney, W. R. (1982). *Power and the profession of obstetrics*. Chicago: University of Chicago Press.

Arenz, S. R., Rückerl, R., Koletzko, B., & von Kries, R. (2004). Breast-feeding and childhood obesity – a systematic review. *International Journal of Obesity, 28*, 1247–1256.

Australian Health Ministers' Conference (2009a). *Primary maternity services in Australia: A framework for implementation*. NSW Department of Health.

Australian Health Ministers' Conference (2009b). *The Australian National Breastfeeding Strategy 2010–2015*. Canberra: Australian Government Department of Health and Ageing.

Australian Institute of Health and Welfare (2011). *Australia's mothers and babies 2009*. Canberra. Retrieved from www.aihw.gov.au/publication-detail/?id=10737420870 (accessed 5 May 2012).

Baïz, N., Slama, R., Béne, M.-C., et al. (2011). Maternal exposure to air pollution before and during pregnancy related to changes in newborn's cord blood lymphocyte subpopulations. The EDEN study cohort. *BMC Pregnancy & Childbirth, 11*(87). Retrieved from http://www.biomedcentral.com/1471-2393/11/87 (accessed 16 May 2012).

Barnes, M., Pratt, J., Finlayson, K., et al. (2008). Learning about baby: what new mothers would like to know. *Journal of Perinatal Education, 17*(3), 33–41.

Barnes, M., Roiko, A., Reed, R., Williams, C., & Willcocks, K. (2012). Outcomes for women and infants following assisted conception: implications for perinatal education, care and support. *Journal of Perinatal Education, 21*(1), 18–23.

Barker, D. (2003). The midwife, the coincidence, and the hypothesis. *British Medical Journal, 327,* 1428–1430.

Beech, B. A. (2008). Ultrasound and the safety myth. *British Journal of Midwifery, 16*(7), 458–459.

Berger, S. L., Kouzarides, T., Shiekhattar, R., & Shilatifard, A. (2009). An operational definition of epigenetics. *Genes & Development, 23,* 781–783.

Birthplace in England Collaborative Group (2011). Perinatal and maternal outcomes by planned place of birth for healthy women with low risk pregnancies: the Birthplace in England national prospective cohort study. *British Medical Journal.* doi 10.1136/bmj.d7400

Bowlby, J. (1969). *Attachment and loss. Vol. 1. Attachment.* New York: Basic Books.

Buckley, S. J. (2004). Undisturbed birth – nature's hormonal blueprint for safety, ease and ecstasy. *MIDIRS Midwifery Digest, 14*(2), 203–209.

Buetow, S. A. (2004). Towards a new understanding of provider continuity. *Annals of Family Medicine, 2*(5), 509–511.

Callister, L. C. (2004). Making meaning: women's birth narratives. *Journal of Obstetric, Gynecologic & Neonatal Nursing, 33*(4), 508–515.

Carolan, M. (2005). The role of stories in understanding life events: poststructural construction of the 'self'. *Collegian: Journal of the Royal College of Nursing, 12*(3), 5–8.

Centers for Disease Control (CDC) (2006). *Preconception health and care.* Atlanta: Department of Health and Human Services.

Cheyney, M. (2011). Reinscribing the birthing body. *Medical Anthropology Quarterly, 25*(4), 519–542.

Cigoli, V., Gilli, G., & Saita, E. (2006). Relational factors in psychopathological responses to childbirth. *Journal of Psychosomatic Obstetrics and Gynecology, 27*(2), 91–97.

Coates, T. (2007). How do they see us? Portrayals of childbirth and the role of the midwife in literature. In L. Davies (Ed.), *The art and soul of midwifery: Creativity in practice, education and research* (pp. 95–110). London: Churchill Livingstone.

Commonwealth of Australia (2008). *Australia: the healthiest country by 2020: A discussion paper.* Barton: Commonwealth of Australia.

Commonwealth of Australia (2009). *Improving maternity services in Australia: The report of the Maternity Services Review.* Barton: Commonwealth of Australia.

Commonwealth of Australia (2011). *National Maternity Services Plan 2010.* Canberra: Commonwealth of Australia.

Cullum, A. (2003). Changing provider practices to enhance preconceptional wellness. *Journal of Obstetric, Gynecologic and Neonatal Nursing, 32*(4), 543–549.

Czarnocka, J. & Slade, P. (2000). Prevalence and predictors of post-traumatic stress symptoms following childbirth. *British Journal of Psychology, 39,* 35–51.

Dahlen, H., Jackson, M., & Stevens, J. (2011). Homebirth, freebirth and doulas: casualty and consequences of a broken maternity system. *Women and Birth, 24*(1), 47–50.

Davis, D., Baddock, S., Pairman, S. et al. (2011). Planned place of birth in New Zealand: does it affect mode of birth and intervention rates among low-risk women? *Birth*, *38*(2), 111–119.

Davis, L. (2004). Tell me a story. *The Practising Midwife*, *7*(7), 22–25.

Endres, L. K., Sharp, L. K., Haney, E., & Dooley, S. (2004). Health literacy and pregnancy preparedness in pregestational diabetes. *Diabetes Care*, *27*, 331–334.

Eriksson, J. G., Forsén, T., Tuomilehto, J., Osmond, C., & Barker, D. (2001). Early growth and coronary disease in later life: a longitudinal study. *British Medical Journal*, *322*, 949–953.

Fabian, H., Rådestad, I., & Waldenström, U. (2005). Childbirth and parenthood education classes in Sweden. Women's opinion and possible outcomes. *Acta Obstetricia et Gynecologica Scandinavica*, *84*, 436–443.

Farley, C. & Widman, S. (2001). The value of birth stories. *International Journal of Childbirth Education*, *16*(3), 22–25.

Forster, D. & McLachlan, H. (2007). Breastfeeding initiation and birth setting practices: a review of the literature. *Journal of Midwifery & Women's Health*, *52*(3), 273–280.

Gagnon, A. J. & Sandall, J. (2011). Individual or group antenatal education for childbirth or parenthood, or both (review). *Cochrane Database of Systematic Reviews*, 2007, Issue 3. Art. No.: CD002869. doi:10.1002/14651858.CD002869.pub2

Godfrey, K. M., Gluck, P. D., & Hanson, M. A. (2010). Developmental origins of metabolic disease: life courses and intergenerational perspectives. *Trends in Endocrinology and Metabolism*, *21*(4), 199–205.

Haggerty, J. L., Reid, R. J., Freeman, G. K., et al. (2003). Continuity of care: a multidisciplinary review. *British Medical Journal*, *327*, 1219–1221.

Halldórsdótti, S. & Karlsdóttir, S. I. (1996). Empowerment or discouragement: women's experience of caring and uncaring encounters during childbirth. *Health Care of Women International*, *17*, 361–379.

Ho, I., Holroyd, E. (2002). Chinese women's perceptions of the effectiveness of antenatal education in the preparation for motherhood. *Journal of Advanced Nursing*, *38*(1), 74–85.

Hofmeyr, G. J., Neilson, J. P., Alfirevic, Z., et al. (2008). *Pregnancy and childbirth: A Cochrane pocketbook*. John Wiley & Sons.

Hoyo, C., Murtha, A. P., Schildkraut, J. M., et al. (2011). Folic acid supplementation before and during pregnancy in the Newborn Epigenetics STudy (NEST). *BMC Public Health*, *11*. Retrieved from http://www.biomedcentral.com/1471-2458/11/46 (accessed 16 May 2012).

Huh, S., Rifas-Shiman, S. L., Zera, C. A., et al. (2012). Delivery by caesarean section and risk of obesity in preschool age children: a prospective cohort study. *Archives of Disease in Childhood.*, doi:10.1136/archdischild-2011-301141

International Confederation of Midwives (2010). The philosophy and model of midwifery care. Retrieved from http://www.internationalmidwives.org/Documentation/CoreDocuments/tabid/322/Default.aspx (accessed 2 May 2012).

International Confederation of Midwives (2011). *ICM International definition of the midwife*. Retrieved from http://www.internationalmidwives.org/Documentation/CoreDocuments/tabid/322/Default.aspx (accessed 2 May 2012).

Kennare, R., Tucker, G., Heard, A., et al. (2007). Risks of adverse outcomes in the next birth after a first cesarean delivery. *Obstetrics and Gynecology, 109*, 270–276.

Kennare, R. M., Keirse, M. J. N. C., Tucker, G. R., et al. (2010). Planned home and hospital birth in South Australia, 1991–2006: differences in outcomes. *Medical Journal of Australia, 192*(2), 76–80.

Kennedy, H. P. & Shannon, M. T. (2004). Keeping birth normal: research findings on midwifery care during childbirth. *Journal of Obstetric, Gynecological and Neonatal Nursing, 33*(5), 554–560.

Kildea, S., Kruske, S., & Sherwood, J. (2010). Life-threatening emergencies. In S. Pairman, S. Tracy, C. Thorogood et al. (Eds.), *Midwifery preparation for practice* (pp. 909–970) (2nd ed.). Elsevier, Sydney: Churchill Livingstone.

Koplin, J., Allen, K., Gurrin, L., et al. (2008). Is caesarean delivery associated with sensitization to food allergens and IgE-mediated food allergy: a systematic review. *Pediatric Allergy and Immunology, 19*, 682–687.

Kramer, M. S. & Kakuma, R. (2012). Optimal duration of exclusive breastfeeding. *Cochrane Database of Systematic Reviews, 15*(8): CD003517. Doi: 10.1002/14651858. CD003517.pub2

Laubereau, B., Filipiak-Pittroff, B., von Berg, A., et al. (2004). Caesarean section and gastrointestinal symptoms, atopic dermatitis, and sensitisation during the first year of life. *Archives of Disease in Childhood, 89*, 993–997.

Lundgren, I. (2005). Swedish women's experience of childbirth 2 years after birth. *Midwifery, 21*, 346–354.

Malaspina, D., Corcoran, C., Kleinhaus, K. R., et al. (2008). Acute maternal stress in pregnancy and schizophrenia in offspring: a cohort study. *BMC Psychiatry, 8*(71), doi:10.1186/1471-244X-8-71

Martino, D. & Prescott, S. (2011). Epigenetics and prenatal influences on asthma and allergic airways disease. *Chest, 139*(3), 640–647.

McLachlan, H. L., Forster, D. A., Davey, M. A., et al. (2012). Effects of continuity of care by a primary midwife (caseload midwifery) on caesarean section rates in women of low obstetric risk: the COSMOS randomised controlled trial. *British Journal of Obstetrics and Gynaecology*, doi: 10.1111/j.1471-0528.2012.03446.x

Meedya, S., Fahy, K., & Kable, A. (2010). Factors that positively influence breastfeeding to 6 months: a literature review. *Women and Birth, 23*, 135–145.

Medical Records Institute (2006). Continuity of care record (CCR). Retrieved from www.medrecinst.com/pages/about.asp?id=54 (accessed 14 January 2007).

MidCentral Health District Health Board (MCDHB) (2005). *Maternity services strategy.* New Zealand: MCDHB, Palmerston North.

Ministry of Health New Zealand (MOH NZ) (2000). *NZ Public Health and Disability Act 2000.* Wellington: MOH NZ.

Ministry of Health, New Zealand Maternity Clinical Indicators (2009). http://www. health.govt.nz/publication/new-zealand-maternity-clinical-indicators-2009-revised-june-2012

Ministry of Health New Zealand (2011). *Maternity snapshot.* New Zealand. Retrieved from http://www.health.govt.nz/publication/maternity-snapshot-2010-provisional-data (accessed 28 June 2012).

Moore, E. R., Anderson, G. C., & Bergman, N. (2007). Early skin-to-skin contact for mothers and their healthy newborn infants. *Cochrane Database of Systematic Reviews*, Issue 4. Art. No.: CD003519. doi: 10.1002/14651858.CD003519.pub2

Moos, M.-K., Dunlop, A. L., Jack, B. W., et al. (2008). Healthier women, healthier reproductive outcomes: recommendations for the routine care of all women of reproductive age. *American Journal of Obstetrics & Gynecology*, *199*(6 Suppl 2), S280–S289.

Napoli, C., Infante, T., & Casamassimi, A. (2011). Maternal–foetal epigenetic interactions in the beginning of cardiovascular damage. *Cardiovascular Research*, *92*, 367–374.

National Breastfeeding Advisory Committee of New Zealand (2009). *National Strategic Plan of Action for Breastfeeding 2008–2012: National Breastfeeding Advisory Committee of New Zealand's advice to the Director-General of Health*. Wellington: Ministry of Health.

Nelson, C. & Bloom, F. (1997). Child development and neuroscience. *Child Development*, *68*(5), 970–987.

New Zealand College of Midwives, Midwifery and Maternity Providers Organisation (2010). *MMPO Midwives 2010 Annual report on care activities and outcomes*. Retrieved from http://www.mmpo.org.nz/site/midwiferyrecruitment/files/Annual%20Reports//2010.pdf (accessed 30 January 2013).

Nunes, C. & Ladeira, S. (2007). Caesarean delivery could be a risk factor for asthma? *Journal of Allergy and Clinical Immunology*, *119*, S164.

Nursing and Midwifery Board of Australia (n.d.). Guidelines and assessment framework for registration standard for eligible midwives and registration standard for endorsed scheduled medicines for eligible midwives. Retrieved from http://www.nursingmidwiferyboard.gov.au/Codes-Guidelines-Statements/Codes-Guidelines.aspx (accessed 2 May 2012).

Nutbeam, D. (1998). Health promotion glossary. *Health Promotion International*, *13*(4), 349–364.

Oddy, W. H. (2004). A review of the effects of breastfeeding on respiratory infections, atopy, and childhood asthma. *Journal of Asthma*, *1*(6), 605–621.

Owen, C., Martin, R., Whincup, P., Smith, G., & Cook, D. (2006). Does breastfeeding influence risk of type 2 diabetes in later life? A quantitative analysis of published evidence. *American Journal of Clinical Nutrition*, *84*(5), 1043–1054.

Passey, M. E., Gale, J. T., & Sanson-Fisher, R. W. (2011). 'It's almost expected': rural Australian Aboriginal women's reflections on smoking initiation and maintenance: a qualitative study. *BMC Women's Health*, *11*(55). Retrieved from http://www.biomedcentral.com/1472-6874/11/55 (accessed 12 June 2012).

Power, M. L. (2012). The human obesity epidemic, the mismatch paradigm, and our modern 'captive' environment. *American Journal of Human Biology*, *24*, 116–122.

Renkert, S. & Nutbeam, D. (2001). Opportunities to improve maternal health literacy through antenatal education: an exploratory study. *Health Promotion International*, *16*(4), 381–388.

Savage, J. (2001). Birth stories: a way of knowing in childbirth. *Journal of Perinatal Education*, *10*(2), 3–7.

Schore, A. (2001). Effects of a secure attachment relationship on right brain development, affect regulation, and infant mental health. *Infant Mental Health Journal, 22*(1–2), 7–66.

Schore, J. & Schore, A. (2008). Modern attachment theory: the central role of affect regulation in development and treatment. *Clinical Social Work Journal, 36*(1), 9–20.

Shieh, C. & Halstead, J. A. (2009). Understanding the impact of health literacy on women's health. *Journal of Obstetric, Gynecological and Neonatal Nursing, 38*(5), 601.

Simpkin, P. (1991). Just another day in a woman's life? Women's long-term perceptions of their first birth experience. Part I. *Birth, 18*(4), 203–211.

Soet, J. E., Brack, G. A., & Dilorio, C. (2003). Prevalence and predictors of women's experiences of psychological trauma during childbirth. *Birth, 30*(1), 36–46.

Souza, J. P., Gülmezoglu, A. M., Lumbiganon, P., et al. (2010). Caesarean section without medical indications is associated with an increased risk of adverse short-term maternal outcomes: the 2004–2008 WHO Global Survey on Maternal and Perinatal Health. *BMC Medicine, 8*(71), doi:10.1186/1741-7015-8-71

Spencer, N. (2000). Social gradients in child health: why do they occur and what can paediatricians do about them? *Ambulatory Child Health, 6*, 191–202.

Sullivan, A., Kean, L., & Cryer, A. (2006). *Midwife's guide to antenatal investigations*. London: Churchill Livingstone: Elsevier.

Suter, M., Ma, J., Harris, A., et al. (2011). Maternal tobacco use modestly alters correlated epigenome-wide placental DNA methylation and gene expression. *Epigenetics, 6*(11), 1284–1294.

Talge, N. M., Neal, C., & Glover, V. (2007). Antenatal maternal stress and long-term effects on child neurodevelopment: how and why? *Journal of Child Psychology and Psychiatry, 48*(3/4), 245–261.

Thavagnanam, S., Fleming, J., Bromley, A., Shields, M., & Cardwell, C. (2008). A meta-analysis of the association between cesarean section and childhood asthma. *Epidemiology of Allergic Disease, 38*, 629–663.

UNICEF/World Health Organization (WHO) (2009). *Baby friendly hospital initiative, revised, updated and expanded for integrated care, Section 1: Background and implementation, preliminary version*. Geneva: WHO.

Wang, Y. A., Chambers, G. M., & Sullivan, E. A. (2011). *Assisted reproductive technology in Australia and New Zealand 2009*. Canberra: Australian Institute of Health and Welfare.

World Health Organization (WHO) (2003). *Global Strategy for Infant and Young Child Feeding*. Geneva: WHO.

World Health Organization (WHO) (2004). *The importance of caregiver–child interactions for the survival and healthy development of children. A review*. Geneva: Department of Child and Adolescent Health and Development, WHO.

World Health Organization (WHO) (2005). *What is the effectiveness of antenatal care? (Supplement)*. Geneva: WHO. Retrieved from http://www.euro.who.int/__data/assets/pdf_file/0005/74660/E87997.pdf (accessed 9 January 2013).

World Health Organization (WHO) (2006). *Neonatal and perinatal mortality: Country, regional and global estimates*. Geneva: WHO.

World Health Organization (WHO) (2012). *Trends in maternal mortality 1990 to 2010: WHO, UNICEF, UNFPA and The World Bank estimates*. Geneva: WHO.

Chapter 7

INFANTS AND THEIR FAMILIES

Jennifer Rowe, Margaret Barnes

LEARNING OUTCOMES

Reading this chapter will help you to:

» identify the knowledge, skills and processes necessary to engage in effective and proactive nursing practice for families with infants

» understand the relationships among infant wellbeing and development, attachment and sensitive, responsive, parenting

» define support and apply the concept to nursing support for early parenting

» critique early parenting support programs

» identify safe, supportive and health promoting practices related to infant feeding

» identify safe, supportive and health promoting practices related to infant settling and sleep

» understand the interactions among sociological, epidemiological and health promotion underpinnings of childhood immunisation.

Introduction

In this chapter some of the challenges that families face during their child's infancy are examined. Infancy is an exciting and challenging time for families, who are shaped by the young child, just as that child is shaped by the family into which they are born. Complex individual, family and community factors interact to influence the quality of caregiving, parenting confidence and adjustment and family dynamics. The child's physical, social and emotional development and wellbeing are likely to be influenced by these dynamics in both the short and the longer term. Early intervention and community health promotion services are embedded in Australian and New Zealand societies to support families during this important transitional time. We present you with a scenario that situates nurses and families with infants in the contemporary, community healthcare context. We then discuss key themes that help you to unpack the scenario and orientate you to the essentials for practice that will support families, and promote infant health and wellbeing, particularly in the areas of attachment parenting, breastfeeding, settling and sleep and immunisation.

Clinical scenario 7.1
Setting the scene

You work in a community, postnatal drop-in service, which seeks to support women with babies aged up to 6 weeks and their families. The service is staffed by a midwife from the local maternity service and a child health nurse. It is 0930 on a Thursday morning. In the open clinic area there are three women with their babies. The husband of one of the women is also present. They are chatting among themselves. You join in their conversation.

Frida is in her late thirties. Her daughter, Katie, is just over 5 weeks old. Frida lives alone with her baby. She has family close by, including her younger sister who has three children. Her partner of 12 years left when she was 5 months pregnant because he did not want to have children. Frida is currently on leave from her executive position. As you listen to the conversation you hear Frida complaining that her baby is difficult as she doesn't sleep for long periods and cries a lot, especially if Frida doesn't pick her up quickly when she wakes.

Roseanne's baby boy was born just 7 days ago. Her 3-year-old son is also with her. She is also on leave from work, this time planning on taking 12 months leave from her government position. Her baby is well and Roseanne is determined to maintain breastfeeding this time. Last time she returned to work after 3 months, and struggled to breastfeed after that point.

The third mother is Asha. Her husband, Kye, has also come today. Their baby girl is now 6 weeks old. She was born at 34 weeks gestation and spent 3 weeks in the special care nursery at the local hospital before being discharged home. A nurse came to visit them in their home during the first week after their baby was discharged home. Asha has just weighed her baby on the scales in the corner of the room. 'Just checking she is doing OK', she comments.

This scenario reflects situations that are played out in a range of services in communities in Australia and New Zealand. It provides a starting point from which to examine services that aim to support families with infants as they transition and adapt to life with a young infant. It is also a point from which to investigate and critique the professional competencies and practices that will be needed to provide effective health care. Services may be universal or targeted and may be provided in community settings or in the homes of individual families. Promoting the health and wellbeing of the infant and their family is the primary aim of such services. How a society provides for the health of its mothers and children has been described as an indicator of social progress represented in the efficacy and availability of the services provided (Wilkinson & Marmot, 2003; World Health Organization, 2010).

For a woman, childbearing and the incorporation of a new infant into a family is a time of dramatic change, and for a family it represents a developmental transition (Deave, Johnson & Ingram, 2008; Salonen, Kaunonen, Åstedt-Kurki et al., 2009). A woman and her family's need for information, support and guidance during this period is potentially great, but it is also individual and influenced by variables such as the infant's health, the family's social situation, past experience of pregnancy and parenting, pre-existing support for the woman and her family, her level of health literacy and also psychological factors. Frida, Roseanne and Asha may each have very different reasons for attending the drop-in clinic. The degree of congruence between their needs and the services provided to them will go a long way towards determining how positive they perceive their experience to be, how well the family transitions and the health and wellbeing of the infant and family members in both the short and the long term (McKellar, Pincombe & Henderson, 2006).

Prior to investigating services and practice in some detail, there are some fundamental understandings about the infant–parent relationship and parenting that provide the necessary groundwork to be able to then assess, plan and deliver care and support.

Responsive parenting and infant development

In Chapter 6 you were introduced to the importance of attachment for a child's neurological and social development and in Chapter 1 you were introduced to the risk and protective factors that may influence the development and wellbeing of children. Among these there are some parenting factors that are significant and that relate to attachment. Sensitive and responsive caregiving helps to develop good attachment relationships that influence later social adjustment and competence in children (Ainsworth, 1979; Landry, Smith & Swank, 2006; WHO, 2004). *Sensitivity* refers to a parent's awareness of their infant's behaviours and *responsiveness* to the ability to respond to those behaviours with timely and appropriate interaction and care.

The links between infants developing attachment styles, their future social and affective skills and parenting have been theorised and researched for many decades. The key theorists in this field, John Bowlby (1969) and Mary Ainsworth (Ainsworth, 1979; Ainsworth, Blehar, Waters & Wall, 1978), have provided a platform for developmental and clinical research, as well as the interventions and professional practice programs that have emerged. Ainsworth suggested that responsiveness '… enables an infant to form expectations, primitive at first, that moderate his or her responses to events, both internal and environmental' (1979, p. 933).

Responsive behaviours on the part of the primary caregiver guide the interactions and allow an infant to develop an understanding, over time, that the caregiver is predictably accessible. This understanding, in turn, appears to influence infant behaviours and developmental competence. The infant's internal regulation, that is, ability to focus, maintain attention and organise behaviours, is influenced (Feeley, Zelkowitz, Westreich & Dunkley, 2011; Landry et al., 2006). Securely attached infants at 12 months are known to display greater degrees of a number of skills than their less secure counterparts – for example, cooperation and accepting help, positive affect, curiosity and exploration (Ainsworth, 1979).

Evidence supporting the link between infant skills and competence and responsive caregiving by the primary caregiver, usually the mother, has been building in recent years through empirical research. More details about what responsive caregiving entails have been tested. The parenting intervention study by Landry et al. (2006), for example, established evidence for a causal link among specific maternal practices and infant developmental competence. These include four areas:

1. being prompt in responding to infant cues
2. being sensitive; for example particularly by using a soothing voice and smiling or displaying positive affect and warmth and, conversely, not displaying detached or negative affect
3. being contingent, that is, appropriate to the infant's signals, for example picking up the crying baby and holding and soothing in a particular way
4. using language in caregiving, for example describing and naming objects and events.

Infants have few primary attachments and are selective so, for most, the mother is the primary attachment figure (Ainsworth, 1979), but it is important to note that it does not have to be the mother. This does not infer that fathers and other significant caregivers, for example grandparents, do not have an important role to play in nurturing the infant through the same kinds of interactions – those that are responsive and timely, warm, soothing and language rich.

Parenting self-efficacy and the parent-infant relationship

The ability to be responsive may be affected by anxiety, self-efficacy or other external or contextual issues (Salonen et al., 2009; WHO, 2004). Parenting self-efficacy (PSE) along with emotional wellbeing, the infant's health status, birth experience and professional care and support in the perinatal period form a complex picture of maternal and family transition during the infant's first year, which influences the dynamics of risk and protection in infancy.

PSE is an important element in understanding a parent's sensitivity and ability to provide responsive care. Self-efficacy concerns the belief or perception that an individual has about their decision making in specific contexts (Bandura, 1977, 1997). PSE is concerned with a parent's belief, and thus confidence, in their decision making around infant care (de Montigny & Lacharité, 2005; Reece & Harkman, 1998; Salonen et al., 2009). Most often the mother is the primary parent caregiver and so maternal self-efficacy has been the subject of significant investigation. Salonen et al. (2009) defined maternal self-efficacy (MSE) as a 'mother's belief in her ability to respond to her infant with behaviours that lead to a desired outcome' (p. 329).

MSE changes over time in the context of the mother–infant relationship. In the perinatal period, soon after an infant's birth, MSE is generally higher than fathers' PSE (Salonen et al., 2009). For mothers, having previously had a child tends to positively influence their confidence as does exclusive breastfeeding. A mother's perception of her infant's temperament also influences MSE over time (Fulton, Mastergeorge, Steele & Hansen, 2012; Salonen et al., 2009). For fathers, good family functioning is thought to be related to PSE (Salonen et al., 2009).

The mother–infant relationship evolves and develops over time, and its quality will be influenced by a range of interacting factors. Maternal psychological health and MSE are two of the more tangible and measurable of these factors that are known to impact parenting behaviours, particularly in being able to demonstrate warmth or positive affect in interactions. In turn, this is thought to have some bearing on longer term child outcomes (Zimmer-Gembeck & Thomas, 2010). The health and wellbeing of the primary caregiver, most usually the mother, is therefore critical. The quality of the infant–mother relationship is important for the infant but also for maternal wellbeing, and so understanding how a mother is feeling about herself, her infant and her ability to parent is a key element in providing effective support (Fulton et al., 2012).

As for women, the transition for men to fatherhood is ongoing and dynamic. The dynamics are similarly complex and involve negotiation and renegotiation of the ideals and realities of care, relationships and other work. Men's transition has received less scrutiny than that of women; however, being involved, believing in their ability to care and having appropriate knowledge and skills appear to be common elements (de Montigny, Lacharité & Devault, 2012). Stress is thought to impact on fathers' perceptions of their competence and there also appears to be an issue that relates to role balance – that is, balancing the demands of being a provider with being available and involved as a carer – that impacts on fathers. Early 1990s' research found that fathers perceived the mother–infant relationship, specifically the breastfeeding interaction, could act as an impediment to their involvement and relationship development with their infant (Bar-Yam & Darby, 1997). However, more recent evidence suggests this may be less of an issue (de Montigny et al., 2012). This change may reflect a generational shift where breastfeeding is more commonly established and maintained today than two decades ago and so is more normalised. For both men and women, successful parenting, marked by acceptance of self and their belief in their ability to be responsive carers, is a cornerstone in family adjustment and thus family strength.

The preterm birth of a baby as experienced by Asha and Kye represents a specific set of stressors for parents as they attempt to transition into parenting roles with a fragile, vulnerable and, sometimes, acutely unwell infant being nursed in a neonatal intensive care or special care nursery. Preterm birth is usually unexpected. The challenge to parents' expectations, the illness of the newborn and the difficulty in undertaking sensitive, responsive caregiving represent significant stressors and challenges for parents (Franck, Cox, Allen & Winter, 2005; Miles et al., 1997). Mothers are often more distressed in the initial period after the birth, but their parenting confidence and efficacy tend to improve more so than that of fathers over time and following their infant's discharge home (Rowe & Jones, 2010). This is particularly true for parents like Asha and Kye whose infant, although preterm, has reasonable gestational maturity (e.g. was born at over 31 weeks gestation and 1500 grams or more) (Feeley et al., 2011; see also fact sheets on the WHO website,

Box 7.1 Research highlight

Helping parents of VLBW and/or preterm infants to address their anxiety and engage with their infants is an important role for nurses and other healthcare providers in neonatal units. Research reported by Feeley et al. (2011) discusses the CUES program, which is an evidence-based program designed in the UK to provide one-on-one intervention for mothers of VLBW infants. The intervention aims to reduce maternal anxiety and enhance maternal sensitivity to their newborn's cues. Six sessions are provided, with most occurring in the neonatal nursery but with telephone support and the final session being provided after the infant's discharge from the hospital. Intervention providers, who are nurses and childbirth educators, receive 35 hours of training. The sessions include learning activities using written materials, observational activities, discussion and video feedback. The program's efficacy is being tested in a randomised controlled trial. Programs that help parents cope with anxiety and stress and that enhance their ability to provide sensitive caregiving in a range of contexts are significant interventions.

See Feeley, N., Zelkowitz, P., Westreich, R., Dunkley, D. (2011) The evidence base for the cues program for mothers of very low birth weight infants: an innovative approach to reduce anxiety and support sensitive interaction. The Journal of Perinatal Education 20(3):142–153, doi: 10.1891/1058-1243.20.3.142

http://www.who.int/mediacentre/factsheets/fs363/en/index.html). Parents of infants who are very preterm or very low birthweight (VLBW) are thought to experience distress and anxiety over longer periods of time, which may in turn affect their caregiving. There is evidence that parenting interventions to promote sensitive and responsive interaction in nursery environments are helpful and also support infants to meet developmental challenges (Feeley et al., 2011; Landry et al., 2006). See an example of research that is investigating the effectiveness of this type of program in Box 7.1.

Whatever the birth and family context, challenges exist for parents as they negotiate the changing demands, needs, priorities and relationships associated with parenting. These challenges, interweaving ones, may give rise to a range of needs and stressors for both mothers and fathers. Thus, for a woman, skills in practical caregiving such as breastfeeding and settling an infant can affirm and confirm her attachment with her infant and assist her sensitivity to her infant's cues and her skills in responsive interaction with her infant. They may also help her confidence in her maternal role and narrative of self as mother. For fathers, knowledge about the importance of attachment, skills in providing warm, language rich care and conversation about role demands may be helpful.

Briefly reflect on the scenario in the light of this information on attachment, responsive parenting and mother–infant relationships. Frida expressed concern that her 5-week-old daughter might be a difficult child because she doesn't sleep in a pattern that Frida expects and is distressed if Frida does not quickly attend to her. This is a reference to infant temperament. It is quite possible that Frida has expectations of her infant that are not realistic for a baby of this age. This, in turn, may impact on her responsiveness to her infant's cues and signals to her mother. Frida's knowledge about infant behaviour, values about what is normal and confidence in her ability to read her baby's cues and make good care decisions could all be topics of conversation at this time. Breastfeeding represents soothing, warm and contingent parenting, and so encouraging Roseanne to breastfeed may enhance her maternal efficacy and support the developing secure attachment of her infant. Conversation with Asha and Kye would begin with finding out more about their experiences in the special care nursery, the stresses that this situation may have created for them as parents and how they coped. In addition, it would be useful to investigate how they view their infant in the light of her prematurity, their expectations for their infant's development and wellbeing and what they believe is important to their parenting. Each of these conversations forms the basis of supporting parenting during this important transitional time.

Supporting parents and families

Supporting parents in the first months of their new baby's life is a significant practice responsibility for health professionals. In both Australia and New Zealand there is a long history of community child health services, reaching out to large proportions of families with babies and young children. Today, such services continue to play a role in promoting health and wellbeing for infants and young children, and now incorporate parenting programs to support parents during early childrearing (Guest & Keatinge, 2009; Rowe & Barnes, 2006). The need to support parents is constant and a vital key to strengthening families, whether health services focus on universal or targeted population groups.

What is support?

Support is an essential aspect of strengths-based and family-centred practice. See Chapter 5 for details of the Australian family strengths framework. One of the fundamental tenets of these approaches, which aligns with health promotion principles, is to enable families to make informed decisions and choose actions that are about things that matter to them. Accepting this assumption is important to the development of services that support families.

Support is conceptualised in various ways in nursing and the social science disciplines. Three types appear frequently: informational, tangible or instrumental and emotional (Heath, 2004). Informational support has two important characteristics: accuracy and relevance (House, 1981). Emotional support is a complex set of interactions, focused on supporting a person's sense of self or value (Heath, 2004; House, 1981), or alleviating emotional responses to stressors (Finfgeld-Connett, 2005). Tangible or instrumental support includes a wide range of concrete actions – those providing goods and services (Finfgeld-Connett, 2005).

Supporting parenting on the basis of these assumptions requires more than providing information or educating parents in parentcraft topics. Based on the assumption that parents are the constant in a young child's life negotiating knowledge and experience and needs, it requires practice that places authority in the hands of parents and accepts that parents bring knowledge and are able to be 'the expert'. It infers practising in such a way as to build the capacity of parents to make decisions and, where able, look after their infant or participate in their infant's care as partners (Rowe & Barnes, 2006). The traditional expert (i.e. the nurse as teacher and authority) is thus replaced by a nurse who is an expert in a number of other practices, including helping parents to:

1. identify and frame their needs and also their strengths
2. reframe their situations
3. access and utilise a range of resources and thus increase adjustment to parenting (e.g. personal/family community resources).

Community-based support and practice

Homer, Henry, Schmied et al. (2009) have argued that, across the childbearing continuum, community services need to be shaped by the needs of that community. This infers that understanding the demographic profile of the community is important. Factors must be considered, such as where clients will be seen (for example in a community centre or in their homes), appropriate timing (for example daytime or evening) and what staff skill will be required to provide effective care and support.

A variety of services and care models may be included. Drop-in clinics, such as the one outlined in the clinical scenario, offer appointment-free access to services such as parental support, advice and information relating to infant growth and development and breastfeeding. Similar outcomes have been reported for these clinics and those that offer appointments; however, drop-in services have been shown to be more resource efficient (Kearney, Fulbrook & Howlett, 2008). A recent evaluation of women's use of a newborn and family drop-in service (NAFDIS) within the Sunshine Coast region of Queensland demonstrated that this type of service was valued for its flexibility and the inherent level of control that women felt they had in accessing the resources it offered (Rowe et al., in press). These findings have been supported elsewhere (Kearney & Fulbrook, 2012).

New parent programs

In community centres support for parents can be generated in programs that connect new parents, often called new mother or new parent programs. They are also known as facilitated peer networking (Barnes, Courtney, Pratt & Walsh, 2004). These are commonly found in public health care maternal/child healthcare services. Privately run versions of this type of parenting support are also common in Australia and New Zealand. New parent programs are generally presented as a set of facilitated meetings, organised through local maternal child health services. The meetings enable mothers (and fathers) to meet other parents, to share information and conversation (Guest & Keatinge, 2009). A partnership model between nurse/midwife and parents is encouraged in most parenting groups, replacing the more traditional expert-to-lay model of earlier decades (Schmied, Donovan, Kruske et al., 2011). The scenario in this chapter demonstrates the potential of making a meeting place available. Parents begin conversations, sharing experiences, concerns and ideas. Both informally and also through more formal sessions that are often part of these programs, there is significant opportunity to encourage attachment parenting and to support the developing mother–infant relationship (Guest & Keatinge, 2009). For example, mothers hear about and can try new activities or witness different practices to their own. They have the opportunity to ask questions and voice their concerns or questions about their infant's behaviours. This sharing attends to both emotional and informational support needs. Women have a space to share the important stories of caregiving minutiae, relationship and family dynamics and reflections on the maternal role. From these interactions, women continue negotiating and confirming their role (Börjesson, Paperin & Lindell, 2004). In addition, it provides the opportunity for anticipatory guidance on caregiving topics such as breastfeeding, settling and sleep, immunisation and important developmental steps for the infants.

Community outreach centres provide interventions, which may be home-based or centre-based. Outreach services may be provided through home visiting from midwives or child health nurses, and they may be universal, such as the Plunkett home visiting service, or they may be targeted. Reflecting on the clinical scenario, the home visit to Asha and Kye may occur within either a universal or targeted service. If they live in an area that provides home visiting to all families with a new baby, it would be considered part of a universal service. If their healthcare service provides a home-based follow-up service for preterm infants and families, it would be considered a targeted service.

Home visiting programs

In today's healthcare policy and service climate, universal home visiting is a population-based healthcare strategy, where it is implemented by state health departments. In New Zealand there is a long history of home visits to families with infants by nurses known as Plunket nurses. The Royal New Zealand Plunket Society (RNZPS), known as Plunket, is the major New Zealand organisation providing community parenting support services. Plunket sees well over 90% of New Zealand's new mothers (Royal New Zealand Plunket Society, n.d., http://www.plunket.org.nz/).

Home visiting represents recognition of the dynamics of protection and risk to infants within families and communities and can be seen as an early intervention strategy designed to identify families at risk of poor outcomes (Schmied et al., 2011). Short-term universal programs aim to connect health services with families with a newborn within the first 2 weeks of birth in order to enhance service continuity from maternity services to child health and community services (Homer et al., 2009). In this type of service, visits may be conducted by nurses or midwives. During the visit, psychosocial assessment, parenting education, identification of resources that may be supportive to the family and basic health assessment/screening of the infant are usually undertaken (Henderson, 2010; Schmied et al., 2011).

Visiting Asha and Kye at home could provide a source of informational and emotional support as they undergo a second important transition in their parenting, moving from the special care nursery, where they were surrounded by health professionals and other staff but would not have been able to fully attach to their infant, to home. At home they can now continue their parenting journey but are without the constant professional and peer support available in the special care nursery environment.

Home visiting programs are best known as intensive or sustained and targeted services (Kemp, Anderson, Travaglia & Harris, 2005). Most often, they are delivered by nurses who visit families in their homes over extended periods of time, usually 12–24 months. The programs aim to influence parenting behaviours so that they positively impact on child outcomes. Evidence for their efficacy has been mounting over the past decade, although it remains mixed. Systematic reviews of home visiting programs in the USA, Canada and the UK have demonstrated that there are some positive outcomes in the environment, and in maternal wellbeing and parenting skill

(Fraser, Armstrong, Morris & Dadds, 2000; Gomby, Culross & Behrman, 1999; Jack, DiCenso & Lohfeld, 2005; Olds, Eckenrode, Henderson et al., 1997; Olds, Kitzman, Cole et al., 2004).

The model that has been most successfully implemented was developed by Olds et al. (1997, 2004) and implemented in at-risk populations of first-time mothers in the USA. There has been some commentary that the availability of a greater range of universal services in countries like Australia and New Zealand accounts for the lower effectiveness of programs implemented in these countries than those found from USA program evaluations (Bayer, Hiscock, Scalzo & Mathers, 2009).

An extended home visiting model in New Zealand was implemented in the early 2000s and evaluated using a randomised trial approach (Fergusson, Grant, Horwood & Ridder, 2006). The program was delivered over a period of 18 months to at-risk families by family health workers, who may or may not be nurses. At 36 months there were positive child outcomes when compared to the control families in terms of improvements in physical health, engagement with early education and exposure to positive parenting and fewer assaults from parents as well as fewer external and internal behaviour issues in the NZ model. However, there were no significant improvements in maternal or family outcomes (see http://www.earlystart.co.nz/pdf/evalreport.pdf).

In the report on the Early Start program the authors make the following important statement:

> ... the results of this evaluation clearly suggest home visitation programmes such as Early Start do not, and perhaps cannot, provide a complete solution to family social and economic problems. This suggests that *such programmes need to be seen as one component of an integrated approach* [emphasis added] to assisting families facing stress and difficulty. (Fergusson, Grant, Horwood & Ridder, 2005, p. 66).

Given what is known about the efficacy of home visiting programs, there are some implications for nurses and health services:

- Promoting attachment parenting and maternal sensitivity needs to be given more priority as the focus has tended to be primarily on behaviour modification in the context of visiting at-risk families (Niccols, 2008; Shepherd, 2011).
- Home visiting nurses need to have adequate and advanced competencies and experience in the range of social and health issues that they will address with families (Fraser et al., 2000; Kearney, York & Deatrick, 2004; Nievar, van Egeren & Pollard, 2010).
- Support for staff in terms of supervision and ongoing training and development in culturally competent care and congruent communication is also recognised as a key ingredient for effective practice (Armstrong, Fraser, Dadds & Morris, 2000; Gomby et al., 1999; Nievar et al., 2010).
- The relationship between visitor and parent is central to positive outcomes (Ammerman, Stevens, Putnam et al., 2006; Jack et al., 2005; Shepherd, 2011).
- In home-visiting situations, acceptance by the mother and family and the development of a respectful relationship and sense of mutuality between visitor and mother will be key requirements (Jack et al., 2005).

From these points it is clear that this service type requires effective assessment and targeting, experienced and specifically educated and trained staff as well as active and ongoing, organisational investment (Kemp et al., 2005). Family-centred practice rather than system-centred practice requires that the maternal and child health nurse practise as a facilitator. Nurses must be well-prepared, have a good knowledge base of risks and protective factors that influence parenting and family adjustment and must have the skills to work with parents so that they might build on existing strengths and their personal, family and other resources. Responsiveness to family-specific situations and needs is important. Further, programs are needed that account for child, parent, family and life events, as well as broader social or community factors. As Fergusson et al. (2006) commented above, there is also need for integration across sectors.

These tensions and concerns extend to the value of a range of activities designed to prevent ill health and promote good health. This knowledge has implications for nurses and the programs that are offered to families during the first year of a child's life. For example, there is good evidence that activities to promote breastfeeding, infant sleep conditions and immunisation are effective. Reflecting on the clinical scenario, these topics were very much in the minds of the women attending the drop-in centre. Everyday life with an infant is very much about feeding and settling. These concerns are directing Frida and Roseanne's attention. Monitoring a baby's health and progress is also important to parents. Asha is doing this by weighing her baby. All of these babies will soon be at the age when their first vaccination would be due.

Infant feeding

In Chapter 6 you were introduced to the benefits of breastfeeding and the ways that health professionals can support women to start breastfeeding. In Australia and New Zealand breastfeeding initiation rates are high but supporting women to continue to breastfeed as recommended remains a challenge. Breastmilk is all an infant needs in the first 6 months of life, after which they can be introduced to family foods. Prior to this time infants are not developmentally ready; however, the earlier introduction of other food is common. Parents may feel that introducing other food will help with sleeping at night, or additional foods are given when breastmilk supply is low. Infants grow rapidly during the first year, and their feeding behaviour changes with their growing needs.

For Frida, Roseanne and Asha attending the drop-in service provides an important support as they transition to the mothering role. The impact of positive support for women to continue breastfeeding is well recognised. In a metasynthesis of qualitative studies exploring women's perceptions and experiences of both peer and professional support for breastfeeding, the type of support provided was found to influence women's perceptions and experience. Not surprisingly, facilitative actions provided in an authentic presence were described as helpful whereas support that was disconnected was not (Sheehan, Schmied, Beake, McCourt & Dykes, 2009). 'Coaching' or providing hands-on, practical support, knowledge sharing and encouragement to meet personal goals have been identified as positive practices that support women's feeding choices (Rowe, Barnes & Sutherns, in press).

Often women find mother-to-mother support very helpful during the early months as they learn from each other and begin to understand normal infant behaviour. Although many informal support groups are formed amongst groups of women, a more formal support program is provided by the Australian Breastfeeding Association (ABA) and Le Leche League in New Zealand. ABA, for example, offers a 24-hour telephone service, local support groups and online information. Consider Roseanne's desire to be successful in breastfeeding over time with her second baby. The ABA would be an option to investigate for Roseanne as they could provide her with ongoing contact with breastfeeding mothers and a range of on-line information.

Encouraging and supporting women to breastfeed is also a wider societal responsibility. Environments that are welcoming to breastfeeding women and infants provide a strong message that breastfeeding is normal and make the task of being a mother feeding an infant easier. However, barriers do remain and accounts of discriminatory practices, particularly around breastfeeding in public, remain.

Settling and infant sleep

Frida expressed concern about her baby's sleep patterns, a concern shared by many parents of infants and young children in developed countries. In the previous 200 years, infant settling and sleep practices in families in western countries have diverged greatly from the practices of history and the majority of the world's population (McKenna, Thoman, Anders et al., 1993). Today, in countries such as Australia and New Zealand, some parents bring their infants to their bed but many parents will be fearful to bedshare, some will keep their young infants in a crib or cot close to their own bed but others prefer their infants to sleep alone. Many believe (and most certainly desire) that an infant of 3 months and older is capable of safely sleeping alone, and through the night.

Whatever the position, settling a baby and getting a baby to sleep are significant issues in the day-to-day lives of parents. Responding to this need becomes integral to child health nursing practice. In addition, promoting safe practices is important as a universal health service, both to promote health and to minimise risk.

A large amount of public health attention is focused on safe infant sleep practices, largely because of sudden infant death syndrome (SIDS; now classified as a type of sudden, unexplained, unexpected death in infancy [SUDI] as distinct from explained, unexpected infant deaths). SIDS was a baffling and devastating event that, until the mid-1990s, claimed the lives of more infants than any other cause, about 2–4 in 1000. The 1990s saw a significant downturn in this statistic in Australia, with an 80% reduction cited over the period 1989–2010 and following the introduction of a public campaign (SIDS and KIDS, 2012). (During this time, further classification and definition of SIDS deaths and clarification of autopsy procedures have occurred, which are also likely to influence the statistics.)

The public health campaign has focused on promoting safe sleeping. The premise of the campaign is that safe sleeping for infants is for them to (SIDS and KIDS, www.sidsandkids.org/safe-sleeping/):

How to Sleep your Baby Safely:

1. Sleep baby on the back from birth, not on the tummy or side
2. Sleep baby with head and face uncovered
3. Keep baby smoke free before birth and after
4. Provide a safe sleeping environment night and day

5. Sleep baby in their own safe sleeping place in the same room as an adult caregiver for the first six to twelve months
6. Breastfeed baby

The fifth point refers to a type of co-sleeping. Co-sleeping is thought to be protective and also promotes secure attachment. It has been defined as '... any situation in which a committed mother sleeps within sensory range of an infant (on the same or different surface) permitting mutual monitoring, sensory access, and physiological regulation, including (but not limited to) the delivery and ingestion of breast milk' (McKenna et al., 1993 cited in Gettler & McKenna, 2011). In this definition a number of things are made clear: that the proximity of mother and baby needs to be sufficiently close to enable a range of physiological and sensory functions to occur and that the arrangement is also linked to infant feeding.

Co-sleeping and bedsharing are terms that are often used interchangeably but it is important to understand the differences between them and also to be able to discuss with parents their practices and values in order to be able to provide effective support that is responsive to their needs and promotes the infant's health and safety. Co-sleeping can include arrangements where the child is in close proximity to the parents on a shared or separate sleeping surface (e.g. a cot beside the bed or a three-sided cot flush against the bed). Bedsharing refers specifically to arrangements in which the infant sleeps in the same bed as the parents.

Although bedsharing is not recommended by the SIDS and KIDS organisation, they provide guidelines for promoting safe bedsharing. These involve following the six safe sleep recommendations as well as ensuring a firm sleep surface, good ventilation, positioning an infant beside one parent, rather than in between both, and not in a place where the infant may become stuck between a mattress and frame or fall out (SIDS and KIDS, 2012).

Nursing practice promoting safe family sleep environments

The challenge for nurses working with families to help them meet the demands they face is not to increase their fears, but rather to provide them with options that are protective, health promoting and nurturing for the infant and their relationship with their infant. Options need to help parents to create realistic and safe sleeping environments for their infant and themselves, according to their specific physical environment and lifestyle needs. To do this, nurses need to first interrogate their own values and ensure that they are guided by evidence and family-centred principles. Evidence suggests the following:

- There is nothing to be gained by an infant sleeping in a solitary place, away from the company of others (McKenna & Joyce n.d.).
- There are some sleep environmental conditions, such as a smoke-free room and use of a firm mattress, either bed or cot, and certain bedclothes, that promote safety (SIDS & KIDS at www.sidsandkids.org/safe-sleeping).
- Back sleeping is a safe position for infants (SIDS & KIDS at www.sidsand kids.org/safe-sleeping).

This and other evidence needs to be incorporated within an individualised, dynamic and negotiated process in which parents are supported to make their own decisions.

To do this, nurses also need to understand how parents appraise their situation. For example, what are parents' assumptions about normal sleep for infants and their own sleep expectations? Frida, for example, seems to have the impression that her baby should sleep for longer periods. Her appraisal that her 5-week-old would sleep for long periods, or even show a sleep pattern or routine, is most likely unrealistic. It is unlikely that her baby has a difficult temperament or behaviours. The baby is clearly signalling to Frida when she awakens, although Frida may not be responsive to her baby's communication cues before she cries loudly. Other communication cues will certainly be used by her baby but may not be recognised as such by Frida. The sixth safe sleeping guideline is to encourage breastfeeding, a protective mechanism for infants. It would be well worth discussing Frida's feeding practice as infant feeding, safe sleep and settling are all intertwined needing sensitivity to the child's needs and responsive caregiving.

Nurses need to assess parents' understanding of their babies' behaviours, and how they interpret what their infants are signalling to them, in order to help them increase their knowledge, where this is needed. Nurses need to help them negotiate their options in ways that promote their relationship with their baby. For example, is there room in the parents' bedroom for a cot for an infant up to 12 months of age? Are there settling strategies they can try? Are there other family or friends who can help, and when and what might they do? Do they link infant feeding with settling and sleep?

Immunisation

The third health promotion area to consider is immunisation. It is beyond the scope of this chapter to provide a detailed analysis of the historical debates and clinical practice guidelines and issues that have surrounded childhood immunisation. Rather, it is the intention here to refer the reader to appropriate information regarding childhood immunisation schedules and to challenge readers to consider and inform themselves about important practice and service factors.

Childhood immunisation coverage rates are measured in Australia at 1, 2 and 6 years. In 2011, they were reported as 91.4%, 92.7% and 90.1%, respectively (Australian Government Medicare, http://www.medicareaustralia.gov.au/provider/patients/acir/statistics.jsp). In New Zealand, the rates were 89.6%, 88.3% and 73.2% in comparative years and, at 2 years, the rate was 77% (Ministry of Health New Zealand, 2011). The standard schedule and vaccines vary in each country but can be easily accessed via the immunisation handbooks for each country, available online.

Immunisation can be provided by health professionals in a range of settings, including general practitioners, hospitals and community health services. Each nurse providing immunisations as part of their clinical practice needs to consider a number of things if they are to promote best practice. We suggest that readers access the handbooks for immunisation for Australia and New Zealand.

- For information on New Zealand childhood immunisation, go to: Ministry of Health New Zealand *Immunisation Handbook 2011*. Retrieved from http://www.health.govt.nz/publication/immunisation-handbook-2011.

- For information on Australian childhood immunisation, go to: Australian Government Department of Health and Ageing. 2008. *The Australian Immunisation Handbook*, 9th ed. Retrieved from http://www.immunise.health.gov.au/internet/immunise/publishing.nsf/Content/Handbook-home.

Use the information in these handbooks to respond to each of the following questions.

1. What diseases is population immunisation combating? How are these diseases transmitted?
2. What is the current immunisation schedule?
3. What are the commonly used vaccine preparations?
4. What is current best practice for vaccine administration?
5. What is current best practice for vaccine storage and transport?
6. What are the adverse effects of immunisations? (*The Australian Immunisation Handbook* provides a useful table identifying disease, method of transmission, effects of disease in type and rate and adverse effects of immunisation in type and rate.)
7. What clinical conditions may delay or contraindicate immunisation?
8. What are the registration and recording procedures for childhood immunisation?

Nurses also need to consider past and present immunisation debates and the issues these raise for parents; in other words, they need to know what the talk on the street is. Informed consent is an important aspect of the immunisation procedure, as it is for other medical treatments. See Chapter 4 for a full discussion of informed consent in treatment and research.

Parents need to have clear and correct information, not only about the vaccine but also about the disease and its adverse effects. They must also be able to interpret their personal experiences as part of their decision making. They have a right to accurate information, provided in a climate of respect for their experience. Resources are available to assist health professionals understand parent concerns and respond to them. See, for example, the National Centre for Immunisation Research (NCIRS) website (http://www.ncirs.edu.au/immunisation/fact-sheets/index.php).

As advocates and change agents, nurses are responsible for individual practice and for health service development. Thus, nurses need to consider the service they work in with regard to immunisation practice:

1. Are current resources for health professionals available to staff?
2. Is appropriate professional development available and valued?
3. Are resources to assist parent/carer knowledge about immunisation available and accessible?

Assessing growth and development

Recall the clinical scenario. Asha and Kye weighed their baby and were keen to know that she was progressing well. This is a common question for parents with infants. For some, objective measurements provide some security. For parents, knowing that a baby is well and progressing along the established norms is often affirmed in data they gather from child health nurses and document in personal health records. Asha and Kye, and indeed all families, will leave maternity services with their newborn and a personal health record for their child. It is known as a 'parent-held' record. In this record, among other things, specific behaviours that are expected at a range of ages as physical, cognitive and motor skills developmental milestones can be mapped out, growth measurements are graphed, potential health problems and symptoms to watch for are identified and schedules for assessment of the child's development and vaccinations are set out.

The record is part of a health surveillance strategy, meaning that it is part of a population-based, systematic approach to measuring growth and development against norms. Health screening and surveillance have been promoted in Australia and New Zealand over a long period of time. Child growth standards are widely used as a tool in public health and medicine and by government and health organisations for monitoring the wellbeing of children and for detecting children or populations who are not growing properly according to measurable norms.

The personal health record is treated as a data archive and growth monitoring, health surveillance and health education tool. Potentially, it provides a history of the child. In Australia and New Zealand, parents can use this record and then access professionals to conduct the appropriate assessments – in child health clinics, general practice rooms and pharmacies, to name a few. See Box 7.2, which highlights the development of growth charts, a central feature of the personal health record.

An evaluation of the use of personal records by parents in the UK revealed that the personal health records functioned best as records and least well as health education tools (Wright & Reynolds, 2006). This evaluation study also found that a more comprehensive education book given to all parents of newborns was also poorly used. A recent literature review undertaken as part of the review of the Victorian Personal Health Record suggested that there was little evidence that personal health records enhanced communication with health professionals or had any impact on population or subgroup health outcomes (Murdoch Children's Research Institute, 2011). The use of personal health records does appear to improve vaccination compliance. Nurses often undertake the regular measurement and assessment of growth and development, and the same review identified issues with the level of training nurses had for accurately measuring and interpreting some of the growth and development measures. This is a serious issue for nurses to address, particularly given the confidence parents place in their skill and also the assumptions that may be made about infants and young children's health and wellbeing based on data in these records.

A trend in personal health records is to provide space for more input by parents and to provide more parenting information. It has some promise as a tool to facilitate communication with parents to support their parenting style and practice.

Conclusion

In this chapter we focused on the importance of caregiving, responsive parenting and parenting support as it influences maternal, family and infant wellbeing and

---

Box 7.2 Practice highlight: Tracking growth

So many babies have had their height and weight tracked through infancy and recorded on growth charts. This practice started in the late nineteenth century and continues to the present day. Charts used through the last decades of the twentieth century were based on norms for children from 1929 to 1975 who were predominantly American middle-class and bottle-fed (Centers for Disease Control and Prevention, 2000). The Centers for Disease Control and Prevention (CDC) in the United States produced more discerning charts in 2000, which are based on norms from both bottle-fed and breastfed infants. These have been widely used. More recently, the World Health Organization (WHO) produced new charts as a single reference point, also establishing breastfed infants as the normative model for growth and development (2006). Information about the WHO child growth standards and their development, as well as the charts, can be accessed on the WHO webpage.

It is interesting to examine these changes, and reflect on the changing social practices and the implications of these for establishing norms for child growth and development and, inevitably, parenting activities. Further, the changes reflect the interactions between epidemiology, science and health policy over time. What does not change is the fact that formula and breastfed infants have different patterns of growth in the first few months of life. Breastfed infants tend to grow more rapidly than formula-fed infants in the first 2 months of life and then more slowly, in comparison, during the third and fourth months.

Implications for nursing practice

It is important that measures such as these are used as reference points, not standards to be met. Measuring growth must be conducted within the context of a health promoting framework, not an isolated test for babies, and their parents, to pass or fail.

Reader activity

The CDC website (www.cdc.gov/growthcharts/) and the WHO website provide comprehensive information on the charts, their use and the basis for changes. Readers are encouraged to spend some time examining this information.

---

development. We examined the range of universal and targeted, health promoting services that can be accessed by families in the community. We identified key characteristics of infant feeding and sleep, and provided guidance in understanding health assessment and immunisation in early childhood. Throughout the discussion, the relevance of health promoting services and nursing practice to the lives and health of families with infants has been demonstrated. For nurses we have argued a role in which we prioritise the expertise of the nurse in facilitation and applying expert knowledge to help families make decisions about caregiving practices for their infants and support parents as they face the significant challenges parenthood brings to everyday life and to their understanding of the needs, priorities and desires of their lives.

CRITICAL QUESTIONS AND REFLECTION

1. Reflect on the health promotion mandate to promote breastfeeding. This may challenge your own experience and beliefs and will certainly be prioritised differently by families you may encounter. To help build your understanding of the issue, and its importance in terms of infant wellbeing and women's rights,

investigate the legislation in your jurisdiction regarding the protection of breastfeeding and safeguards against discrimination.

2. Reflect on the clinical scenario presented at the beginning of the chapter. Frida's baby is 5 weeks old, Roseanne's is 1 week and Asha and Kye's is 6 weeks, but having been born at 34 weeks gestation has a corrected age of 2 weeks (that is the age she would be if born on her due date). Access and review a reliable and current source of developmental milestones and consider what social and physical behaviours and communications you might expect of each of these babies. Consider what cues parents could be encouraged to be aware of, anticipate and respond to in their caregiving.

References

Ainsworth, M. D. (1979). Infant–mother attachment. *American Psychologist*, *34*(10), 932–937.

Ainsworth, M. D., Blehar, M. C., Waters, E., & Wall, S. (1978). *Patterns of attachment: A psychological study of the strange situation*. Hillsdale, NJ: Erlbaum.

Ammerman, R., Stevens, J., Putnam, F., et al. (2006). Predictors of early engagement in home visitation. *Journal of Family Violence*, *21*(2), 105–115.

Armstrong, K., Fraser, J., Dadds, M., & Morris, J. (2000). Promoting secure attachment, maternal mood and child health in a vulnerable population. *Journal of Paediatrics and Child Health*, *36*, 555–562.

Bandura, A. (1977). Self-efficacy: toward a unifying theory of behavioural change. *Psychological Review*, *84*(2), 191–215.

Bandura, A. (1997). *Self-efficacy: The exercise of control*. New York: WH Freeman and Company.

Barnes, M., Courtney, M., Pratt, J., & Walsh, A. (2004). The roles, responsibilities and professional development needs of child health nurses. *Focus on Health Professional Education*, *6*(1), 52–63.

Bar-Yam, N. B. & Darby, L. (1997). Father and breastfeeding: a review of the literature. *Journal of Human Lactation*, *13*(1), 45–50.

Bayer, J., Hiscock, H., Scalzo, K., & Mathers, M. (2009). Systematic review of preventive interventions for children's mental health: what would work in Australian contexts? *Australian and New Zealand Journal of Psychiatry*, *43*, 695–710.

Börjesson, B., Paperin, C., & Lindell, M. (2004). Maternal support during the first year of infancy. *Journal of Advanced Nursing*, *45*(6), 588–594.

Bowlby, J. (1969). *Attachment and loss: Vol. 1. Attachment*. New York: Basic Books.

Centers for Disease Control and Prevention (CDC) (2000). Clinical growth charts. Retrieved from http://www.cdc.gov/growthcharts/clinical_charts.htm (accessed 1 February 2013).

Deave, T., Johnson, D., & Ingram, J. (2008). Transition to parenthood: the needs of parents in pregnancy and early parenthood. *BMC Pregnancy and Childhood*, *8*, 30, doi:10.1186/1471-2393-8-30 retrieved from http://www.biomedcentral.com/1471-2393/8/30 (accessed 14 January 2013).

de Montigny, F. & Lacharité, C. (2005). Perceived parental efficacy: concept analysis. *Journal of Advanced Nursing, 49*(4), 387–396.

de Montigny, F., Lacharité, C., & Devault, A. (2012). Transition to fatherhood: modeling the experience of fathers of breastfed infants. *Advances in Nursing Science, 35*(3), E11–E22.

Department of Child and Adolescent Health and Development, World Health Organization (2004). *The importance of caregiver–child interactions for the survival and healthy development of young children.* WHO. Retrieved from http://whqlibdoc. who.int/publications/2004/924159134X.pdf (accessed 14 January 2013).

Feeley, N., Zelkowitz, P., Westreich, R., & Dunkley, D. (2011). The evidence base for the cues program for mothers of very low birth weight infants: an innovative approach to reduce anxiety and support sensitive interaction. *The Journal of Perinatal Education, 20*(3), 142–153, doi: 10.1891/1058-1243.20.3.142

Fergusson, D., Grant, H., Horwood, J., & Ridder, E. (2005). *Early Start. Evaluation Report.* Christchurch School of Medicine and Health Sciences. Retrieved from http://www.msd.govt.nz/documents/about-msd-and-our-work/publications-resources/evaluation/early-start-evaluation-report.pdf (accessed 22 January 2013).

Fergusson, D., Grant, H., Horwood, J., et al. (2006). Randomized trial of the Early Start program of home visitation: parent and family outcomes. *Pediatrics, 117,* 781–786.

Finfgeld-Connett, D. (2005). Clarification of social support. *Journal of Nursing Scholarship, 37*(1), 4–9.

Franck, L. S., Cox, S., Allen, A., & Winter, I. (2005). Measuring neonatal intensive care unit-related parental stress. *Journal of Advanced Nursing, 49*(6), 608–615, doi: 10.1111/j.1365-2648.2004.03336.x

Fraser, J., Armstrong, K., Morris, J., & Dadds, M. (2000). Home visiting intervention for vulnerable families with newborns: follow up results of a randomised controlled trial. *Child Abuse and Neglect, 24*(11), 1399–1429.

Fulton, J., Mastergeorge, A., Steele, J., & Hansen, R. (2012). Maternal perceptions of the infant: maternal self-efficacy during the first six weeks' postpartum. *Infant Mental Health, 33,* 329–338.

Gettler, L. & McKenna, J. (2011). Evolutionary perspectives on mother–infant sleep proximity and breastfeeding in a laboratory setting. *American Journal of Physical Anthropology, 144,* 454–462.

Gomby, S., Culross, P., & Behrman, R. (1999). Home visiting: recent program evaluations – analysis and recommendations. *The Future of Children, 9*(1), 4–26.

Guest, E. & Keatinge, D. (2009). The value of new parent groups in child and family nursing. *Journal of Perinatal Education, 18*(3), 12–22.

Heath, H. (2004). Assessing and delivering parent support. In M. Hoghughi & N. Long (Eds.), *Handbook of parenting. Theory and research for practice* (pp. 311–333). London: Sage.

Henderson, S. (2010). Community child health (CCH) nurses' experience of home visiting for new mothers: a quality improvement project. *Contemporary Nurse, 34*(1), 66–76.

Homer, C., Henry, K., Schmied, V., et al. (2009). 'It looks good on paper': Transitions of care between midwives and child and family health nurses in New South Wales. *Women and Birth, 22*, 64–72.

House, J. (1981). *Work stress and social support*. Massachusetts: Addison-Wesley, Reading.

Jack, S., DiCenso, A., & Lohfeld, L. (2005). A theory of maternal engagement with public health nurses and family visitors. *Journal of Advanced Nursing, 49*(2), 182–190.

Kearney, L. & Fulbrook, P. (2012). Open-access community child health clinics: the everyday experience of parents and child health nurses. *Journal of Child Health Care, 16*(1), 5–14.

Kearney, L., Fulbrook, P., & Howlett, L. (2008). 'Drop-in' clinics compared with individual appointment clinics: an outcome evaluation of an innovative group model of care for parents with infants aged 0–18 months. *The Australian Journal of Child and Family Nursing, 5*(1), 8–16.

Kearney, M. H., York, R., & Deatrick, A. (2004). Effects of home visits to vulnerable young families. *Journal of Nursing Scholarship, 32*(4), 369–375.

Kemp, L., Anderson, T., Travaglia, J., & Harris, E. (2005). Sustained nurse home visiting in early childhood: exploring Australian nursing competencies. *Public Health Nursing, 22*(3), 254–259.

Landry, S., Smith, K., & Swank, P. (2006). Responsive parenting: establishing early foundations for social, communication, and independent problem-solving skills. *Developmental Psychology, 42*(4), 627–642.

McKellar, L. V., Pincombe, J. I., & Henderson, A. M. (2006). Insights from Australian parents into educational experiences in the early postnatal period. *Midwifery, 22*, 356–364.

McKenna, J. J. & Joyce, E. P. (n.d.). *Mother–baby behavioral sleep laboratory*. Indiana: Department of Anthropology, University of Notre Dame. Retrieved from http://cosleeping.nd.edu/ (accessed 22 January 2013).

McKenna, J. J., Thoman, E., Anders, T., et al. (1993). Infant–parent co-sleeping in an evolutionary perspective: implications for understanding infant sleep development and the sudden infant death syndrome. *Sleep, 16*(3), 263–282.

Miles, M. S. & Holditch-Davis, D. (1997). Parenting the prematurely born child: pathways of influence. *Seminars in Perinatology, 21*(3), 254–266.

Ministry of Health New Zealand (2011). *Immunisation Handbook 2011*. Retrieved from http://www.health.govt.nz/publication/immunisation-handbook-2011 (accessed 14 January 2013).

Murdoch Children's Research Institute (2011). *Child health record literature review*. State Government of Victoria: Department of Education and Early Childhood Development.

Niccols, A. (2008). 'Right from the Start': randomized trial comparing an attachment group intervention to supportive home visiting. *Journal of Child Psychology and Psychiatry, 49*(7), 754–764.

Nievar, M., van Egeren, L., & Pollard, S. (2010). A meta-analysis of home visiting programs: moderators of improvement in maternal behaviour. *Infant Mental Health Journal, 31*(5), 499–520.

Olds, D.L., Eckenrode, J., Henderson, C. R., Jr., et al. (1997). Long-term effects of home visitation on maternal life course and child abuse and neglect: fifteen-year follow-up of a randomized trial. *Journal of the American Medical Association, 78*(8), 637–643.

Olds, D. L., Kitzman, H., Cole, R., et al. (2004). Effects of nurse home-visiting on maternal life course and child development: age 6 follow-up results of a randomized trial. *Pediatrics, 114*(6), 1550–1559.

Reece, S. M. & Harkless, G. (1998). Self-efficacy, stress, and parental adaptation: applications to the care of childbearing families. *Journal of Family Nursing, 4,* 198–215.

Rowe, J. & Barnes, M. (2006). The role of child health nurses in enhancing mothering know-how. *Collegian, 13*(4), 22–26.

Rowe, J., Barnes, M., & Sutherns, S. (in press) Supporting maternal transition: continuity, coaching and control. *Journal of Perinatal Education.*

Rowe, J. & Jones, L. (2010). Discharge and beyond: a longitudinal study comparing stress and coping in parents of preterm infants. *Journal of Neonatal Nursing, 16,* 258–266, doi: 10.1016/j.jnn.2010.07.018.13(4):22–6

Salonen, A., Kaunonen, M., Åstedt-Kurki, P., et al. (2009). Parenting self-efficacy after childbirth. *Journal of Advanced Nursing, 65*(11), 2324–2336, doi: 10.1111/j.1365-2648.2009.05113.x

Schmied, V., Donovan, J., Kruske, S., et al. (2011). A review of Australian state and territory maternity and child health policies. *Contemporary Nurse, 40*(1), 106–117.

Sheehan, A., Schmied, V., Beake, S., McCourt, C., & Dykes, F. (2009). A meta-synthesis of women's perceptions and experiences of breastfeeding support. *JBI Library of systematic reviews, 7*(14), 583–614.

Shepherd, M. (2011). Behind the scales: child and family health nurses taking care of women's emotional wellbeing. *Contemporary Nurse, 37*(2), 137–148.

SIDS and KIDS (2012). Fast facts. Retrieved from http://www.sidsandkids.org/research/ (accessed 14 January 2013).

Wilkinson R & Marmot M (Eds.), (2003). *Social determinants of health. The solid facts* (2nd ed.). World Health Organization. Retrieved from http://www.euro.who.int/__data/assets/pdf_file/0005/98438/e81384.pdf (accessed 14 January 2013).

World Health Organization (WHO) (2006). *WHO Child growth standards: Length/height-for-age, weight-for-age, weight-for-length, weight-for-height and body mass index-for-age: Methods and development.* Geneva: WHO. Retrieved from http://www.who.int/childgrowth/en/ (accessed 1 February 2013).

World Health Organization (WHO) (2010). *The World Health Report.* Geneva: WHO. Retrieved from http://www.who.int/whr/2010/en/index.html (accessed 1 February 2013).

Wright, C. & Reynolds, L. (2006). How widely are personal child health records used and are they effective health education tools? A comparison of two records. *Child Care, Health and Development, 32*(1), 55–61.

Zimmer-Gembeck, M. J. & Thomas, R. (2010). Parents, parenting and toddler adaption: evidence from a longitudinal study of Australian children. *Infant Behaviour and Development, 33*(4), 518–529. Retrieved from http://dx.doi.org/10.1016/j.infbeh.2010.07.004 (accessed 1 February 2013).

Chapter 8

HEALTH PROMOTION THROUGH EARLY CHILDHOOD

Anne Tietzel, Avril Rose

LEARNING OUTCOMES

Reading this chapter will help you to:

» define health promotion in the early years of education and care

» explore development, health and wellbeing in the early years

» understand the influence of early childhood education and care environments on children's development, health and wellbeing

» appreciate the role of nurses and health promotion in education and care environments

» develop an understanding of principles of practice that strengthens the development, health, wellbeing and education of young children and their families.

Introduction

Early childhood is the stage of life when families, communities, organisations and governments focus on children's development, health and wellbeing in a range of contexts such as playgroups, long day care and kindergarten. Contemporary research and policy initiatives in health and education highlight the need for collaborative partnerships that promote children's healthy development and holistic wellbeing in order to provide children with the best start to life and learning. Contemporary images of children view them as being competent individuals who contribute to families and communities through their own voice and agency. Children living in Australian and New Zealand communities are considered capable of understanding and expressing their development, health, wellbeing and education needs within supportive environments and relationships.

In this chapter early childhood is defined as the period of growth and development that spans from toddlerhood to starting school: 18 months to 5 years. The reader is provided with an overview of contemporary children's capabilities, interests and social and cultural environmental contexts. Major sources of influences on social, cultural and political contexts are outlined as these may impact children's development, health, wellbeing and education. An integrated approach to health promoting activities in early childhood education and care and health services is discussed.

A history of holistic views on development, health, wellbeing, care and education

Rebecca, the child health nurse in the clinical scenario, finds that early childhood education and care has a long history of implementing holistic approaches to children's development, health, wellbeing and learning, recognising the need to cater for the whole child and their family. Early models of care and education were founded on medical and maternal health principles, acknowledging that meeting a child's basic physical needs was essential for their ongoing social, psychological and cognitive development.

In the early 1900s an American doctor, Arnold Gesell, became concerned about children's growth and development. He believed that maturation was an innate and powerful force in determining children's development. He conducted quantitative studies of child development, observing and measuring children's growth and development between infancy and adolescence. Gesell developed norms that described what was appropriate growth and development at a particular age and stage in the child's life. Gesell's intent was to reassure parents that a child's growth and development were beyond their control and that their role was to assist nature to take its course. The research conducted by Gesell in the 1920s sparked interest in a child study movement, with a common focus on children's development, health, wellbeing and education, and drew together the disciplines of health, education and psychology (Charlesworth, 2011; Gordon & Browne, 2011).

At about the same time Maria Montessori, the first Italian woman to become a medical doctor, worked with young children with intellectual disabilities whom she

---

Clinical scenario 8.1
Setting the scene: Holistic early childhood health and wellbeing

Rebecca is a child health nurse employed in a child and family community health service located in the inner suburbs of a large regional city. Over the past few years Rebecca has become aware of the growing trend among families of enquiring if the child health service operates outside of business hours or if they visit children in other settings, such as long day care centres and kindergartens. During this period Rebecca has also noted that there has been an increasing number of early childhood educators calling the child and family health service to discuss child development, health and parenting issues. More regularly, she is being invited to speak at early childhood education and care professional development sessions and to early childhood education students.

At a community child and family event, Rebecca observes that there is a range of early childhood development, health, wellbeing and early learning services and organisations represented. Her attention is drawn to the banner and brochure of one early childhood education and care centre that is promoting their holistic and integrated child- and family-related services. On reading the brochure she discovers they offer a broad range of services from playgroups to toy libraries to breastfeeding clinics and parenting classes. The centre employs specialist health practitioners, including maternal and child health nurses, to promote early childhood development, health and wellbeing. They are open extended hours and offer evening child health and parenting support. The centre markets itself as the 'one stop shop for children and families'.

While attending a national child and family health conference, Rebecca mentions the changes she has noted in child, family and community dynamics and needs. She ascertains that other child health nurses across the country are noticing similar trends. One colleague comments that a local long day care centre often sends home brochures and newsletters containing health-related matters, including information on immunisation, diet and nutrition, toilet training and games to play to promote strong healthy growing bodies. Rebecca also learns that many of her colleagues are participating in multidisciplinary healthy early years strategies.

Rebecca decides to do some research on the changing needs of children and families and the role of early childhood education and care settings in promoting the development of health and wellbeing. Her findings show that early childhood education and care settings have a long history of providing for young children's development, health and wellbeing as well as their early learning needs. Contemporary policy and practice recognise early childhood education and care settings as providing a universal platform from which to initiate and build on programs that promote health, wellbeing, child development and nurturing relationships. She notes that, at present, the early childhood education and care sector is increasingly being influenced by the fields of health and medicine, neurobiological science, psychology and mental health. In her discussions with early childhood educators and health practitioners employed in multidisciplinary services, Rebecca determines that these changes are shaping the contemporary care and education of young children and the view of children and families within communities. She notes that more services are looking towards developing holistic, multidisciplinary partnership approaches to providing children and families with the best start to life.

---

believed would benefit from care and education supports rather than just medical intervention. In 1907 Montessori was asked by the housing authority of the City of Rome to take charge of a children's day nursery with the aim of keeping young children safe from harm and off the streets. She founded *Casa di Bambini*, a centre for children aged 2 to 5 years, who all received two meals a day, a daily bath and medical treatment (Gordon & Browne, 2011). Montessori developed methods that encouraged the children to engage in life skills play, which sought to foster independence and self-discipline. She determined that there were times or 'sensitive periods' in which children were most ready to attend to specific tasks through sensory exploration and discrimination tasks (Catron & Allen, 2008). Montessori's methods proved that young children were capable of managing their own self-help skills if instruction was provided at sensitive periods in children's growth and development. She developed child-sized equipment and sequential learning materials to assist children develop and learn in a series of small steps within a supportive environment (Gordon & Browne, 2011).

These international models of providing for children's development, health and wellbeing influenced Australia's early history of service development. The Sydney Day Nursery, which commenced operating in 1905, is one of Australia's earliest community-based children's services and was established to care for children aged from birth to 3 years while their parents worked. In the first 30–40 years of operation the nurseries were run by matrons and nursing staff whose primary concern was for the children's health (SDN Children's Services, 2012). In 1940 the Commonwealth Department of Health established demonstration centres in each capital city of Australia. The centres were named after the wife of the Governor-General, Lady Gowrie, in honour of her support in lobbying for the establishment of demonstration centres for the care and wellbeing of young children (Lady Gowrie Inc., 2012). The centres aimed to improve the health and wellbeing of Australian children, particularly disadvantaged children. Each centre was required to study children's physical growth, nutrition and development as well as testing and demonstrating methods of care and instruction of young children. Most of the six centres established employed a registered nurse, a social worker, a teacher and a cook–housekeeper. The children were provided with a hot meal and primary health care each day.

Contemporary children, families and communities

In contemporary society the needs of children and families are changing with many parents juggling paid employment and family responsibilities. The rapid changes in society have seen twice as many families with both parents entering the paid workforce (Centre for Community Child Health, 2006) and more children attending early childhood education and care services (Office for Early Childhood Education and Care, 2010). Researchers have found that families are under increased stress, trying to balance their children's care and health, social and educational outcomes while meeting their employment commitments (Centre for Community Child Health, 2006). Policymakers and practitioners across care and education services are considering reforms and program initiatives that will assist 21st century families support their health, wellbeing and social needs as well as children's development and learning.

Developmental milestones for healthy growth and wellbeing still feature within the policy directions for early childhood education and care; however, contemporary philosophy and practices adopt a more sociocultural approach to child development.

Age and stage norms still provide health and education providers with a gauge for normal development, but it is becoming more widely recognised that they do not account for family, social or cultural diversity in the many contexts in which early development occurs (Gordon & Browne, 2011). Sociocultural approaches acknowledge that children live in diverse family, social and cultural contexts and that there are multiple ways of understanding children's development, health, wellbeing and learning (Arthur, Beecher, Death, Dockett & Farmer, 2012). Sociocultural theories highlight the way children develop and learn behaviours through social interaction within their families and communities and that understanding children involves understanding their social and cultural contexts (Rogoff, 2003). Contemporary early childhood philosophy supports collaborative approaches to assessing and collating data on children's development, health, wellbeing and learning. Participants in each child's social and cultural context, such as family members, health and inclusion support professionals and educators, are all given a voice in assessing and gathering information that provides insights into the child's progression and achievements. The child's view on their own emerging physical, social, emotional and cognitive capabilities and expectations are valued and included in the data collections (Arthur et al., 2012).

Bronfenbrenner's (2005) bioecological theory suggests that children's development is influenced by the system of relationships and contexts in which they live and that children themselves impact their own development and wellbeing through their interactions within these contexts. Bronfenbrenner describes different layers of context or environments that impact the lives of children, ranging from those closest to the child to the outermost broader social, cultural, economic and political contexts – the micro, meso, exo and chrono systems. As children move between contexts such as home, health and education services, they will modify their interactions, behaviours and communication. Bronfenbrenner's theory purports that the child's interactions with social, economic and political layers of the systems, or contexts, are dynamic and will change over time, producing and affecting a range of developmental outcomes for the child. He advocates that, when making decisions for children about their needs, environment and experiences, families, health professionals, educators and policy makers need to consider that children will respond differently in varied contexts and that no two children share the same development, health and wellbeing characteristics or contexts.

Contemporary images of children's development

In her discussions with early childhood educators, Rebecca determines that dominant images of children, crafted by the society in which they live, create conceptual meanings that can carry powerful emotions that dictate how children will be cared for and responded to. The National Research Council (2000) reported that a child's capacity for learning is not determined at birth. Throughout these vital foundation years young children attain the physical, emotional, social and intellectual skills that they will build on throughout their life. Children develop and acquire knowledge through investigation and discovery, taking in information through their senses. It is critical that children have the opportunity to learn through active participation in their environment. During the early years there is a focus on learning through play, body mastery and skills development (Oates, Currow & Hu, 2001).

   Throughout history various ideologies have been attached to childhood, such as playfulness, innocence, victimisation and even bad behaviour, all of which have an impact on the way children are treated (Holland, 2004). The contemporary image of the child reflected by postmodern social constructionists is one that views the child as 'rich in potential, strong, powerful, competent and, most of all connected to adults and to other children' (Dahlberg, Moss & Pence, 2007; Malaguzzi, 1993). Other postmodernist theories contest images that reflect young children as lacking, passive, waiting to be acted upon or following a predetermined path set out by adults and/or innate development. Rinaldi (in Fraser, 2012) suggests those espousing contemporary practices of care and education based on theory and research should see that an emphasis is placed on considering children as unique individuals with rights rather than simply needs. She reminds us that children have potential, plasticity, the desire to grow, curiosity, the ability to be amazed and the desires to relate to other people and to communicate. These contemporary images of childhood have become a catalyst for parents, care providers and educators to provide children increased autonomy. Berk (2006) claims there can be cultural variations in infant-rearing practices that affect motor development (p. 145). It is, however, highly beneficial for those charged with designing and implementing healthcare and education programs to share a common vision of what a young child is really like and capable of achieving.

Physical and intellectual achievements

After the rapid pace of the first 2 years, growth slows to a steadier rate and generally follows a predictable pattern. Changes in physical–motor development are the most obvious. The sequences of motor development are known as principles. The cephalocaudal principle, also described as head-to-tail physical–motor development, acknowledges that very young children gain control over their head and neck movements first and that control of their feet comes later. The proximodistal, or centre-to-edge principle, states that children gain gross motor development control from the body midline, chest, shoulders and upper arms before they gain fine motor control of the hands and feet. These principles can be seen to operate in nearly all children in all cultures (Bentzen, 2009). Healthy children move through major milestones, developing gross motor skills and fine motor skills. Children share several characteristics and needs, demonstrating high levels of physical activity as their large muscles continue to grow and become more advanced. High activity needs to be balanced with rest and reflection time. Play becomes more focused on physical skills, intellectual ability and fantasy. Typically, the preschooler is active running, jumping and learning how to balance by riding a tricycle or bike with training wheels. As a result of high levels of physical activity, this age group needs periodic rest periods. Fine motor skill control is demonstrated when they hold a pencil to draw, use scissors to cut, use a computer mouse, tap a keyboard or deliberately balance blocks while building a tower. It is a time of wonder and awe that is characterised by a thousand 'why' questions. Children's vocabulary has increased and they are able to construct sentences, recount recent events and state their name and address. They may count by rote to 20 or more and know and can sing nursery rhymes and mimic popular songs. Strickland, Morrow, Neuman et al. (2004) reinforce that the link between supportive parental investment and children's early literacy development is essential (Box 8.1).

During the critical early years of learning and development, everything that adults do to support children's language and literacy counts (Hart & Risley, 1995). See Box 8.2 for details of a reading program aimed at this particular age group.

Box 8.1 Practice highlight: Key implications for parents and educators

Strickland et al. (2004) suggest the following:

» Take time to listen and respond to children.
» Talk *to* and *with* children, not *at* them.
» Engage children in extended conversations about events, storybooks and a variety of other print media.
» Explain things to children.
» Use sophisticated and unusual words in everyday talk with children, when they are appropriate to the conversation (p. 87).

Think about the language you use and the responses you make when working with children. Are you taking time to listen and engage children in conversations?

Box 8.2 Practice highlight: The Let's Read Program

The Let's Read Program is run by the Royal Children's Hospital, Melbourne's Centre for Community Child Health. Designed as a sustainable community-based program, it facilitates early child health and development through promoting reading in the 4–6 months to 5-year age group, particularly in disadvantaged groups. The rationale for the program is the important research evidence linking brain development and language and literacy skill development, and also the ongoing relationship between literacy, life chances and self-esteem. The program has two components:

1. training key community-based professionals, such as child health nurses
2. providing resource materials, including reading guidelines and books for community-based groups.

Read about it on the website at www.rch.org.au/ccch/research/index. cfm?doc_id=5821#about.

Questions
1. Look at the risk and protective factors in Table 1.1 in Chapter 1. How does a program like this interact with this balance of risk and protective factors in ways that might strengthen a child's wellbeing and future?
2. Have you ever thought that helping improve language and emergent literacy for young children could be a major health promoting role for you to undertake?
3. More generally, how could you use reading and picture books with children and their families in health promoting activities?

Perhaps you could build an archive of useful titles. Don't forget that appropriate, accessible and affordable are key elements to consider.

Social and emotional achievements

It is healthy and normal behaviour for children to assert their own will and challenge authority as they begin to express their individuality. Play is the vehicle for learning, particularly dramatic play and inquiry-based discovery learning, where the child explores their role and place in the environment through hands-on experiences. Social interactions take the form of playing alongside others, which evolves into more cooperative play with rules as the child matures. Generally, children try to abide by rules and please others and are mostly independent in self-care activities. 'Play gives opportunities to try out what is not allowed, to test boundaries and be aware of what can happen if they are broken. Rather than seeing, in children's actions and play, fear of authority, children show what they know about, how to deal with authorities and how to gain authority' (Lofdahl, in Bruce, 2004, p. 144).

Young children who are securely attached and living in supportive environments become increasingly more autonomous and independent. Sheridan (1994) and Wong, Perry and Hockenberry (2006) suggest that the child's interaction with the family goes from rebellion, frustration and being argumentative to getting on well with parents and seeking them out for reassurance and security, especially when starting preschool and school. Self-concept and body image begin to be influenced by peers, but positive experiences can be promoted by family and other adults or organisations. A positive self-concept leads to self-respect and self-confidence (Wong et al., 2006). Rituals and conforming increasingly become a major focus in early childhood. Team play emerges and peer interaction with rules and referees provide opportunities for the child to make judgements, plan strategies and assess the strengths of their own skills within the team. Psychologists and educators alike accept that Vygotsky's sociocultural theory (1978) reflects that it is through relationships with others that the next generation is being shaped by the values, beliefs, skills and traditions that are within their 'zone of proximal development' (McLeod, 2010). Traditional discourses on development have been expanded to accommodate a greater awareness of the significance of sociocultural contexts impacting on children (Fraser, 2012).

Diverse developmental achievements

The view of what a child is, and ought to be, has deep roots in the culture, society and family values of the people involved in the care and wellbeing of the child. Dahlberg et al. (1999), Arthur, Beecher, Harrison & Morandini (2003), Lenz Taguchi (2006) and Fraser (2012) all argue that, not only is the image of the child being contested, but so too is the image of families and community. They challenge us to move beyond simplistic assumptions and stereotypes and acknowledge the diversity of patterns of interactions, experiences and goals of families and, in so doing, recognise the complex and changing reality of families within the Australian context. Within the context of their families and communities children grow and learn the cultural tools of their world. A celebration of childhood for its unique richness and recognition of the vital role that families and community play in the child's holistic development strengthens partnerships and supports and validates children.

According to Shonkoff and Phillips (2000, p. 219), the 'environment provided by the child's first caregivers has a profound effect on virtually every facet of early development ranging from health and integrity of the baby at birth to the child's readiness to start school at age 5'. They believe that children's family, home, care and early childhood education contexts profoundly affect children's capabilities, beliefs and expectations as well as their social relationships. Vecchi (2010) claims that, based on research that has been undertaken since the 1990s, attention is increasingly being paid to the critical role the environment plays in nurturing the child. She stresses the importance of sensory qualities (light, colour, sound and microclimate) as a means of influencing people's perceptions and overall quality of living. The care and education environments created should, therefore, correspond to the image of the child (Vecchi, 2010, p. 89). The child's early contexts for development and learning lay the foundations for their differing passages as they move into middle childhood years.

Social, cultural and economic policy contexts for health promotion in early childhood

The changing images of and increasing diversity in children, families and communities are reflected in contemporary health promotion initiatives and government policies. Both Australian and New Zealand governments have reviewed their social, cultural and economic policies for early childhood development, health, wellbeing and education over the past decade. Drawing on international research and evidence-based practice, governments have developed a system of policies and initiatives that focus more holistically on the interrelated nature of children's development, health, wellbeing and education. New policy directions reflect research in neurobiology highlighting the importance of interactions between genetics and early childhood experiences in shaping the architecture of the brain and the recognition that the early years of a child's life profoundly impact their future development, health, wellbeing and learning (Shonkoff & Phillips, 2000). Increasingly, governments and communities are recognising that connecting a range of services that children and families need to access, such as maternal, child and family health care, support for parents and play-based early childhood education and care, promotes improved outcomes for children and families.

New Zealand

The New Zealand *Pathways to the Future: Ngā Huarani Arataki* 2002–2012 Strategic Plan for the early childhood education and care sector called for better collaboration and cooperation between services including parent support, health and social services, early development and learning and education settings. The interconnected strategies and goals of the Plan called for early childhood education and care to be more responsive to the holistic needs of children, families and communities (Ministry of Education, New Zealand, 2002). The Public Health Advisory Committee (PHAC) 2010 Report, *The Best Start in Life: Achieving Effective Action on Child Health and Wellbeing,* calls for New Zealand to consider an integrated approach to service delivery for children as a way of improving children's health and wellbeing. The PHAC proposed increasing investment in public health initiatives such as developing programs and guidelines to promote physical activity, safety, hygiene, healthy eating and mental health and wellbeing in early childhood education and care and community settings. The Report recognises that children spend a great deal of time in early childhood education and care settings and that these settings should be used more widely in health promotion (Public Health Advisory Committee, Ministry of Health, New Zealand, 2010).

Australia

The Australian *National Early Childhood Development Strategy – Investing in the Early Years* was endorsed by the Council of Australian Governments in 2009. The Strategy vision for 2010–20 sets out a 10-year action plan for strengthening early childhood and family services with the aim of providing the best start to life for all children. The Strategy focuses on children's development and learning in the first 8 years of life including physical, social, emotional, cognitive and cultural aspects of development. It promotes prevention and early intervention initiatives in the early years, such as secure attachment relationships, good nutrition and equitable access to health and education services, to ensure children have a healthy start to life and positive future development, health and wellbeing (Commonwealth of Australia, 2009).

The Strategy recognises the critical role of parents, communities, non-government and government organisations and the need to work collaboratively to provide good outcomes for children (see Box 8.3).

In order to determine if Australian children have benefited over time from the National Early Development Strategy a longitudinal study will be conducted. The Australian Early Childhood Development Index (AEDI) will collect waves of data every three years measuring children's development across five domains: physical health and wellbeing, social competence, emotional maturity, language and cognitive skills (school-based) and communication skills and general knowledge (Box 8.4). The AEDI, conducted in partnership by the Centre for Community Child Health, Melbourne (at the Royal Children's Hospital and a key research centre of the

---

Box 8.3 Practice highlight: Outcomes for children

The Strategy identifies seven key outcomes:

1. Children are born and remain healthy.
2. Children's environments are nurturing, culturally appropriate and safe.
3. Children have the knowledge and skills for life and learning.
4. Children benefit from better social inclusion and reduced disadvantage, especially Indigenous children.
5. Children are engaged in and benefiting from educational opportunities.
6. Families are confident and have the capabilities to support their children's development.
7. Quality early childhood development services support the workforce participation choices of families (*Supporting the development of young children in Australia: 2009: A snapshot*).

How could the Strategy influence the promotion of child health and development initiatives in urban, regional, rural and remote communities?

In 2009 the first report on AEDI data collection was released, providing a snapshot of early childhood development outcomes in Australian communities. The report, *A Snapshot of Early Childhood in Australia*, detailed how children in local communities had developed across the five AEDI developmental domains by the time they started school. The key findings report that the majority of children are developing well across the AEDI domains with 23.5% of children being identified as developmentally vulnerable in one or more domains and 11.8% of children identified as developmentally vulnerable in two or more domains.

The report enables communities to access scores for each AEDI domain to gauge how many of their children are considered 'on track', 'at risk' and 'developmentally vulnerable'. The AEDI also reports on the communities' socioeconomic status, location, gender and language factors as well as developmental differences. It aims to assist communities understand how local children are developing compared with children nationally and how communities could provide a range of early childhood services to improve outcomes for local children.

Reader activity

Consider how the findings of the research could influence, contribute to and be integrated in practice. Readers are encouraged to spend some time examining the developmental data for their community and/or state or territory. Visit the nation-wide AEDI results at http://maps.aedi.org.au/.

Murdoch Children's Research Institute) and the Telethon Institute of Children's Health Research, Perth, will collect information from local community groups of children who are in their first year of full-time schooling (Royal Children's Hospital Melbourne, 2012).

According to Shonkoff and Phillips (2000), numerous studies and research findings link the quality of early childhood education and care to every measure of early childhood development and long-term outcomes. As part of Australia's national reform agenda for early childhood development, a range of initiatives has been implemented to focus on the quality of early childhood education and care. A *National Quality Framework for Early Childhood Education and Care* has been developed to drive evidence-based changes in the early years of children's lives and their present and future development, health and wellbeing (Australian Children's Education and Care Quality Authority, 2009). The *National Quality Framework* aims to ensure children's safety, health and wellbeing while attending early childhood education and care settings and that these settings improve the children's educational and developmental outcomes. The settings will be assessed against seven quality areas outlined in a National Quality Standard, including a quality area that explicitly rates the setting's ability to provide for children's safety, health and wellbeing. Early childhood educators have a responsibility to ensure children's environments are responsive, safe and hygienic and that illness and injury are managed within health guidelines. Educators must work collaboratively with families, communities and other professional services, such as maternal, child and family health providers, to promote and support children's health needs, healthy eating practices, physical activity, rest and relaxation and their personal safety (Australian Children's Education and Care Quality Authority, 2011).

Setting the scene: Integrated approaches to promoting development, health, wellbeing and education

Through her research Rebecca learned that, in Australia and New Zealand, services for children and families are increasingly moving towards a universal, integrated and interdisciplinary approach to promoting children's development, health, wellbeing and education with the aim of preventing problems later in life. Research evidence suggests that integrated place-based approaches to providing social supports, health and education services are more effective in providing holistic support for children, families and communities (Centre for Community Child Health, 2011). The PHAC report states that integrated service delivery should have 'a comprehensive focus on the whole child and, in most cases, the whole family' (p. 32). The PHAC believes that integrated approaches empower children and families to make decisions about what is a child's best start to life based on a range of milestones in development, health, wellbeing and learning. Integrated approaches (Box 8.5) provide opportunities to work in partnership to address a range of social, cultural, health and education

---

Box 8.5 Practice highlight: Integrated service delivery models

Across communities in Australia and New Zealand, non-government and government organisations are implementing models of integrated service delivery to assist children and families access development, health and wellbeing supports that enhance present and future life and learning outcomes:

» In Australia, through *Closing the Gap: National Partnership Agreement on Indigenous Early Childhood Development*, integrated children and family centres are being established to provide a dynamic mix of services that are responsive to community needs, including early childhood education and care, antenatal services, child and maternal health services and parent and family support services (see http://www.federalfinancialrelations.gov.au/content/npa/education/ctg-early-childhood/national_partnership.pdf).
» In Queensland, four early years centres have been established to assist children and their families to access integrated early childhood education and care, parenting and family support and selected health services in one location (see http://deta.qld.gov.au/earlychildhood/families/early-years-centres.html).
» In South Australia, CaFE Enfield Children's Centre provides integrated early years services where educators, families and the local community work together to support children's development, health, wellbeing and education (see www.childrenscentres.sa.gov.au/pages/cafeenfield/home/?reFlag=1).
» In New Zealand, Barnardos are involved in a number of community development hubs that deliver integrated services including early childhood education and care, antenatal and well child services, parenting support and home visiting programs (see www.barnardos.org.nz/Child-and-Family-Services/Community/Hubs.htm).

What is the role of nurses in promoting integrated service delivery for children, families and communities?

influences and avoid any 'unintentional negative consequences' in the lives of children (Ministry for Heath NZ).

An integrated and partnership approach to promoting children's development, health and wellbeing in early childhood education and care

The holistic integrated and interdisciplinary approach to promoting children's development, health and wellbeing is reflected broadly in early childhood policy and in learning frameworks in both Australia and New Zealand. In Australia the *National Quality Framework* includes a new *Education and Care Services National Law 2011*, which mandates that early childhood education and care centres must have educators who hold approved first aid, asthma management and anaphylaxis management qualifications present at all times. The *National Quality Framework* sets out a National Quality Standard with a specific Quality Area relating to *Children's Health and Safety*. This Quality Area requires early childhood educators to demonstrate that they are providing for, and supporting, children's health needs, including promoting healthy eating and physical activity, as well as managing medical conditions and implementing effective hygiene practices.

This policy requirement is bringing together the departments of health and education across Australia in order for children's health needs to be effectively supported while they attend an early childhood education and care setting. The Queensland Departments of Health and Education and Training along with Workplace Health and Safety Queensland have developed a collaborative project to provide training to early childhood educators to enhance health and hygiene practices in early childhood education and care centres (Queensland Government, 2012). The *Healthy Early Years Training Strategy* is a registered training package that aligns with key health resources, the National Quality Standard and the *Early Years Learning Framework for Australia*. In June 2012 the Queensland Population Health Unit, in consultation with registered training organisations and education and care services, developed publications to promote and provide information on immunisation in early childhood education and care. The National Health and Medical Research Council has now released the fifth edition of *Staying healthy: Preventing infectious diseases in early childhood education and care services* (National Health and Medical Research Council, 2012).

The *Early Years Learning Framework for Australia*, for children aged from birth to 5 years, has been designed with the intent of bringing together children's development, health, wellbeing and learning outcomes within the home and community and early childhood education and care settings. The aim is to support the Council of Australian Governments' vision that 'All children have the best start in life to create a better future for themselves and for the nation' (National Early Childhood Development Strategy) and provide young children with opportunities to maximise their potential and develop a foundation for future success. The *Early Years Learning Framework for Australia* reinforces the principles of the United Nations *Convention on* the Rights of the Child and sets out the goals for fundamental daily practice in early childhood education and care services that enhance children's development, health, wellbeing and learning. The Framework recognises that care and education are dynamic, complex and holistic and advocates that children's physical, social, emotional, personal, spiritual, creative, cognitive and linguistic development are all interrelated (Department of Education, Employment and Workplace Relations, 2009).

In the Framework's outcome 3: 'Children have a strong sense of wellbeing', children's wellbeing is defined as achieving good physical health, feelings of happiness, satisfaction and successful social functioning. It states that having a strong sense of wellbeing will endow children with confidence and optimism, maximising their learning potential and providing them with resilience and the capacity to cope with day-to-day stress and challenges. Outcome 3 explicitly focuses on, and promotes, physical, social and emotional wellbeing, including good nutrition, personal hygiene, physical fitness and cooperative, trusting relationships acknowledging that wellbeing contributes to children's abilities in life and learning.

The New Zealand early childhood curriculum, Te Whàriki, also promotes that development, health, wellbeing and learning begin at home, and that early childhood settings and communities to which each child belongs play a significant role in laying the foundations for successful future life and learning. The curriculum asserts that adults working with children should have knowledge and understanding of health and wellbeing and what this means in practice and, particularly, Māori definitions of cultural norms. The curriculum's 'Strand 1 – Wellbeing' states that all children 'have a right to health, to protection from harm and anxiety, and to harmony, consistency, affection, firmness, warmth, and sensitivity' (Ministry of Education, New Zealand, 1996, p. 46). The goals of this strand aim to collaboratively assist children understand their bodies and how they function; develop knowledge about how to keep themselves healthy through teaching self-help and self-care skills for eating, drinking, food preparation, toileting, resting, sleeping, washing and dressing; and promote positive attitudes to life and learning. The strand acknowledges that the early childhood years and social and cultural contexts all play a critical role in children's developing health, wellbeing and learning.

Healthy early years strategies: Promoting health and wellbeing in early childhood

Rebecca contacts other delegates who attended the child and family health conference to determine how they are contributing to promoting healthy early years strategies as outlined in the national quality agenda. She aims to determine how best she can initiate, build on and contribute to contemporary multidisciplinary policy and practice directions for young children and their families. Rebecca acknowledges Australia and New Zealand's serious legal obligations in developing and implementing policies, such as the NZ Agenda for Children and A Head Start for Australia, and the role of governments in actively seeking to build effective alliances with children by 'increasing children's participating in policy action, awareness raising and advocacy' (New South Wales and Queensland Commission for Children and Young People, 2004). Rebecca already has an understanding of Australia and New Zealand's obligations under the United Nations *Convention on the Rights of the Child*. Therefore, she appreciates that their governments and organisations must demonstrate an ethical responsibility towards children by focusing on the developmental health and wellbeing of children (United Nations, 1989; United Nations General Assembly, 2002).

Children, their families and the broader society all benefit when early childhood health and development are promoted. McCain and Mustard (1999) claim there is evidence that good nutrition, nurturing and responsive care in the first few years of life improve outcomes for children's learning and behaviour and physical and mental health throughout life. More recently Foley, Goldfeld, McLoughlin et al. (2000), Stanley (2001), Leseman (2002) and Brooks-Gunn (2002) concluded that high quality cost-effective early childhood developmental programs, particularly those associated with quality early childhood services that targeted high-risk families, produced positive results in health and wellbeing. Children in these programs demonstrated improved readiness to learn and positive social skills. Research conducted by van der Gaag (2002) described pathways linking early childhood development to human development whereas further research in early childhood development indicated immediate benefits for children, long-term adult benefits and benefits for society. In short, when quality early childhood development programs were implemented effectively children, adults and society all showed positive outcomes in health, social capital, education and equality.

Two major health promotion initiatives being implemented are the *Healthy Kids Check* and the accompanying *Get set 4 Life – Habits for Healthy Kids Guide*. The *Healthy Kids Check* is available for all 4-year-old children who are permanent residents in Australia or who are covered by a reciprocal healthcare arrangement. The Guide provides families with practical information on key areas of health and development such as: healthy eating, regular exercise, speech and language, oral health, skin and sun protection, hygiene and sleep patterns. The interactive resources have been specifically developed to assist parents/carers interact with their children to develop and reinforce the importance of establishing healthy life habits.

The Queensland State Government collaborative initiative involving the departments of Education and Training, Communities – Sport and Recreation and Queensland Health implements the *Smart Moves* physical activity program in Queensland state schools. *Smart Moves* aims to increase student participation in physical activity and to improve the quality of that activity. *Smart Moves* is also a key strategy in the *Toward Q2: Tomorrow's Queensland 2020* healthy children target to reduce obesity by one-third. A similar initiative for children aged 2.5–6 years is the physio-designed multi-sport exercise program *readysteadygokids* (http://www.readysteadygokids.com.au). Programs such as these are designed to promote healthy lifestyles by developing a lifelong passion for physical activity, increasing children's confidence, building positive self-esteem, preventing overweight and obesity concerns in young children and encouraging participation in the broader community.

Whereas physical health is critical, positive mental health is essential for children to flourish. Adverse trends identified by Stanley (2001) included that the rate of mental health morbidities has risen among young people with 15% of children aged 4–17 years scoring in the clinical range for somatic complaints, delinquent behaviour, attention problems and aggressive behaviour. Strengths-based programs such as the Australian mental health initiative *KidsMatter* include promotion, prevention and early intervention initiatives to support children. *KidsMatter* has been developed in collaboration with the Commonwealth Government Department of Health and Ageing, beyondblue: The national depression initiative, the Australian Psychological Society and the Australian Principals Associations Professional Development Council (APAPDC) and is supported by the Australian Rotary Health Research Fund. The program aims to improve the mental health and wellbeing of children by reducing anxiety, depression and behavioural problems. The program encourages greater community support and assistance for children experiencing mental health problems. The *Seasons for Growth* program, developed out of grief theory and related to the work of psychologist J. William Wordon, targets and supports children who have experienced significant change, loss and grief as a consequence of family breakdown, separation, divorce or death. The strategies and techniques within the program are informed by a cognitive behavioural and educational framework. Community-based organisations can help provide support for young children via programs like the Life Education van and Healthy Harold. The Healthy Harold program uses electronic resources and Healthy Harold's humour to deliver non-threatening tips on maintaining a healthy life style. The mobile program helps children develop knowledge and skills to identify risks and make informed decisions to support healthy physical, emotional and mental health.

Evidence by Jolley and Masters (2004) suggests strengths-based programs empower children by assisting them to develop a positive identity and positive view of their personal future. Given the fact that good nutrition, nurturing and responsive care in the first years of life improve outcomes for children's physical and mental health, behaviour and learning throughout life (McCain & Mustard, 1999; Young, 2002), families, primary healthcare providers and educators have a moral responsibility to strengthen their capacity to work collectively to provide supportive environments for young children that will send a clear message to all children that they are citizens of a community that cherishes and values them. Across Australia, early childhood education and care, and school, settings are recognised as the starting point for promoting healthy, active and productive citizenship where knowledge and skills for lifelong learning and pro-social behaviour will enhance individual potential to contribute to a healthy, active Australian society (Ministerial Council on Education, Employment, Training and Youth Affairs, 2008).

Conclusion

Children living in contemporary Australian and New Zealand communities are viewed as capable, competent and confident individuals who are influenced by and contribute to their social and cultural contexts for development, health, wellbeing and learning. Adopting holistic practices to foster development, health, wellbeing and learning is widely recognised by health professionals, educators and policymakers as the most effective means of providing children the best start to life and positive future outcomes. Health, education and community services are increasingly working in partnership to promote and enhance children's development, health and wellbeing. Research indicates that integrated systems and approaches to implementing health, education and social support services strengthen children's, families' and communities' participation in active, healthy lifestyles and promote positive attitudes to life and learning.

KEY POINTS

» Early childhood education and care environments are natural settings for health promotion.
» Early childhood is a critical time of life when development is rapid and interrelated with health and wellbeing.
» Collaborative partnerships with parents, health care providers, educators and communities in socially and culturally supportive and responsive environments promote children's healthy development and wellbeing.

CRITICAL QUESTIONS AND REFLECTIONS

1. Why is it important for nurses to know about initiatives for physically active play, health and wellbeing that are implemented in early childhood education and care settings?

2. How can nurses and educators work in partnership to promote children's development, health and wellbeing?

3. How do children's development, health and wellbeing impact their learning in the early years?

4. What is your view of a holistic approach to integrated service delivery for children aged from birth to 8 years?

USEFUL RESOURCES

Australian Early Development Index (AEDI) National Report 2009 *A snapshot of early childhood development in Australia*: www.rch.org.au/aedi/media/Snapshot_of_ Early_Childhood_DevelopmentinAustralia_AEDI_National_Report.pdf

National Health Committee 2010 *The best start in life: Achieving effective action on child health and wellbeing*, Wellington, Ministry of Health: http://nhc.health.govt. nz/resources/publications/best-start-life-achieving-effective-action-child-health-and-wellbeing

Our kids, our present and our future, New Zealand Agenda for Children: www.msd.govt.nz

Queensland Health, *Immunisation recommendations for early childhood educators and staff*: http://www.health.qld.gov.au/immunisation/documents/earlychild-imm-broch.pdf

Seasons for Growth: www.goodgrief.org.au

Supporting the development of young children in Australia 2009: A snapshot: http://deewr.gov.au/information-national-early-childhood-development-strategy

References

Arthur, L., Beecher, B., Death, E., Dockett, S., & Farmer, S. (2012). *Programming and planning in early childhood settings* (5th ed.). South Melbourne, Victoria: Cengage Learning Australia.

Arthur, L., Beecher, B., Harrison, C., & Morandini, C. (2003). Sharing the lived experiences of children. *Australian Journal of Early Childhood, 28*(2), 8–13.

Australian Children's Education and Care Quality Authority (2009). *National Quality Framework for Early Childhood Education and Care.* Retrieved from http://acecqa.gov.au/national-quality-framework/ (accessed 23 May 2012).

Australian Children's Education and Care Quality Authority (2011). *Guide to the National Quality Standard.* Retrieved from http://acecqa.gov.au/national-quality-framework/national-quality-standard/ (accessed 30 April 2012).

Bentzen, W. (2009). *Seeing young children: A guide to observing and recording behaviour* (6th ed.). Belmont, CA: Delmar Cengage Learning.

Berk, L. E. (2006). *Child development* (7th ed.). USA: Pearson Education, Inc.

Bronfenbrenner, U. (Ed.), (2005). *Making human beings human: Bioecological perspectives on human development.* Thousand Oaks, CA: Sage Publications.

Brooks-Gunn, J. (2002). *Do you believe in magic? What we can expect from early childhood interventions programs. Social Policy Report Vol XVII, No. 1.* Ann Arbor MI: Society for Research in Child Development.

Bruce, T. (2004). *Developing learning in early childhood 0–8 years.* London: Sage Publications.

Catron, C. E., & Allen, J. (2008). *Early childhood curriculum: A creative-play model* (4th ed.). Upper Saddle River, NJ: Pearson Education Inc.

Centre for Community Child Health, Royal Children's Hospital Melbourne (2006). Policy Brief 3. Retrieved from http://www.rch.org.au/ccch/policybrief/ (accessed 22 January 2013).

Centre for Community Child Health, Royal Children's Hospital Melbourne (2011). Policy Brief 23. Retrieved from http://www.rch.org.au/ccch/policybrief/ (accessed 22 January 2013).

Charlesworth, R. (2011). *Understanding child development* (8th ed.). Belmont, CA: Wadsworth Cengage Learning.

Commonwealth of Australia (2009). *National Early Childhood Development Strategy – Investing in the Early Years.* Retrieved from http://www.coag.gov.au/node/205 (accessed 22 January 2013).

Dahlberg, G., Moss, P., & Pence, A. (2007). *Beyond quality in early childhood education and care. Languages of evaluation* (2nd ed.). London: Routledge.

Dahlberg, G., Moss, P., & Pence, A. (1999). *Beyond quality in early childhood education and care. Postmodern perspectives.* London: Routledge.

Department of Education, Employment and Workplace Relations (2009). *Early Years Learning Framework for Australia.* Canberra: Commonwealth of Australia.

Foley, D., Goldfeld, S., McLoughlin, J., et al. (2000). *A review in the early childhood literature.* Canberra: Commonwealth of Australia.

Fraser, S. (2012). *Authentic childhood: Experiencing Reggio Emilia in the classroom* (3rd ed.). Canada: Nelson Education.

Gordon, A. M., & Browne, K. W. (2011). *Beginnings and beyond. Foundations in early childhood education* (8th ed.). Belmont, CA: Wadsworth Cengage Learning.

Hart, T. R., & Risley, B. (1995). *Meaningful differences in the early experience of young American children*. Baltimore: Brooks.

Holland, P. (2004). *Picturing childhood: The myth of the child in popular imagery.* New York: I. B. Tauris & Co Ltd.

Jolley, G., & Masters, S. (2004). *Seasons for growth: Evaluation report on the South Australian Primary schools program.* Adelaide: South Australia Community Health Research Unit.

Lady Gowrie Inc (2012). *History of Lady Gowrie Centres.* Retrieved from http://www.gowrievictoria.org.au/AboutUs/History.aspx (accessed 14 January 2013).

Lenz Taguchi, H. (2006). *Reconceptualising early childhood education: Challenging taken-for-granted ideas in Nordic childhoods and early education.* In J. Einarsdottir & J. T. Wagner Greenwich (Eds.), *Nordic childhoods and early education. Philosophy, research, policy and practice in Denmark, Finland, Iceland, Norway and Sweden.* Connecticut: Information Age Publishing.

Leseman, P. P. M. (2002). *Early childhood education and care for children from low-income or minority backgrounds.* Oslo: Paper presented at the OECD Oslo Workshop.

Malaguzzi, L. (1993). For an education based on relationships. *Young Children, 49*(1): 9–12.

McCain, M. N., & Mustard, F. (1999). *Reversing the brain drain: Early study: Final report.* Toronto: Ontario Children's Secretariat.

McLeod, S. A. (2010). *Simply psychology, zone of proximal development.* Retrieved from http://www.simplypsychology.org/Zone-of-Proximal-Dvelopment.html (accessed 30 May 2012).

Ministerial Council on Education, Employment, Training and Youth Affairs (2008). *Melbourne Declaration on Educational Goals for Young Australians.* Retrieved from http://www.mceecdya.edu.au/verve/_resources/National_Declaration_on_the_Educational_Goals_for_Young_Australians.pdf (accessed 23 May 2012).

Ministry of Education, New Zealand (1996). *Te Whàriki: He Whàriki Màtauranga mò ngà Mokopuna o Aotearoa Early Childhood Curriculum.* Wellington: Learning Media Ltd.

Ministry of Education, New Zealand (2002). *Pathways to the Future: Ng Huarahi Arataki 2002–2012: A Ten Year Strategy for Early Childhood Education.* Retrieved from http://www.educate.ece.govt.nz/Programmes/CentresOfInnovation/DocumentsandResources/ServiceSpecific/NgaTakohangaeWha.aspx (accessed 21 May 2012).

National Health and Medical Research Council (2012). *Staying healthy: Preventing infectious diseases in early childhood education and care services* (5th ed.). Retrieved from http://www.nhmrc.gov.au/guidelines/publications/ch55 (accessed 6 February 2013).

National Research Council (2000). *How people learn: Brain, mind, experience and school.* Washington: National Academy Press.

New South Wales and Queensland Commission for Children and Young People (2004). *A head start for Australia: An early years framework.* Retrieved from http://www.ccypcg.qld.gov.au/resources/publications/headStart04.html (accessed 22 January 2013).

Oates, K., Currow, K., & Hu, W. (2001). *Child health. A practical manual for general practice.* Sydney: MacLennan & Petty.

Office for Early Childhood Education and Care (2010). *State of child care in Australia.* Department of Education, Employment and Workplace Relations, Australian Government. Retrieved from foi.deewr.gov.au/system/files/doc/other/state_of_child_care_in_australia.pdf (accessed 22 January 2013).

Public Health Advisory Committee, Ministry of Health, New Zealand (2010). *The best start in life: Achieving effective action on child health and wellbeing.* Wellington: Ministry of Health. Retrieved from http://nhc.health.govt.nz/publications/phac-pre-2011 (accessed 14 January 2013).

Queensland Government (2012). *Early childhood education and care skilling strategy: Healthy early years training strategy* fact sheet. Retrieved from http://www.childcaresupport.org.au (accessed 21 May 2012).

Rogoff, B. (2003). *The cultural nature of human development.* Oxford: Oxford University Press.

Royal Children's Hospital Melbourne (2012). *Australian Early Development Index.* Retrieved from http://www.rch.org.au/aedi/index.cfm?doc_id=1305 (accessed 30 April 2012).

SDN Children's Services (2012). *History of Sydney Day Nursery.* Retrieved from http://www.sdn.org.au/about/history/ (accessed 23 May 2012).

Sheridan, M. D. (1994). *From birth to five years. Children's developmental progress.* Melbourne: ACER.

Shonkoff, J. & Phillips, D. (Eds.), (2000). *Neurons to neighborhoods: The science of early childhood.* Washington DC: National Academy Press.

Stanley, F. (2001). *Developmental health and wellbeing: Australia's Future into the 21st century.* Paper presented at the Prime Minister's Science, Engineering and Innovation Council Seventh Meeting.

Strickland, D., Morrow, L., Neuman, S., et al. (2004). Distinguished educator: the role of literacy in early childhood education. *The Reading Teacher, 58*(1), 86–100.

United Nations (1989). *Convention on the Rights of the Child.* Geneva: Office of the United Nations High Commissioner for Human Rights.

United Nations General Assembly (2002). *A world fit for children.* Retrieved from http://www.worldlii.org/int/other/UNGARsn/2002/34.pdf (accessed 1 February 2013).

van der Gaag, J. (2002). From child development to human development. In M. E. Young (Ed.), *2002 From early childhood development to human development: Investing in our children's future.* Retrieved from http://books.google.com.au/books?hl=en&lr=&id=RuS_BIxS8sEC&oi=fnd&pg=PT88&dq=van+der+Gaag+in+young+2002&ots=4_sehTFoNF&sig=O9iWkh3rqMjT4OOFSvCBflAKus4#v=onepage&q&f=false (accessed 6 February 2013).

Vecchi, V. (2010). *Art and creativity in Reggio Emilia: Exploring the role and potential of ateliers in early childhood education*. New York: Routledge.

Vygotsky, L. S. (1978). *Interaction between learning and development* (M Lopez-Morillas, trans). In M. Cole, V. John-Steiner, S. Scribner, et al. (Eds.), *Mind in society: The development of higher psychological processes* (pp. 79–91). Cambridge MA: Harvard University Press.

Wong, D., Perry, S., & Hockenberry, M. (2006). *Maternal child nursing care* (3rd ed.). St Louis: Mosby Elsevier.

Young, M. E. (Ed.), (2002). *From early childhood development to human development: Investing in our children's future*. Washington DC: The World Bank.

Chapter 9

ACUTE ILLNESS: THE CHILD AND THEIR FAMILY

Anne Walsh, Penelope Harrison

LEARNING OUTCOMES

Reading this chapter will help you to:

» understand the diversity of middle childhood

» identify common causes and settings of injury and differentiate between intentional and unintentional injury

» critique the role of child-centred care within a family-centred framework in regard to caring for the injured or acutely ill child in the family

» summarise the characteristics of the diverse age group that includes middle childhood by locating sources including population demographics

» understand the range of resources parents access for child health information including the role of practice nurses in child health care.

Introduction

During the ages of 5–12 years, children continue to develop cognitively, socially, emotionally and physically and overall tend to be relatively healthy. Cognitively, this period is called the '*sensitive period*', due to the active role new experiences play in cognitive development (Knudsen, 2004). Children's gross and fine motor skills continue to be refined, and they are able to ride bikes and skateboards, climb trees and generally enjoy testing their physical boundaries, often beyond their capabilities (Erikson, 1963). Middle childhood is an exciting time, a period in life when children gain independence from their parents through attending school and participation in sporting activities. In terms of health care, middle childhood is an area where there has been little research, representing the '*forgotten years*' (Mah & Ford-Jones, 2012).

This chapter explores the reasons for the middle child's contact with the health profession, injury and acute illnesses, and the impact these have on parents, siblings and the family in general. The forgotten years cover a broad area of childhood development from the 5-year-old with beginnings of independence in activities of daily living, such as dressing and bathing without supervision, to the pre-adolescent 12-year-old. With this comes the struggle over independence in activities where parents perceive a need for continued supervision and children strive for independence; sometimes there are negative outcomes. Injury is the main health concern in this age group: injury at home, school and sporting events, everywhere really. Through two scenarios, we will explore the impacts of common causes of injury and acute illnesses, their influences on children and their families. Engagement of children and family with the healthcare system is addressed through exploration of family-centred care, child-centred care and caring for a middle child and their family in both the community and hospital setting.

Middle-aged children and their families: Australia and New Zealand

On 30 June 2010, 10% of Australians were children aged between 5 and 12 years (Australian Institute of Health and Welfare, 2011). This equates to 1.4 million Australian children aged between 5 and 12 years. Ruby (see Clinical scenario 9.1) would have fallen within the 6% of these who were Australian children aged between 5 and 9 years (30 June 2010) (Australian Institute of Health and Welfare, 2011). The other 4% of these children were between 10 and 12 years of age. Most of these children lived in homes in major cities (66.0%). One-fifth (20.8%) were living in inner regional areas and one-tenth (10.3%) in outer regional areas, with smaller numbers living in remote and very remote areas of Australia (1.8% and 1.1%, respectively) (Australian Institute of Health and Welfare, 2011).

As families grow many difficulties are encountered. Sometimes, this results in divorce with children living between parents. In 2007 in Australia, Ruby would have been included in one of the 18.9% of single parent families in Australia (Australian Institute of Health and Welfare, 2011). There is s similar story in New Zealand where the steadily declining birth rate over the past 40 years has seen the estimated

Clinical scenario 9.1
Setting the scene: Injuries are common in middle childhood

Injuries can occur at any time in any place with children in their middle childhood years. Ruby is no exception. The scenario below describes a common occurrence in middle childhood.

School

Ruby Rodriguez is a 9-year-old girl in year 5 at her local primary school. Her parents, Claire and Joseph, are separated and Ruby lives with either parent on alternate weeks. This is Claire's week. While waiting for her mother to pick her up after school, Ruby decided to have one last play on the monkey bars before going to the school gates to be picked up. Unfortunately, Ruby lost her grip and fell awkwardly from the monkey bars putting out her left hand to break her fall. Immediately upon landing on the ground, she felt a sharp pain in her left arm and began to cry. Crying and trying to support her sore arm, while also dragging her school bag, Ruby walked to the school gate. When Claire arrived and saw Ruby's distress and then her distorted arm, she panicked. What should she do? Finally, after carefully settling Ruby in the back seat of the car, she drove Ruby straight to the local district general hospital.

Hospital

Upon arriving at the emergency department, Ruby was reviewed by Sally, the triage nurse, who instructed Claire that Ruby should not eat or drink until a doctor had seen her. Sally applied a sling to Ruby's arm and encouraged her to rest her arm on a pillow. Ruby was reviewed by one of the doctors on duty and had an X-ray, confirming displaced fractures of her left radius and ulna. It was determined that a specialist doctor should review Ruby.

The orthopaedic surgeon informed Claire that Ruby needed to have an anaesthetic to enable him to realign the fractures and apply a plaster cast on her left arm. Claire now realised she would need to contact her estranged husband, Joseph. Upon receiving the news, Joseph left work immediately and came up to the hospital. Ruby went to the operating theatre soon after he arrived.

When Ruby recovered from the anaesthetic she transferred to the paediatric ward, arriving there at 11 pm. Ruby was asleep and unaware of her new surroundings. The ward nurse orientated Claire and Joseph to the ward and explained to them the ward policy of allowing only one parent to stay overnight at the bedside. It was decided that Claire would stay, as it was her week with Ruby.

Ruby recovered quickly. The next morning, following a healthy breakfast, the orthopaedic surgeon reviewed Ruby and discharged her. Claire received home care advice regarding plaster care and pain management and a discharge letter to take to her local general practitioner. Ruby was not to attend school until reviewed by the orthopaedic surgeon in the fracture clinic in one week's time (on a Wednesday).

Home and community

Claire took this day and the following 2 days off work to care for Ruby, taking them to the weekend. Joseph negotiated time off work for the following week to continue to care for the injured Ruby until she could return to school the following Thursday. On Saturday, Ruby changed residences and stayed with her father. Claire gave Joseph all the literature she had received from the hospital. On Sunday morning, Joseph was concerned because Ruby was complaining of pain in her arm; however, he did not feel confident in giving Ruby the pain relief tablets Claire had left with him. He decided to ring the 1300 CHILDHEALTH line and discussed his concern with the nurse, who informed him of the potential side effects and the benefits of the pain medication. Following this, he felt confident to reduce Ruby's pain without causing her any harm from the tablets.

proportion of children aged from birth to 14 years drop from 32.1% of the total population in 1969 to 20.5% in 2009, 892,600 children (Bascand, 2010).

Injury

Injury is common among this age group, often resulting from greater perceptions of their capabilities rather than their actual abilities and/or the influence of peers. Most of these injuries are unintentional or accidental, as Ruby's was. Injuries most commonly occur in transport-related settings: in a car, as a passenger, sitting in the front seat (where they are anatomically, incorrectly supported by the seat belt or air cushion); riding a bike for fun or to and from school; and as a pedestrian at any time. Recreational injuries are common and include, as previously mentioned, bikes and quad (all terrain bikes) bikes, but they also occur in playgrounds, on skates, skateboards and skis and playing sport, e.g. football, tennis, horse riding (Australian Bureau of Statistics [ABS], 2010a; Centre for Community Child Health, 2006).

Unintentional and intentional injuries are the major cause of hospitalisation and death in middle-aged children in both Australia and New Zealand. For example, in Australia more children die as a result of transport accidents, drowning or assault (36%) than from neoplasm (19%) and other diseases of the nervous system combined (11%) (Australian Bureau of Statistics, 2006). In New Zealand, there is a similar story with fatal and serious non-fatal injuries from falls, motor vehicle accidents, pedestrian accidents etc (Gulliver, Cryer & Davie, 2010). The Injury Prevention Strategy in New Zealand has been effective in reducing the risk of fatal injuries from 14.0 to 11.4 per 100,000 person years from 1994 to 2007 (Statistics New Zealand, 2011). However, the risk of a serious non-fatal injury has increased from 55.7 to 72.9 per 100,000 person years from 1994 to 2009 (Statistics New Zealand, 2011). Between 2006 and 2007 in Australia there were 1462 per 100,000 children aged 0–14 years hospitalised for an unintentional injury (Australian Institute of Health and Welfare, 2009). In New Zealand 4976 children per total population were hospitalised in the public system during 2007–08 for unintentional injury.

Common causes

Falls continue to be the most significant cause of injury and hospital admission for this age group. With their belief in their ability to climb, children fall from bunk beds, trees, playground equipment or during sporting activities. Recreational equipment is involved in most injuries: climbing apparatus and monkey bars followed by trampolines, slides, swings and flying foxes (Kreisfeld & Harrison, 2010). Children aged 5–9 years are more prone to falls from playground equipment and three times more likely to be hospitalised than 10–14-year-olds. Children aged 5–9 years have the highest proportion of fractures, intracranial injuries, dislocations, sprains and strains, with fractures of the forearm the most frequent type of fracture (Helps & Pointer, 2006).

Drowning, thought to be a cause of injury and death in younger children, persists in this age group as they play in rivers, creeks and unsupervised in swimming pools and go fishing and boating. Burns also continue to occur though from different sources than in the earlier years. These burns are likely to be from experimentation and/or exposure to ignitable and flammable substances (school or play) (Australian Bureau of Statistics, 2006, 2010; Barker, Heiring, Spinks & Pitt, 2008a).

As little environmentalists, children interact with nature exposing themselves to potential risks from tics and insect and snake bites, for example. In Queensland in 2007, 2311 children under 14 years of age were treated for spider bites; redback spiders accounted for 29% and only 1 bite was from a funnel web spider (Barker, Heiring, Krahn, Spinks & Pitt, 2008b). Australia's insects and animals are amongst the most venomous in the world. New Zealand has a small number of venomous creatures biting children. The white-tailed spider arrived from Australia in the late 19th century. In 1980 the redback spider arrived (Slaughter, Beasley, Lambie & Schep, 2009). Both countries have venomous and dangerous marine creatures, a problem in countries where people have a love of water sports.

Children living on farms have a different injury profile. From the age of 5 years, they present with injuries from motorcycles and riding animals or being an occupant of an animal-drawn vehicle. Head injuries and lacerations are most common for children aged 5–9 years, and these children tend to stay in hospital for farm-related injuries for an average 2.8 days (Kreisfeld & Harrison, 2010).

Injury in middle childhood causes angst for parents. How do they keep their children safe while letting them experiment and trial their advancing skills? However, there are fewer resources available to parents of these children. Potential avenues for support include the school setting through parenting programs, previously formed groups from child health settings and work colleagues, family and friends. They also seek information online. Which of these sources provide evidence-based information?

School as a setting for injury

Ruby becomes a statistic. She was in the one-fifth of children injured at school every year. In 2008, 20% of all injuries to children aged between 5 and 13 years happened in a school setting. Falling was the most common cause of these injuries, accounting for two-thirds of all school injuries; of these, one quarter fell more than 1 m. Play equipment, as in the scenario, is a major culprit: 20% of school injuries happen on play equipment (Barker et al., 2008b). Ruby is a perfect example of this – 'just one more play'. In the scenario, it is clear to Claire that Ruby needs urgent medical assistance. She was fortunate to have access to appropriate hospital and specialist services.

Another cause of injury in the Australian school setting is through intentional injury – bullying. In 2008, 3% of all primary school injuries were the result of bullying. Some 19–27% of Australian schoolchildren report being bullied at some time during their schooling. Primary school students, those in their middle childhood, are more likely to be bullied face-to-face, which can involve verbal or physical assault such as punching or kicking, necessitating children have contact with the healthcare system. Unseen outcomes from bullying can include psychological and/or emotional trauma (Ministerial Council for Education, 2011). Cyberbullying, with associated psychological/emotional trauma, is more common with high school students (Ministerial Council for Education, 2011). Please refer to Chapter 12 for further information about mental health needs in middle childhood.

Intentional injury

In Australia in 2006–07, the rate of hospitalisation for children aged 5 to 12 years relating to intentional injury was 20 per 100,000 (Australian Institute of Health and Welfare, 2009). Intentional injury includes injury from bullying, abuse and/or self-harm. In 2006–07, intentional self-harm was the reason for the hospital admission of 41 per 100,000 Australian children 10–14 years of age (Australian Institute of Health and Welfare, 2009). New Zealand children are at similar risk of intentional injury. There has been no change in the risks of serious fatal or non-fatal intentional injury from 1994 to 2007 (5.4 and 5.4 per 100,000 person years, respectively) (Statistics New Zealand, 2011).

There is a strong causal relationship between the health and wellbeing of children and the environment in which they grow up. The complex nature of child abuse and neglect has been widely acknowledged, nationally and globally, with governments developing strategies to address this. In their response to the need to protect Australian children the government, in collaboration with all states and territories, developed a National Framework for Protecting Australian Children (Council of Australian Governments, 2009). The New Zealand government worked in collaboration with regions and districts to develop the New Zealand Injury Prevention Strategy (Gulliver et al., 2010). When implemented, these strategies promote proactive, preventative practices and initiatives to improve children's safety and wellbeing.

Nurses and intentional injury

Intentional injury is an area where nurses not only have a duty to care for the child and family, they also have a duty of care to report any suspected child abuse and/or neglect (Australian Institute of Family Studies, 2012). This can be an uncomfortable position for a nurse to be in, caring for the child and family when suspecting the family as the reason the child is now in their care. Often, intentional injuries go unreported or incorrectly identified as accidental and thus poorly investigated. Of concern is the shorter length of stay of children in the hospital system, limiting the opportunity for nurses to conduct a complete assessment and observation of *at-risk children* and/or their family.

Mandatory reporting of suspected child abuse and neglect is now a legal requirement. Those mandated to report child abuse vary across Australian states and territories. It is therefore imperative that nurses caring for these children are cognisant of their state legislation relating to child abuse and neglect. Prior to the legislated mandatory reporting, Piltz and Wachtel (2009) found that, even though reporting suspected child abuse was a mandatory requirement of all healthcare professionals, nurses who work in emergency departments were hesitant to report any suspicious injuries to Child Protection Services. The lack of education and experience in reporting their suspicions were the main explanations for emergency nurses' hesitancy to formally report or even record their concerns in patient notes. The emergency nurses interviewed in this study reported they feared for their own safety and that of their family and did not trust Child Protection Services to act appropriately. Similar traits were found among community-based nurses who reported role conflict as the rationale for their hesitancy to report suspicions. They argued that reporting clients to Child Protection Services would impinge on their role to implement strategies to assist and support the family (Piltz & Wachtel, 2009). In Australia in the early 2000s, police, school personnel, parents and guardians, friends, neighbours and other relatives were more likely to report cases of suspected child abuse than nurses (Australian Bureau of Statistics, 2003). Refer to Chapter 4 for a detailed explanation of advocacy and the legal implications of nursing children.

Family-centred care: implications for middle childhood and families

Family-centred care is an approach to planning, implementing and evaluating health care for children and adolescents; it is a partnership between healthcare professionals and families (Dunst & Trivette, 2009). As a concept it was originally concerned with paediatric hospital services; more recently, it has been adopted in community settings by many healthcare professionals (Frank & Callery, 2004). The concept of family-centred care is composed of:

- respect for the child and family
- appreciation of the importance of the family to the child's wellbeing
- recognition of the importance of creating a partnership between the family and the healthcare team. (Frank & Callery, 2004).

It is a process of mutual respect. Family-centred care is for care planned around the family unit rather than the individual child (Shields, Mamun, Pereira, O'Nions & Chaney, 2011).

Nethercott (1993) recognised the necessity for the family needs to be viewed in context, and that there was a difference between parental involvement and parent participation. Lee (2004) argues for two approaches to family-centred care, functional and holistic. The functional model relates to the care directed by the nurse, who determines the parent's involvement in their child's care. The alternative is a holistic approach; this approach empowers the parents to be able to negotiate care decisions.

It is important to ensure parents are not intimidated by the unfamiliar hospital environment or daunted by the technology attached to their child. Ruby was admitted to hospital straight after her accident; Claire was very worried and concerned about Ruby. Parents often have no clear understanding of what is expected of them in the hospital setting (Frank & Callery, 2004; Young, McCann, Watson et al., 2006). Through family-centred care, roles and responsibilities are negotiated between parents and nurses. After being orientated and having ward policies explained, Claire and Joseph felt confident in participating in Ruby's care. This was demonstrated by Claire and Joseph's willingness for Claire to stay with Ruby; Joseph was happy going home knowing that he was acknowledged as one of Ruby's carers.

Some parents want to be actively involved in their child's care. Sometimes parents have cared for their sick child at home for days prior to the child's hospitalisation, and they may be exhausted and in need of sleep. Parents can feel resentful when nurses do things for their child that they would like to do, or vice versa. This could be due to miscommunication or the parents' belief that nurses expect them to do everything (Jolley & Shields, 2009). Resentment may be exaggerated by the parent's difficulty defining their role due to the ambiguous boundaries of responsibility. Misunderstandings can usually be resolved; family and health professionals both want what is best for the child. Claire was scared of hurting Ruby and did not want to wash her after she returned from theatre. Fortunately, the ward nurse was understanding and demonstrated to Claire how to dress and undress Ruby while her arm was in a plaster cast. However, this is not always the case. At the end of the day family-centred care is a process of constant negotiation of roles and expectations, a partnership between the family and health professionals.

Parents

It is important to respect parents' knowledge about their child and the current health issue. Parents are alert to variations in their child's behaviour, changes from the norm, when to seek help. Health professionals must acknowledge parents' expertise in knowing their child. Sharing information between parents and health professionals empowers the family and strengthens their therapeutic relationship with the health profession (Frank & Callery, 2004). The formation of a therapeutic relationship assists in ensuring that the child and their family are appropriately informed about how to care for their child in both the hospital setting and when they return home, in the community setting, and that they are aware of available resources to assist them with their child's health care. This relationship is built on mutual respect and maintained dignity (Lundqvist & Nilstun, 2007). The child's trusting relationship within their family must be valued and maintained during any period of acute illness or injury (Jolley & Shields, 2009). It is in the child's best interest to have their family involved in their care. Nurses, however, must also be alert to inconsistencies and incongruities that may indicate abuse and/or neglect or a need for education/assistance.

Child-centred care: is the child important?

Paediatric care: child-centred or family-centred? This a common debate in paediatric health services. Child-centred care not only acknowledges the importance of family involvement in a child's care but is intrinsically focused on the child's needs (O'Hare & Blackford, 2005). Family-centred care purports that the care of the child is a collaborative process between the health service and the child's family, assuming that parents will act in the child's best interest. However, this model does not always address the interests of the child (Kerridge, Lowe & McPhee, 2005).

Concern for the child's ability to determine care and to make decisions is a contentious issue. For those in middle childhood this issue becomes more obvious. Autonomy disappears when children enter any health setting (Lundqvist & Nilstun, 2007). However, children in the 5–12 years age group, particularly at the higher end of this spectrum, are able to make judgements on their desired outcomes when provided with information in a manner they can comprehend (Erikson, 1963). For example, something as simple as allowing Ruby to determine when she has a bath and who will assist her. A 12-year-old Ruby beginning puberty may not want her father to bathe her. Despite not having the legal ability to consent to treatment, their involvement in determining aspects of their care and assenting to care must be encouraged (O'Hare, 2005). There is a fundamental need for health professionals to support and encourage their child client's involvement in all decision making relating to their health.

Contexts of care: hospital, community and home

Most care of children occurs in the home and the community. In the community nurses in general practice settings, 'practice nurses' and general practitioners provide parents with child health and development assistance (Walsh & Mitchell, in press). Tertiary care tends to be for injury and elective surgery, an acute illness or to address chronic conditions such as cystic fibrosis or cancer. Therefore, most will enter the hospital through emergency departments for 24-hour centralised service, as did Ruby.

Care in the hospital

Most communities in Australia and New Zealand are serviced by hospitals treating both adults and children. Only in metropolitan areas (capital cities) are there hospitals designed to exclusively treat children. Larger regional hospitals often have a specialist ward and services specifically targeting paediatric care. Ruby required specialist attention and admission due to her fracture.

Developments in technology and treatment have resulted in children experiencing more day procedures and earlier discharge from hospital with community follow-up programs including treatment and assessment by community child health services, practice nurses, nurse practitioners and general practitioners (Aylott, 2006; Smith & Coleman, 2010). This process assumes that the services will be available and pertinent information transferred between health sectors in a timely manner. Practice nurses report a gap in the translation of knowledge from hospital to community (Walsh & Barnes, 2012).

The nature of childhood admissions through injury and acute illness allows little preparation for hospitalisation, or for preparation of parents for caring for their injured/ill child once discharged. However, there are resources available to parents to prepare a child for hospitalisation, for example the Royal Children's Hospital, Melbourne, virtual hospital tour (http://ww2.rch.org.au/info/tour.cfm) and children's books about hospital and hospitalisation.

HOSPITAL SETTING: NEEDS OF PARENTS AND FAMILY MEMBERS

Every family responds to hospitalisation differently. Some take it in their stride but, for most, their experience will be fraught with varied levels of anxiety as it is a stressful life event. Reasons for anxiety include confrontation with a novel situation, fear of the unknown and separation from normality (school and home). Orientation of the child and family to the ward environment can assist in allaying fears and concerns and address any myths and misconceptions about hospital care (Weaver & Groves, 2010).

THE CHILD

The hospital environment, with its strange sights, sounds and smells, is alien to most children (Crole, 2002). Children need a sense of normality in their environment through personal belongings and knowing the rules and their boundaries. Younger children in middle childhood, 5- to 7-year-olds, thrive on rules with their good–bad, reward–punishment morality; boundaries such as when the television will be turned off and maintaining their normal bedtime routine need to be implemented (Boom, 2011).

It is important to maintain a child's pride and positive self-image. In a healthcare setting, they are often at risk of losing their dignity, restrained for often-painful procedures all in the name of their wellbeing. They may lose any sense of self and privacy for their maturing and sometimes suddenly changed body. In their eyes, they may be disfigured from scars or surgical incisions or proud of a plaster cast. Their autonomy disappears when they enter any health setting, which is a frightening experience, be it only for a short time (Lundqvist & Nilstun, 2007). However, children are resilient; they have a strong sense of a positive future (Zolkoski & Bullock, 2012).

PARENTS/CAREGIVERS

When an acutely unwell or injured child is hospitalised, it can cause great stress for the child's parents and other family members (see Box 9.1). The speed at which their child changes from normal to a state of injury or illness, requiring hospitalisation, can vary from minutes to days. As in the scenario, Claire met an

---

Box 9.1 Research highlight: The hospital experience

Parents experience emotional stress when their child has an acute illness or injury and caring for the acutely unwell or injured child has a significant impact. The role of carer changes and they have to adopt increased responsibilities, making immediate healthcare decisions for their child. There is no opportunity to comprehensively research their child's health problem or access the usual support systems for information and advice (e.g. from friends or extended family).

How do parents and children rate the care they receive in hospital? A study by Pelander and Leino-Kilpi (2010) found children reported negative aspects of hospitalisation to include pain and painful procedures, long waiting times for appointments, illness symptoms and separation from family and friends. Children in isolation rooms negatively rated their restricted ability to explore their environment and to interact with other children. There is a need for isolation; the impact on the children's quality of life while in isolation requires exploring. Little research addresses this problem. Interestingly, parents in this study rated waiting times as the most negative hospital experience. These findings highlight the need to keep children occupied and ensure pain management is timely and appropriate; hospitalised children need to maintain contact with the outside world.

injured and unhappy Ruby at the end of the school day. There was no opportunity for preparation; Claire simply had to respond.

Parents frequently face financial stress when they have a sick or injured child. In both nuclear and blended families it is common for both parents to work. The work environment is complex and varied. Some families can access their sick and/or family leave. However, the recent trend of casual or fixed contract employment means that these employees do not have access to entitlements such as sick leave (Australian Bureau of Statistics, 2010). As a result, families may be financially disadvantaged having to take time off work to stay with a hospitalised child and/or remaining at home to care for the sick or injured child.

Parents need to feel competent to care for their child at home. Hospital stays are generally short with restricted time for parent education. To address this, discharge preparation must begin on admission. Approaches to discharge planning come in many forms; it is important for health professionals to target education towards parents' needs. It has been established that the most effective form of discharge education is a combination of verbal and written information (Johnson & Sandford, 2005).

Community setting: needs of child, parents and family members

Most care of children in this age group occurs in the home, recovering from injuries or during acute self-limiting viral illnesses. The school setting is a perfect breeding ground for cross-infection.

Clinical scenario 9.2
Setting the scene: Care of an acutely ill child in the home

Albert, a 5-year-old, lives with his parents, Phoebe and Kevin, and his 2-month-old baby sister, Lulu. Phoebe is breastfeeding Lulu and on maternity leave for another month. Albert is generally a healthy child. However, he has been unwell for the past 2 days and Phoebe has kept him home from school. He has had a 'high fever' of 38.5°C, his appetite has been poor and he has been 'clingy'. Phoebe is concerned and googles Albert's symptoms. Phoebe and Kevin's neighbour's 1-year-old infant had a febrile convulsion last month; his parents were terrified at the time and thought he might die. He is perfectly well now, having recovered from a self-limiting viral infection.

Fortunately, today is Lulu's 2-month appointment at the child health clinic. While there, Phoebe asks the nurse for some advice about caring for a very miserable Albert. The nurse questions Phoebe about Albert's symptoms and asks what she has been doing to care for him. Phoebe is reassured that she is caring for Albert correctly; the nurse repeats what Phoebe has read on the paediatric hospital website on the Internet: keep him comfortable, push fluids and watch his overall condition for signs of deterioration and, if this should happen, take him to see his general practitioner. When told that his temperature is really only mild Phoebe is confused; she thought a normal temperature was 37.0°C and Albert's temperature of 38.5°C was much higher. Phoebe is relieved to be told it is not 'very high'.

PRIMARY HEALTH CARE

In the community setting these middle childhood children do not generally go to child health clinics, though they are available to them in some states. In Queensland, the care of children from birth to 18 years is available through community-based government-funded child health clinics. However, these clinics are generally utilised by parents with children from birth to 18 months of age (Kearney & Fulbrook, 2012). Middle childhood children often receive community-based primary health care in general practice settings, by practice nurses (Walsh & Barnes, 2012; Walsh & Mitchell, in press).

In the home

Middle children can undertake some of their own healthcare needs, such as bathing, eating and entertaining themselves and are used to being active and stimulated. When sick or injured they may regress and prefer their parents to attend to some of their usual activities, such as making their bed, getting snacks ready etc. This will increase the parents' workload in addition to caring for the child's specific health needs. In both scenarios, Albert and Ruby are in need of assistance. Albert is unwell and wanting his mother's company for comfort. Ruby needs assistance with many activities of daily living due to her immobile left arm.

Box 9.2 Practice highlight: Primary care nursing as a speciality

In acknowledgement of the care provided by nurses in primary health care, general practice settings, a new nursing speciality has been identified and developed through the national Nursing in General Practice 2001 initiative (NiGP) (Jolley & Shields, 2009; Watts, Bell, Byrne, Jones & Davis, 2008). In 2001 the Australian Practice Nurses' Association was formed (Watts et al., 2004). Through this program there was reimbursement from the Australian government to the general practice for specific care nurses provide to clients (Jolley & Shields, 2009; Watts et al., 2008). Initially, NiGP focused on chronic disease management in remote and rural settings to ensure equitable access to primary health care across Australia. The success of the program saw support for practice nurses in general practice in provincial and, finally, metropolitan areas. This was such a successful initiative that there has been continued expansion through both government initiatives and patient demographics (Jolly, 2007).

A move into the care of children and families came with the release of Medicare Benefit Schedule item numbers for immunisation and wound care in 2004 (Pascoe, Foley, Hutchinson et al., 2005). Further expansion occurred in 2008, through The Healthy Kids Check initiative, as the basic 4-year-old child health checks significantly extended practice nurses' care of well and sick children (Department of Health and Ageing, 2010). Practice nurses, however, come from a wide range of nursing backgrounds and very few Australian practice nurses (14.9%) have experience with child patients, their developmental and healthcare needs or the needs of their parents (Walsh & Barnes, 2012; Walsh & Mitchell, in press). Practice nurses report their role to include phone and practice triage of children (86.7%); they provide care for asthma management (58%), fever (66.6%), wounds (79.4%) and immunisation (95.6%) and refer children (and parents) to appropriate community services and advise/counsel parents about behavioural problems (e.g. bullying, eating practices) (Walsh & Barnes, 2012).

Caring for these children in the home is both easier and more difficult than caring for younger children. They can entertain themselves with many different sedentary activities, such as computer games, watching movies, texting friends etc. Having a sick or injured child has a significant influence on family functioning. The child may need attention regularly through the day and night, interrupting sleep and increasing parental fatigue. Other children may feel neglected through the increased attention given to one child. Parents are in a new position, having to devote more time to the sick or injured child, and how to manage this can be challenging, incorporating it into normal activities of daily living and work. Parents report fatigue and relationship stress when children are acutely ill/injured; they worry about missing work, financial losses and the need to also care for other children (Walsh, 2007). They look to health professionals for advice on how to care for their child. Advice, as mentioned earlier, given in more than one medium (e.g. oral and printed form) is helpful.

FEVER

Caring for the child with a febrile illness *can bring back bad memories*. Albert is 5 years old, the upper age group where febrile convulsions occur, though it would be rare for a first febrile convulsion to occur at this age (Sillanpää, Camfield, Camfield et al., 2008). Phoebe and Kevin were worried about febrile convulsions. Though it is unlikely Albert would have a febrile convulsion, fears and phobias are common (Walsh, Edwards & Fraser, 2007). Nurses are ideally placed to alert parents to the benefits of fever in increasing the immunological processes to produce antibodies against the invading organism (Blatteis, 2006). When Albert is febrile, he must stay home from school to allow him to rest, so that his body can fight the infectious illness and to prevent spread of his illness to his classmates, teachers and friends (see Box 9.3).

Phoebe is not alone in her search for child health information. Parents seek information on how to care for an ill or injured child from many sources; they ask friends with children and their own parents (Walsh, 2007). More recently, the norm is to search online for information; parents do this for their own health (Walsh, Hyde, Hamilton & White, 2012). Parents look online for a number of reasons. Is their child sick enough to need to go to the doctor or could they wait till the morning? Following a medical consultation, parents search online to gain a better understanding of their child's diagnosis and treatment. They need reassurance that they are actually doing the right thing for their child (Walsh, 2007; Walsh et al., in press).

Considering the dubious quality of some available online information, parent-reported actions following accessing online health information are concerning for health professionals. Parents report using online information to diagnose (43%) and treat (33%) their sick child; in an Australian study, 18% of parents reported altering their child's health management to align with online information (Wainstein, Sterling-Levis, Baker, Taitz & Brydon, 2006). Younger parents, aged 20 to 35 years, are more likely to report using online information, with more women than men likely to engage in seeking health information online (Ybarra & Suman, 2008). In 2008, 9% of Australian parents reported the Internet as the least, greatly trusted child health information source (Khoo, Bolt, Babl, Jury & Goldman, 2008). The incongruence in this research highlights the urgent need for health professionals to provide evidence-based health sites to parents when advising them on how to care for their child.

Box 9.3 Research highlight: Changing our understanding of the way parents manage childhood fever

In an Australian study Walsh (2007) found that, when their child was febrile, parents had several concerns. These were about: the possibility of febrile convulsions, the underlying cause of the fever, whether the illness was serious/fatal or their child's overall wellbeing.

A majority of parents also thought that fevers of 39.0°C or lower, medically considered a mild fever, were harmful or even very harmful. Despite concerns about the harmful effects of antipyretic medications causing a range of illnesses including liver damage, overdosing or stomach or kidney damage, parents used a range of medications to reduce fever. Parents reported using accurate doses; some alternated types of medication and some administered medicines more frequently than the 4-hourly recommended dosage interval.

This study used the theory of planned behaviour (Ajzen, 1991) to explore the predictors of parents' intentions to reduce their child's next fever. Their attitudes about fever, opinion of others and whether the child took medicine easily were influencing factors. Interestingly, those parents whose child did not take medications easily had more positive attitudes towards fever (fever is beneficial) and were less influenced by normative pressure.

These findings have provided evidence to guide nurses and other health professionals in their interactions with parents about fever management. It is recommended that you access this paper, to read the full research process and details of the results.

See Walsh A (2007) *Parents' management of childhood fever*. School of Nursing QUT, Brisbane, p. 413.

Indigenous children

Indigenous children are over-represented in injury prevalence and associated morbidity and mortality in developed countries throughout the world, including Australia and New Zealand. Despite this, there is relatively limited research into this area and implementation of the recommendations and strategies from reports (Lennon, Haworth, Titchener et al., 2009). New Zealand children, overall, have poorer health than those in any other developed OECD country and children of Māori and Pacific Islander descent have poorer health than those of European descent. Māori and Pacific Islander children have higher rates of hospitalisation for serious infections, respiratory illnesses, acute rheumatic fever (*50 times more likely*) and meningococcal disease than other New Zealand children (New Zealand and Ministry of Pacific Island Affairs, 2011). Of concern is that many of these illnesses, for which these children are hospitalised, are preventable through primary healthcare interventions and improved housing conditions.

It is important to protect cultural safety and connection to country, language and culture in indigenous families with acutely unwell and/or injured children (Schmied et al., 2011). Indigenous families, such as New Zealand's Pacific Island and Māori families, come from a strong socially cohesive society with high levels of social connectedness and strong participation in church life and volunteering. This cohesion promotes strength in feelings of belongingness; it has some protective health and social effects evidenced through the lower levels of considered and attempted suicide (Stanfeld, 2006). Social connectedness builds resilient and supportive communities and provides useful foundations for community health interventions (New Zealand and Ministry of Pacific Island Affairs, 2011).

Indigenous families living in remote regions of Australia face isolation and community separation if they need to leave their community to access tertiary-based services. This may result in cultural shock. Those who have moved from a predominantly indigenous community find themselves in a place where their cultural norms and mores are neither supported nor acknowledged (Tanner, Agius & Darbyshire, 2005). When cultural safety is practised there is support for the principal of solution-focused nursing, whereby family strengths are acknowledged and nurses focus on the values and resilience of the client and their family rather than on cultural differences (Barnes & Rowe, 2007). By identifying and supporting strengths, nurses can endeavour to support cultural fortitude rather than cultural shame.

Cultural differences and cultural misunderstandings often result from poor communication, poor care and/or a dysfunctional nurse–client relationship. However, by appreciating cultural differences health services, irrespective of the setting (hospital or community), can provide support for cultural needs in the diverse cultural client populations. Providing a safe environment when families may be experiencing a traumatic life event is paramount.

Conclusion

Middle childhood is a period of rapid growth and development when the transition from a child to an emerging adolescent occurs. These children are experiencing rapid expansion of their cognition, skills and knowledge. The school environment addresses many of their developmental needs through education, sports and social interactions. These team players are blossoming. Their social network expands, parents are no longer the centre/controller of all knowledge, peers become very important and teachers know best. Through new friendships, the need to conform is confronted and social norms are challenged. As an individual or member of a peer group, they are in harm's way, with injury just waiting to occur as they test their developing skills and generally play.

Injury is their main reason for any contact with health professionals. Infectious diseases are on the decline due to the national goals of countries for immunisation and the continual development of new vaccines. Health care is generally community-based, with practice nurses and general practitioners, and visits to hospital for injury and complex or serious acute illnesses are few. Parents are therefore the primary carers of sick or injured children.

When children are in contact with health professionals, a family strengths model for care is essential. These children are beginning to care for their own health; we must build on their strengths and continue to educate and advise them for optimum health. The child must not be ignored through a family-centred orientation; child-centred care must remain a priority – it must be incorporated into the family-centred care model. There is an urgent need for research in this area to ensure these children receive the best possible care from the nurses with whom they are in contact. Most research is this area targets hospitalised children, yet these children receive the bulk of their care in the community.

Community involvement in acute care and higher acuity levels of hospitalised patients have resulted in increased parental responsibility. This increases parental fatigue and work-related pressures where a parent needs to take leave from work to care for a sick or injured child. The need to access sick/family leave can increase parental stress. With more parents working there is a need for policy and attitude changes to enable parents to provide care for their children, and have access to paid leave when they themselves are ill. Meeting the healthcare needs of the middle child is complex. Health services must support family strengths and develop collaborative approaches to care.

KEY POINTS

» Children in their middle years are generally healthy.

» Medical/nursing assistance is more likely for injury than an acute illness.

» The needs of the hospitalised child are important to ensure independence and involvement in health decision making.

» They may be injured anywhere: school, home, sports, community.

» They are subjected to intentional injury at school through bullying and at home.

CRITICAL QUESTIONS

1.   What are the needs of an acutely ill child in different settings? Are they different? If so why; if not why?

2.   What is the impact on parents when their middle-aged child is injured?

3.   What is the impact on parents when their middle-aged child is acutely ill?

4.   What is the impact on families when a middle-aged child is ill/injured? How does this differ from the impact on the parents?

5.   Explain the difference between family- and child-centred care.

6.   Why is the middle childhood age group called 'the forgotten years'?

7.   How do these children's needs differ in the general practice setting and the hospital setting?

USEFUL RESOURCES

Australian Bureau of Statistics: http://www.abs.gov.au/

Australian College of Children and Young People's Nurses (ACCYPN): http://www.accypn.org.au/

Australian Government Children's Health: http://australia.gov.au/topics/health-and-safety/childrens-health

Australian Indigenous Health*Info*Net: http://www.healthinfonet.ecu.edu.au/?gclid=CLCRp-CkyLECFaRMpgodkksADg

Australian Institute of Health and Welfare (AIHW), 2009 *A picture of Australia's children, 2009.* AIHW, Canberra: www.aihw.gov.au/publication-detail/?id=6442468252

Commission for children and young people and child guardians: http://www.ccypcg.qld.gov.au/index.aspx

Kidsafe Australia: http://www.kidsafe.com.au/

Kidsafe New Zealand: http://www.safekids.org.nz/

Ministry of Health New Zealand Child Health: http://www.health.govt.nz/our-work/life-stages/child-health

New Zealand Office of Children's Commissioner: http://www.occ.org.nz/

Queensland Injury Surveillance Unit: http://www.qisu.org.au/ModCoreFrontEnd/index.asp?pageid=109

Raising Children in New Zealand: http://www.raisingchildren.org.nz/

Raising Children Network the Australian parenting website: http://raisingchildren.net.au/

Royal Children's Hospital Melbourne: www.rch.org.au/

Safe Schools – The National Safe Schools Framework: http://www.deewr.gov.au/schooling/nationalsafeschools/Pages/overview.aspx

Starship Children's Health, Auckland: https://www.starship.org.nz

Statistics New Zealand: http://www.stats.govt.nz/

The Children's Social Health Monitor New Zealand: http://www.nzchildren.co.nz/

References

Ajzen, I. (1991). The theory of planned behavior. *Organisational Behavior and Human Decision Processes, 50,* 179–211.

Australian Bureau of Statistics (ABS) (2003). *Australian Social Trends 2003* (Family and Community Services and Assistance: Child Protection). Retrieved from http://www.abs.gov.au (accessed 19 June 2012).

Australian Bureau of Statistics (ABS) (2006). *Year book Australia, 2006* [Cat. No. 1301.0]. Canberra: ABS.

Australian Bureau of Statistics (ABS) (2010a). *Year book Australia, 2009–10* [Cat. No. 1301.0]. Canberra: ABS.

Australian Bureau of Statistics (ABS) (2010b). *Work: Casual employees: Measures of Australia's Progress* [Cat. No.1370.0]. Canberra: ABS.

Australian Institute of Family Studies (2012). Mandatory reporting of child abuse and neglect. Retrieved from http://www.aifs.gov.au/cfca/pubs/factsheets/01/index.html (accessed 21 June 2012).

Australian Institute of Health and Welfare (AIHW) (2009). *A picture of Australia's children, 2009.* Canberra: AIHW.

Australian Institute of Health and Welfare (AIHW) (2011). *Headline indicators: For children's health, development and wellbeing, 2011.* Canberra: AIHW.

Aylott, M. (2006). Observing the sick child: part 2a respiratory assessment. *Paediatric Nursing, 18*(9), 38–44.

Barker, R., Heiring, C., Krahn, D., Spinks, D., & Pitt, R. (2008a). Injuries related to bunk bed use in Queensland. *Injury Bulletin*. Brisbane: Queensland Injury Surveillance Unit.

Barker, R., Heiring, C., Krahn, D., Spinks, D., & Pitt, R. (2008b). Injuries in primary school children. *Injury Bulletin*. Brisbane: Queensland Injury Surveillance Unit.

Barnes, M. & Rowe, J. (2007). Introduction. In M. Barnes & J. Rowe (Eds.), *Child, youth and family health: Strengthening communities*. Chatswood: Churchill Livingstone.

Bascand, G. (2010). *National population estimates: December 2009 Quarter. Hot Off the Press*. Statistics New Zealand Tatauranga Aotearoa.

Blatteis, C. (2006). Endotoxic fever: new concepts of its regulation suggest new approaches to its management. *Pharmacology & Therapeutics, 111*, 194–223.

Boom, J. (2011). Egocentrism in moral development: Gibbs, Piaget, Kohlberg. *New Ideas in Psychology, 29*, 355–363.

Centre for Community Child Health (2006). *Preventing injury: Practice resource*. Retrieved from http://www.rch.org.au/ccch/profdev/Preventing_Injury_Practice_ Resource/ (accessed 14 January 2013).

Council of Australian Governments (2009). *Protecting Children is Everyone's Business National Framework for Protecting Australia's Children 2009–2020*. Canberra: Australian Government.

Crole, N. (2002). Examining the phases of nursing care of the hospitalised child. *Australian Nursing Journal, 9*(8), 30–31.

Department of Health and Ageing (2010). *Medicare Benefits Schedule (MBS) healthy kids check provided by a practice nurse or registered Aboriginal health worker. MBS Item 10986 Fact Sheet*. Canberra: Australian Government.

Dunst, C. J. & Trivette, C. (2009). Meta-analytic structural equation modelling of the influences of family-centred care on parent and child psychological health. *International Journal of Paediatrics 2009*: Article ID 576840, doi:10.1155/2009/576840

Erikson, E. (1963). *Childhood and Society*. New York: Norton.

Frank, L. & Callery, P. (2004). Re-thinking family-centred care across the continuum of children's healthcare. *Child: Care, Health & Development, 30*(3), 265–277.

Gulliver, P., Cryer, C., & Davie, G. (2010). *A chart book of the New Zealand Injury Prevention Strategy Serious Outcome Indicators for Children 1994–2009*. Wellington: New Zealand Government.

Helps, Y. & Pointer, S. (2006). *Child injury due to falls from playground equipment, Australia 2002–2004*. Canberra: AIHW.

Johnson, A. & Sandford, J. (2005). Written and verbal information versus information only for patients being discharged from acute hospital settings to home: systematic review. *Health Education Research, 20*(4), 423–429.

Jolley, J. & Shields, L. (2009). The evolution of family-centred care. *Journal of Pediatric Nursing, 24*(2), 164–170.

Jolly, R. (2007). *Practice nursing in Australia*. Research paper No. 10. 2007–08. Canberra: Parliament of Australia.

Kearney, L. & Fullbrook, P. (2012). Open-access community child health clinics: the everyday experiences of parents and child health nurses. *Journal of Child Health Care, 16*(1), 5–14.

Kerridge, I., Lowe, M., & McPhee, J. (2005). *Ethics and law for the health professions.* Leichhardt: The Federation Press.

Khoo, K., Bolt, P., Babl, F., Jury, S., & Goldman, R. (2008). Health information seeking by parents in the internet age. *Journal of Paediatrics and Child Health, 44,* 419–423.

Kreisfeld, R. & Harrison, E. (2010). *Hospital separations due to injury and poisoning 2005–06. Injury Research and Statistics Series.* Canberra: AIHW.

Knudsen, E. (2004). Sensitive periods in the development of the brain and behaviour. *Journal of Cognitive Neuroscience, 16*(8), 1412–1425.

Lee, P. (2004). Family involvement: are we asking too much? *Paediatric Nursing, 16*(10), 37–41.

Lennon, A., Haworth, N., Titchener, K., et al. (2009). *Injury prevention in Queensland: report to Queensland Injury Prevention Council. QUT: The Centre for Accident Research and Road Safety-Queensland.* Brisbane: QUT.

Lundqvist, A. & Nilstun, T. (2007). Human dignity in paediatrics: the effects of health care. *Nursing Ethics, 14,* 2215–2228.

Mah, V. K. & Ford-Jones, E. L. (2012). Spotlight on middle childhood: rejuvenating the 'forgotten years'. *Paediatric Child Health, 17*(2), 81–83.

Ministerial Council for Education (2011). National safe schools framework resource manual. Retrieved from www.Safeschools.deewr.gov.au (accessed 19 June 2012).

Nethercott, J. (1993). A concept for all the family. Family-centred care: a concept analysis. *Professional Nurse, 8*(12), 794–797.

New Zealand and Ministry of Pacific Island Affairs (2011). *Health and Pacific peoples in New Zealand: Pacific progress.* Wellington: Statistics New Zealand and Ministry of Pacific Island Affairs.

O'Hare, S. B. & Blackford, J. C. (2005). Nurses' moral agency in negotiating parental participation in care. *International Journal of Nursing Practice, 11*(6), 250–256.

Pascoe, T., Foley, E., Hutchinson, R., et al. (2005). The changing face of nurses in Australian general practice. *Australian Journal of Advanced Nursing, 23*(1), 44–50.

Pelander, T. & Leino-Kilpi, H. (2010). Children's best and worst experiences during hospitalisation. *Scandinavian Journal of Caring Sciences, 24*(4), 726–733.

Piltz, A. & Wachtel, T. (2009). Barriers that inhibit nurses reporting suspected cases of child abuse and neglect. *Australian Journal of Advanced Nursing, 26*(3), 93–100.

Schmied, V., Donovan, J., Kruske, S., et al. (2011). Commonalities and challenges: a review of Australian state and territory maternity and child health policies. *Contemporary Nurse, 40*(1), 106–117.

Shields, L., Mamun, A., Pereira, S., O'Nions, P., & Chaney, G. (2011). Measuring family-centred care: working with children and their parents in a tertiary hospital. *The International Journal of Person Centred Medicine, 1*(1), 155–160.

Sillanpää, M., Camfield, P. R., Camfield, C. S., et al. (2008). Inconsistency between prospectively and retrospectively reported febrile seizures. *Developmental Medicine and Child Neurology, 50*(1), 25–28.

Slaughter, R., Beasley, D., Lambie, B., & Schep, L. (2009). *New Zealand's venomous creatures. The New Zealand Medical Journal.* Christchurch: New Zealand Medical Association.

Smith, L. & Coleman, V. (2010). *Child and family-centred healthcare.* Houndmills: Palgrave.

Stanfeld, S. (2006). Social support and social cohesion. In M. Marmot & R. Wilkinson (Eds.), *Social determinants of health.* New York: Oxford University Press.

Statistics New Zealand (2011). *Serious injury outcome injuries for children, 1994–2010. Monitoring the New Zealand Injury Prevention Strategy.* Wellington: Statistics New Zealand.

Tanner, L., Agius, K., & Darbyshire, P. (2005). 'Sometime they run away that's how scared they feel': the paediatric hospitalisation experience of indigenous families from remote areas of Australia. *Contemporary Nurse, 18*(1–2), 2–17.

Wainstein, B., Sterling-Levis, K., Baker, S., Taitz, J., & Brydon, M. (2006). Use of the internet by parents of paediatric patients. *Journal of Paediatrics and Child Health, 42,* 528–532.

Walsh, A. (2007). *Parents' management of childhood fever. School of Nursing* (p. 413). Brisbane: QUT.

Walsh, A. & Barnes, M. (2012). Nurses in Australian general practice settings: expanding role in child health and wellbeing. *Primary Times, 12*(1), 30.

Walsh, A., Edwards, H., & Fraser, J. (2007). Influences of parents' fever management: beliefs, experiences and information sources. *Journal of Clinical Nursing, 16*(12), 2331–2340.

Walsh, A., Hyde, M., Hamilton, K., & White, K. (2012). Predictive modelling: parents' decision making to use online child health information to increase their understanding and/or diagnose or treat their child's health. *BMC Medical Informatics and Decision Making, 12, 144.* Retrieved from http://www.biomedcentral.com/1472-6947/12/144 (accessed 12 March 2013).

Walsh, A. & Mitchell, A. (in press). A pilot study exploring Australian general practice nurses roles, and responsibilities and professional development needs in well and sick child care. *Neonatal Paediatric and Child Health Nursing.*

Watts, I., Foley, E., Hutchinson, R., et al. (2004). *General practice nursing in Australia.* Australia: Royal College of General Practitioners and Royal College of Nursing.

Watts, K., Bell, L., Byrne, S., Jones, T., & Davis, E. (2008). Waist circumference predicts cardiovascular risk in young Australian children. *Journal of Paediatrics and Child Health, 11,* 709–715.

Weaver, K., & Groves, J. (2010). Play provision for children in hospital. In A. Glasper, M. Aylott, & C. Battrick (Eds.), *Developing practical skills for nursing children and young people* (pp. 72–88). London: Hodder Arnold.

Ybarra, M. & Suman, M. (2008). Reasons, assessments and actions taken: sex and age differences in uses of internet health information. *Health Education Research, 23,* 512–521.

Young, J., McCann, D., Watson, K., et al. (2006). Negotiation of health care for a hospitalised child: parental perspectives. *Neonatal, Paediatric and Child Health Nursing, 9*(2), 4–13.

Zolkoski, S. M. & Bullock, L. M. (2012). Resilience in children and youth: a review. *Children and Youth Services Review, 34*(12), 2295–2303.

Chapter 10

THE YOUNG PERSON

Lindsay Smith

LEARNING OUTCOMES

Reading this chapter will help you to:

» understand the importance of the bioecological context of the young person

» review key indicators of health and wellbeing for the young person in Australia and New Zealand

» discuss a range of protective factors that support health and development for the young person

» discuss a range of risks threatening the health and development of young people

» describe how nurses promote health and support optimal outcomes for the young person in the community.

Introduction

> The plasticity (potential for systematic change) associated with the engagement of the active individual with his or her active context legitimates an optimistic approach to the possibility that applications of developmental science may improve the course and contexts of human life. (Lerner, 2005, p. ix).

This chapter explores nursing the young person within the context of their family and their community. The focus of this chapter is to understand how nurses promote health and wellbeing for the young person, establishing successful and altering harmful developmental pathways across the bioecological context. The life stage between late childhood and young adulthood (approximately 10–24 years old) is together termed the 'young person' in this chapter. Our understanding of this period of life is changing, especially in relation to adolescence. Many children are moving out of the innocence and dependence of childhood at a younger age. Likewise, it may take longer for adolescents to move fully away from semi-dependence on their family. Thus, nursing young people is not bound by age and hormonal changes of the person (as much as these bring significant biological factors that need to be considered), rather nursing is concerned with helping young people fulfil their personal goals and autonomy within specific sociocultural contexts and health concerns.

The young person lives through an exciting period of life that is characterised by transitions. Through these transitions, from one developmental achievement to the next, challenges surface that the young person needs to address successfully so they emerge as a young adult established for a successful life journey. These transitions are all about potential – potential of what the young person may achieve and become. Young people who experience chronic illness, family separation, isolation, homelessness and other significant stress during this transition period can face additional developmental challenges, often as a result of insufficient broader community support and an inability to fulfil developmental aspirations of emerging adulthood (Johnstone & Lee, 2012). Nurses have a significant role during these transitions in empowering young people to take control of their health care and transition to young adulthood, especially within the community where most nursing and health care for this group occurs. Positive communication and a family-focused approach are necessary to facilitate a solution-focused approach to health care with young people. See Chapter 5 for a detailed discussion of communication approaches and strategies.

While reading this chapter, reflect on this scenario and consider how the issues discussed relate to Becky (see Clinical scenario 10.1) and your nursing. We will return to Becky throughout this chapter.

Health and wellbeing of young people

Childhood is often experienced as a period of delight and joy. This delight, however, can be interrupted by the onset of developmental changes that create

Clinical scenario 10.1
Setting the scene

As a community health nurse working in a rural community health centre, you receive a referral from the local high school. Becky, a 14-year-old female, is legally competent to give consent for her own health care and has accepted the referral (see Chapter 4 for further information about informed consent and young people). Becky has been referred following noticeable behavioural changes that are negatively affecting her relationships with the teachers and other students. Her appearance has become increasingly 'scruffy' and her language has become nonchalant and at times offensive.

Becky has not previously been reported for disruptive behaviour at school. Becky was the highest achiever in year 8 science last year. In primary school, Becky was the year 6 representative on the student council. As a young child, Becky played well with all her friends and was an excellent mentor to the kindergarten children.

Becky lives with her mother, Jill, and older brother. Her parents divorced late last year. She has not seen her father since, as he relocated interstate; yet, they speak on the telephone monthly. Becky did enjoy talking to her mum after school; however, 3 months ago her mum re-entered the workforce taking a position as an evening waitress, involving long hours in the night and regular absences from home in the afternoon when Becky gets home. She misses sitting with her mum around the kitchen table.

You spend time listening to Becky tell you her life story and start to develop a relationship with her. Becky starts by telling you 'things at home and school haven't been good this year and I've had some thoughts lately that are really scary. The thoughts started shortly after I broke up with my boyfriend. I don't like school anymore and I take everything out on mum. I just don't know what to do anymore.' Becky asks, 'Can you help me cope, please?' You also discover that she broke off with her boyfriend after her best friend started seeing him. Becky's mum recently arranged a medical appointment for Becky to review her chronic yet usually controlled asthma following recent episodes of coughing at night. Becky has been neglecting to self-administer her asthma preventers saying, 'What's the point? We all die of something.'

Becky's family and relationship losses are distressing her. You ask Becky to draw a genogram, a diagram that depicts family relationships (McMurray & Clendon, 2011), and then you use this to identify important relationships in her life. Since Becky is autonomous in seeking health care in this situation, you ask her how she would like your relationship to progress. You let Becky know that she is free to direct what her needs are and when she would like to meet with you. Becky decides that she would like to get together next week, and says she really liked talking to you about her life without being told what to do.

At your next visit, you further explore her family and personal strengths, and together you identify where Becky would like to be in 2 months' time. Becky identifies that she wants to continue with her schooling and to make some new friends. She also wants to find some time to talk to her mum more. A visit to her dad also seems a nice idea to her, perhaps in the summer holidays.

challenges for the upper primary child and adolescent. The joys of childhood can be quickly forgotten when the tumultuous years of change appear. Despite community concerns over perceived increasingly negative outcomes of late childhood and adolescence, developmental indicators in both Australia (Australian Institute of Health and Welfare [AIHW], 2011) and New Zealand (Wauchop, 2010) indicate that the majority of young people experience good health, enjoy strong relationships with family members and friends, contribute positively to their community and succeed in their transition into young adulthood. For example, New Zealand youth in 2007 reported a greater level of satisfaction in life, fewer depressive symptoms and fewer thoughts about and attempts to kill themselves compared to in 2001 (Adolescent Health Research Group, 2008, p. 104). In Australia the AIHW (2011, p. vii) reports statistics for young people aged 12–24 years reflect 'large declines in death rates (mostly due to declines in injury deaths) … favourable trends in some risk and protective factors, such as declines in smoking and illicit substance use, and most Year 10 and Year 12 students using contraception'. Many young people are ambassadors for charities, promote real tolerance of others and champion for justice, equality and sustainable living. The world is definitely a better place because of the enthusiasm and passions of youth.

Despite the generally pleasing youth health and wellbeing trends, there is conjecture that there is too high a proportion of young people who are not doing as well as could be expected across a range of developmental health and wellbeing measures when compared to young people in other countries (Australian Research Alliance for Children and Youth [ARACY], 2008). These areas of concern reported by ARACY include: levels of young people living in poverty and with deprivation, injury (including poisoning and suicide), mental health issues, alcohol and illicit drug use, abuse and neglect, poor educational outcomes, youth crime and teenage pregnancy. In the Australian Temperament Project (see Box 10.1), up to 23% of study participants reported the experience of maltreatment, which had a significant association to higher levels of depression and higher levels of anxiety

---

Box 10.1 Research highlight: Australian Temperament Project (ATP)

The ATP is a longitudinal study that aims to investigate the contribution of personal, family and environmental factors to development and wellbeing. The study recruited 2443 children aged 4–8 months, who were a representative sample of Victorian children, and their parents in 1982–83. The study fills the gap in Australian research exploring the associations between childhood experiences and adolescent and young adult life outcomes. Following 15 waves of data collection, there has been analysis of the data and many of the subsequent publications are available through the ATP website (http://www.aifs.gov.au/atp/about/about.html).

As the cohort now emerges from adolescence to young adulthood, further analysis exploring the associations between adolescence and young adult outcomes is available. In one publication, Hawkins et al. (2012) report that positive adolescent outcomes are predictive of young adult outcomes of emotional health, physical wellbeing, friendship quality and antisocial behaviour. O'Connor, Sanson, Hawkins et al. (2011) have reported on the predictors of positive development in emerging adulthood. Their findings highlight the importance of helping young people to develop strong family and peer relationships, the ability to self-regulate and their connectedness to school and community. Such evidence identified through the ATP strengthens the impetus for programs in the community that encourage positive adolescent development, such as adolescent mental health and parenting programs. The nursing profession may need to rediscover their role in the multidisciplinary field of adolescent and young adult health as well as embed this evidence into their familiar child health and parenting role.

(Price-Robertson, Smart & Bromfield, 2010). Carlisle, Henderson and Hanlon (2009) have identified that, in modern Western cultures, vulnerable young people may experience a 'growing sense of individual alienation, social fragmentation and civic disengagement and decline of more spiritual, moral and ethical aspects of life' (p. 1556).

Aboriginal and Torres Strait Islander young people in Australia and Taitamariki Māori (Māori young people) and Pacific Islander young people in New Zealand suffer from inequalities and injustices, which result in higher preventable mortality and morbidity rates than for non-indigenous and European youth (Australian Institute of Health and Welfare, 2011, p. 171; Clark, Robinson, Crengle et al., 2008, p. 5; Statistics New Zealand and Ministry of Pacific Island Affairs, 2011, p. 13). The Australian Institute of Health and Welfare (2011, p. vii) concluded 'many young Australians are faring well according to the national indicators … however, there is considerable scope for further gains particularly among Aboriginal and Torres Strait Islander young people'. This trend of a coexisting increase in social inequalities and decrease in development indicators for vulnerable youth at a time of unprecedented prosperity within modern societies has been recognised as 'modernity's paradox' (Li, McMurray & Stanley, 2008; Wyn, 2009). Evidence is mounting as to the potential detrimental effects of modern living on the formation of secure relationships, which in turn progressively undermine the human development potential of vulnerable youth (Bronfenbrenner & Morris, 1998). Such indicators highlight the modern shift from biological causes of morbidity and mortality among youth to ecological causes (Keating & Hertzman, 1999). It is encouraging that most young people in Australia and New Zealand are faring well, but it remains a concern that not all youth make the transition into adulthood reasonably well and some carry scars, living lives of latent if not lost potential.

Young people and their family

Chapter 1 presented a detailed description of family types as well as family factors that may influence the health and wellbeing of children and young people. The resilience of the family to remain and to function well serves a protective function for young people (Hayes, 2008). It is often depicted that young people are in a constant state of tension with their family. Research on how families influence health outcomes of young people, however, has focused on family cohesion – the emotional bonds that connect family members together. Price-Robertson, Smart and Bromfield (2010, p. 15) concluded 'close, loving and encouraging childhood relationships with parents lays a strong foundation for thriving in young adulthood and may also buffer young people from mental health problems'. Two useful indicators of family connectedness are the number of times per week the family enjoy eating their main meal of the day together and a young person's reporting of parents spending time 'just talking' with them. Australians aged 15 years report that only 70.98% eat more than one main meal a week with their parents and only 51.13% spend time with their parents just talking more than once a week (Australian Research Alliance for Children and Youth, 2008). Australian families rank 21 out of 27 and 18 out of 27 OECD nations on these two indicators, respectively. Strengthening family connectedness and cohesion should underpin all endeavours to promote young people's developmental health outcomes.

Clinical scenario 10.1
continued

At your next appointment with Becky, you ask her if it would be OK for her mother to join you for a short while in an appointment so you can start to explore with Becky her family strengths using the AFS Nursing Assessment Guide (see Table 5.1 in Chapter 5). Becky agrees and you arrange a suitable time for all to meet. During this appointment, both Becky and Jill discuss their family strengths and discover that they still have many strengths that they cherish. They also identify that they would like to find time to share an evening meal together and they set the goal of identifying, at the start of each week, one evening when they will have dinner together and spend the evening at home to 'just talk'. Becky agrees to ask her older brother if he would have dinner with them once a week as well.

The young person in a bioecological context

Recent developmental research discoveries have indicated that genetic make-up does not solely determine human traits and achievement; rather, positive developmental outcomes require genetic messages interacting with positive and complementary environmental experiences (Australian Institute of Health and Welfare, 2012). Genetic material contains blueprints for potential; however, they do not contain all necessary processes. Human interactions are the primary mechanism through which human genetic potential is actualised (Bronfenbrenner, 2001). Thus, development occurs through interactions between the individual and the interacting systems around them (Rutter, 2006). These interactions, which become effective if occurring regularly over time, are bi-directional. The ecology changes the person and the person changes the ecology. Therefore, the individual is active in their own development through selective patterns of attention, action and responses with people, objects and symbols.

The bioecological theory of human development proposes that, by enhancing human interactions and environments, it is possible to increase the extent of genetic potential realised into development (Bronfenbrenner, 2001; Bronfenbrenner & Ceci, 1994, p. 568). The bioecological theory focuses on the mechanisms of development alongside the ecological context as equal determinants of development. This establishes the basis for understanding the young person within their environment as an active participant in their own development. It also establishes that, in human development, the influential environment is not merely the immediate context in which the developing young person resides; rather, it also includes interactions between people in various settings and influences from larger surroundings (Green, 2010). Understanding bioecological determinants of development, health and wellbeing assists nurses to promote optimal outcomes for the young person.

The bioecological theory of human development argues that inherent potential is not static. Rather, potential increases for the young person who is well supported by their family, school, church, community and all levels of government. For many young people, peers are also an important aspect of their life. Benefits from stable

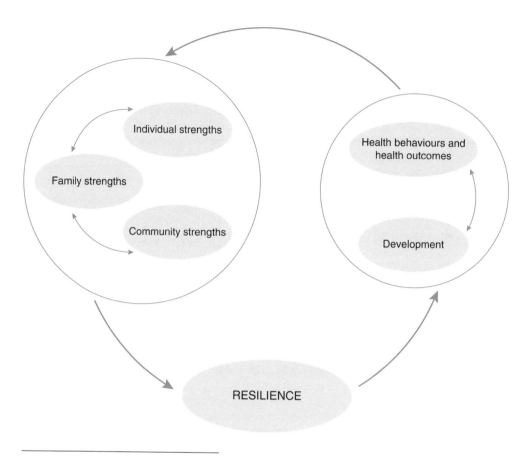

FIGURE 10.1 The resilience cycle

peer relationships can significantly increase developmental outcomes. However, these same peer relationships can create tension for the young person and their family.

Using an interacting systems approach, bioecological determinants of health and wellbeing can be grouped under three domains – individual (biological and relational), family and community – providing a framework guiding nursing intervention that promotes young people's strengths and moderates risk factors across all three domains. The enhanced health and development outcomes influence the individual, family and community strengths, thus creating a positive cycle in the bioecological determinants (see Figure 10.1). For example, families who completed family development programs demonstrate greater cohesion and better communication, and the young people involved in the program continued to report very low participation in alcohol, tobacco and other drugs 6 months after completing the full program (Riesch, Brown, Anderson et al., 2012). Similarly, in Australia and New Zealand, the Triple P – Positive Parenting Program is offered in many different settings: nurses in government health clinics may train for one-on-one consultations; psychologists in private practice may offer it to their patients; school guidance officers or community program officers may conduct group courses or seminars in local settings; and Triple P can also be done from home with the self-help books and

DVDs (Sanders, 2008). A referral to a local Triple P – Positive Parenting Program may help strengthen Becky's family and may also reduce various risks for Becky.

Protective factors, risk factors and developmental health outcomes

Research has shown that many health and wellbeing outcomes are vulnerable to various risk factors and amenable to protective factors (Hunter, 2012). Risk as a research term means 'the probability that an event will occur' (Young, 2005, p. 177). Risk, however, is commonly conceived of as the likelihood of a negative outcome rather than the likelihood of a positive one. To clarify this concept, protective factors increase the likelihood of a positive outcome and risk factors increase the likelihood of a negative outcome. The effect of some protective factors is strong, with evidence to support the conclusion that higher numbers of protective factors, regardless of the number of risk factors, lower the risk of reduced developmental health outcomes (Blum & Ireland, 2004; Wilkinson & Marmot, 2003).

This discourse on risk and protective factors, however, is not without criticism. Some risks known to have strong correlations to negative health outcomes for some young people may be mediated through other factors that negate the risk for other young people (Godin, 2006). Although protective factors can modify the effects of risk factors and generate wellbeing, the ways in which protective and risk factors interact are not well known. Placing restrictions on young people because of a known risk, based on assumptions that may not be generalisable, is problematic.

Green (2010) believes that understandings of youth remain dominated by the notions of danger and risk constructed through social, cultural and political processes. This is disempowering to the individual and allows allocation of blame based on association with subjectively determined risk-taking. Lupton (1999) argues that risk findings tend to categorise groups of people as 'problems' without any effort to understand the individuals within these groups. For example, being an adolescent is often seen as a risk itself, one that is resolved by obtaining the status of an adult. Males (2009), however, identified that statistics demonstrate young people do not take excessive risks compared to adults and that adolescent risk-taking is often associated strongly with ecological conditions beyond their control and prevailing local adult behaviours.

Although it is understood there is a potential to stigmatise young people through the discourse of risk, historically the risk framework has stimulated research exploring pathways and outcomes of behaviour. Such research exploring risks often identified protective factors and strengths in people's lives – moving towards an understanding of resilience. Strengthening resilience from a holistic interacting systems approach may prove to be most effective means of promoting long lasting developmental health outcomes. See Table 1.1 in Chapter 1 for a list of individual, family and community risk and protective factors that influence early childhood health, and see Table 12.1 in Chapter 12 for risk and protective factors for mental health in children and young people.

Returning to Becky briefly, using positive communication strategies identified by Carlsson, Bramhagen, Jansson and Dykes (2011) in Chapter 5, it would be important to empower Becky through helping her describe any risk-taking behaviour she may be involved in that she would like to change rather than pointing out risky behaviours you think Becky should avoid. Finding the solution herself and helping Becky to act to solve the issue will empower her to promote her own developmental health outcomes. For example, given the opportunity, Becky may identify the disruptive behaviour at school as an issue to address or raise an issue related to her sexual health and her past boyfriend.

Spiritual wellbeing and developmental health outcomes

Perhaps one of the most controversial and least understood protective factors is spiritual wellbeing. Modernity, and its healthcare system, is criticised for its rhetoric of inclusivity yet insistence on rejecting spirituality and traditions as no longer relevant (Ahern, 2010). Yet, in a national study of New Zealand young people aged 10–15 years, around 60% report a belief in a higher power and about 50% agree that 'spiritual beliefs make you stronger' (Wauchop, 2010). Likewise Mason, Singleton and Webber (2007) report in Australia 41% of young people are engaged with their stated spirituality type. Research clearly identifies spiritual wellbeing as a health promoting and protective factor for young people (Roehlkepartain, Benson, Scales, Kimball & King, 2008). For example, adolescents with higher levels of spiritual wellbeing displayed fewer depressive symptoms and engaged in fewer risk-taking behaviours (Cotton, Larkin, Hoopes, Cromer & Rosenthal, 2005). Lerner, Alberts, Anderson and Dowling (2006, p. 65) concluded that 'contemporary scholars of adolescent development are pointing to the implications of religiosity and spirituality on positive youth development'. The strength of this protection, however, is at times disputed.

A few explanations as to why spiritual matters contribute towards positive developmental outcomes have been proposed. Spiritual expression in Australian 16–20-year-olds is reported to enhance connectedness to family and friends and promotes a sense of self-worth, helping young people to find meaning and purpose (de Souza, Cartwright & McGilp, 2004). Regular engagement with religious activities has been shown to be positively related to life satisfaction and wellbeing through building of social networks (Stoll, Michaelson & Seaford, 2012).

In a recent Australian case study of spiritual wellbeing and its relationship to adolescent resilience, Smith (2011) identified four areas where spiritual matters contribute towards positive developmental outcomes for young people. Firstly, families implementing spiritual practices together reported enhanced family connectedness and cohesion. Joshua, 24 years old, identified in the study that implementing spiritual practices had the benefit of strengthening his family connectedness through creating some vulnerability with one another. Joshua said:

> I have always loved praying as a family. It is the communal side of this that I think draws me to it. A common understanding and almost that vulnerability of letting out our spiritual side in front of each other.

Secondly, spiritually active families encouraged young people to develop strong connections with members of their church outside the family unit. These wider relationships provided a way of securing support during life crises and times of stress. Thirdly, in an endeavour to strengthen their spiritual wellbeing, young people modified their behaviour to include regular spiritual practices and reduce known

Box 10.2 Practice highlight

The young people in the previously mentioned study undertaken by Smith (2011) predominantly focus their spirituality on developing relationships. As a result of their spiritual wellbeing and relationships with others, the young people in the study reported a sense of peace and life satisfaction. Many young people may not respond to words that describe spirituality and religiosity or be able to talk easily about their spiritual wellbeing. Yet young people may recognise their level of spiritual wellbeing in terms of their satisfaction with life, or the peace they experience. In healthcare interactions with young people, inquiring about peace or satisfaction with life the young person is feeling may facilitate conversations and encourage connections that strengthen resilience.

risky behaviours. In the study Joshua is explicit in how spiritual wellbeing influenced his life choices:

> Spiritual wellbeing sets guideposts for my life. Tells me when I should stop. And I know inside if I have gone too far, i.e. sex, swearing, hate, love, being friendly, lust, how and when I spend my money.

Finally, the study reported that young people who enjoyed a sense of spiritual wellbeing also reported a sense of peace and satisfaction in life. In the study Ben said 'to have spiritual wellbeing is to have inner peace and a sense of connection'. This finding is consistent with research on spiritual wellbeing by Rowold (2011), who reported that aspects of spiritual wellbeing in a group of university students (mean age 24.16 years, SD = 9.49) are related to subsequent happiness.

The associations between spiritual matters and positive youth outcomes are many; however, they are at times variable in strength and direction. No doubt some young people are harmed through their association with religion, and tension can arise within families over differing spiritual beliefs and practices as young people establish their own spiritual beliefs. Research evidence, however, does demonstrate consistently positive correlations between spiritual matters and developmental health outcomes for many young people (Myers, 2008). This protective factor may be strongest for those whose spiritual wellbeing is strong and their spirituality and religious beliefs are salient. See the practice highlight in Box 10.2 for practice suggestions.

Promoting resilience

Over recent years resilience has gained increasing popularity in the literature, research and popular media for its promise to help develop positive developmental outcomes from life, especially following adversity. A classic feature of a resilient person is his or her ability to bounce back, cope and deal with stressful or challenging situations. Initially, resilience was seen as a characteristic of an exceptional individual, and focused on individual personality and variations in response to adversity. Adding a promotive and protective framework to the known personal characteristics of the resilient person led to the understanding that factors that promote resilience could be nurtured prior to adversity within everyone (Masten, Monn & Supkoff, 2011). Resilience is understood as a dynamic process by which individuals utilise available personal characteristics and ecological resources to successfully reflect on and negotiate life as it is faced. Thus, resilient people are able to negotiate their life journey along pathways that lead to positive outcomes and optimal developmental health despite inevitably encountering some form of adversity at some point of time.

Understanding the two broad domains of resilience is important when promoting resilience in practice with individuals and with groups. Firstly, resilience researchers have identified beneficial *personal attributes* including patterns of thought, personality traits, social skills, coping mechanisms, perceptions and decision-making ability in response to stressful situations (Agaibi & Wilson, 2005). Some personal attributes can be learnt; others appear to be inherent and reside at the level of the individual's biology. Such personal attributes enable competent functioning through bidirectional relationships. The second broad domain of resilience is at the level of *interacting systems*, often described as social capital. These systems include the family, friends, school, local community, governance and cultural attributes (Semo, 2011).

Experiencing the benefits of high levels of social cohesion and social capital during childhood and adolescence has been linked to 'better health, improved education outcomes, lower rates of child abuse, lower crime rates, increased productivity, and civic participation' (Semo, 2011, p. 2). Adolescent resilience promotes health over time through strengthening resources beneficial to positive health outcomes both internally (such as interpersonal skills) and externally (enhancing connectedness to family, other caring adults, school and other community groups) (Ahern, 2006; Semo, 2011). Montgomery-Andersen and Borup (2012) identified that social networks are highly developed in indigenous populations where members of the community allow themselves to be adopted by children and young people without large family networks. Such kinship relations help strengthen resilience and should be recognised during health care.

Developing resilience involves the successful adoption of protective factors and the management of risk factors across the interconnected system at the personal, family and community level (Hunter, 2012). Promoting attributes of resilience provides the ecological circumstances and personal skills that permit positive growth over time to occur. Interventions aimed at optimising developmental outcomes of youth through strengthening resilience include: developing interpersonal and communication skills, improving relationships between young people and their parents, assisting families to remain intact, assisting parents to develop parenting skills and finding ways to enhance connectedness at school (Edwards, Mumford & Serra-Roldan, 2007; Masten et al., 2011).

One important finding from resilience research is that neither available resources nor individual skills alone can promote positive youth outcomes and thriving. Individuals access available support systems and resources through effective interpersonal skills and sustained bidirectional relations over time. Resources are necessary, but without the personal skills or means to effectively access these resources, they remain unutilised. Understanding the positive outcomes resilience affords makes it a much needed attribute that should be actively promoted in the lives of young people, families and communities.

Health promotion with young people

A health promotion framework of increasing protective factors while decreasing risk factors provides positive direction for promoting health and wellbeing in young people. Blum as long ago as 1998 (p. 373) noted that risk reduction approaches to health promotion alone do not appear to work, especially with young people, and risk-focused deficit models should change to asset-focused strengths models of health promotion. Risk-reduction health promotion models focus on what not to do, yet provide little guidance about what young people and health professionals can do to optimise positive outcomes. Likewise, enhancing protective factors and addressing risk factors at only one system level, for example focusing on personal behaviours, is unlikely to achieve lasting benefits as the interacting forces from other systems re-establish their influence and mitigate the newly established healthy behaviours. Nonetheless, protective factors and strengths demonstrate powerful moderating ability and reveal that reducing risk factors and increasing protective factors (strengths) enhance developmental outcomes (Blum, McNeely & Nonnemaker, 2002).

The greatest achievements in promoting health for young people and establishing pathways towards positive young adult outcomes can be gained through strengthening family cohesion and reducing the incidence of abuse and maltreatment. Other health promoting activities need to promote broad ecological factors including the availability of caring non-parental adults, positive relationships between young people and teachers, strong cultural identity and a sense of collective belonging within the communities young people belong to (Fourie & Theron, 2012). McMurray and Clendon (2011, p. 222) identify seven major health issues affecting adolescents that health promotion activities should address to 'create healthy pathways to adulthood that overcome risk and promote resilience':

1. mental and emotional health and maturity
2. physical health and wellbeing
3. minimisation of conditions that create risks to health and wellbeing
4. sustainable lifestyle habits
5. healthy environments
6. adolescent-appropriate nursing and health services
7. empowering structures and processes for successive generations.

Promoting strengths and positive attributes focuses on what is working rather than what is going wrong: salutogenic qualities rather than pathogenic ones, resilience over weakness. It examines the strengths that young people, families and communities display, and ways in which they interconnect to act as protective factors and support optimal development and health outcomes. However, without contextualisation, all health-promoting activities may be ineffective since resilience is a contextually specific and culturally based construct.

Clinical focus for nursing the young person

Developing connections in partnership between the nurse, the young person and their family is a key strategy for nursing care of the young person. These connections are particularly important in promoting adolescent health and wellbeing, as they recognise the autonomy of the young person and promote empowering partnerships. In an empowering relationship, the nurse uses their power (skills, knowledge and will) for the other and rejects using power to control others (Balswick, King & Reimer, 2005). Nursing care of the young person attempts to enable the family and the young person in their decision making related to health care. While enabling the family in this process, the nurse needs to remain aware of the struggle for autonomy that the young person is attempting to manage, while they need support from their loved ones when faced with health issues.

The family-strengths perspective (see Chapter 5) lends itself particularly well to nursing young people. Don't let the stereotype that all young people are disengaged from their family delude you. All young people have strength and families are important to young people. Young people, however, can feel disconnected from their family and some are alienated. Parents may feel despondent, worn out and challenged by the transitions and choices of the young person. It is most important for nurses to help young people identify their place in their family, as well as helping families identify their functioning (past and present) strengths and facilitate their further development. These decisions are complicated when the young person is estranged from their parents or hesitant to include them in the decision. When promoting lifestyle choices in health promotion activities, an enabling approach facilitates empowerment and significantly increases the likelihood of long-term benefits being achieved.

Helping young people to be more aware of their connectedness to their family enhances their resilience. The young person should be explicitly asked to identify their family strengths. Identifying and documenting a history of family strengths can act as a significant means of helping the young person and their family draw on their strengths during stressful times (Sittner, DeFrain & Hudson, 2005). Adopting a positive perception of adversity inspires and encourages the young person to know that they have the strength to be resilient, to withstand stressors and to recognise that growth occurs from experiencing stressful conditions and transitions (Wright & Leahey, 2009).

Returning to Becky from our clinical scenario, we can see how important it is that the connections she has in her life are further strengthened and developing the personal skills of problem solving, goal setting and positive cognition. Her connections with her parents, her brother, her friends and her school have been challenged recently. Through a family-strengths perspective, these challenges and stresses can be reframed as transitions that are leading to growth in some relationships while others may be coming to an end. It is through enhancing the strengths in Becky's life across all areas (individual, family and community, as shown in the resilience cycle in Figure 10.1) that resilience is strengthened and her health and wellbeing outcomes are protected and enhanced.

Further challenges that Becky may encounter associated with adolescence include her body image and self-esteem and her ability to be resistant to the misuse of drugs and alcohol. What actions Becky could take are dependent on many factors not identified within this scenario. For now, ensuring Becky feels connected to her family, friends and community is a high priority.

Conclusion

Nursing the young person can incorporate a family-strengths perspective as a basis of nursing care. Nursing actions and attitudes that enable the young person and the family, build connections and relationships and help mobilise strengths are the most effective nursing strategies for enhancing health and development. Nurses increase connectedness to the young person through spending time developing a relationship with the young person, talking about things that matter to them and including the young person and the family in the decision-making process as much as they are able and willing.

The literature indicates that young people face a number of issues that can threaten their health and wellbeing. Some are buffered from these challenges by the family and community strengths and by their own spiritual wellbeing and resilience. Other young people are not so fortunate. The challenge that may impact on youth potential the most is childhood abuse in its many forms. The persistent rate of young Australians experiencing disadvantage and abuse is alarming and unacceptable. A strong society must protect its children and strengthen its young people. A strong society should also protect the children and youth of others – in nations around the world and refugees on their own doorstep. Optimal and acceptable developmental youth outcomes are built on the nurturing and nature of childhood. Concurring with Lerner's (2005) opening statement, developmental plasticity strengthened through protective factors combined with the exuberant engagement of young people in their community leads to the optimistic hope that all young people may one day thrive.

KEY POINTS

Nurses caring for the young person from a family-strengths perspective will seek to:

» look for healthy intentions in the young person and in their family

» support the young person's courage in taking actions towards their desired goals

» collaborate with the whole family (where appropriate) in a partnership that seeks to maintain the family's coherence

» enable the young person through active participation in decision making whenever appropriate (as determined by the young person and the family) and if possible (ensuring negotiation, safe preparation and education has occurred).

CRITICAL QUESTIONS AND REFLECTIONS

1. Assessing family strengths and the young person: utilising the Australian Family Strengths Nursing Assessment Guide found in Chapter 5, Table 5.1, engage in a conversation with a young person whom you know about their family's strengths and how their family functions across the strengths qualities. Explore what goals the young person is currently striving towards concerning their health, wellbeing and family.

2. Do you think that young people under the age of 18 years should have a say in decisions impacting on their health outcomes?

3. If Becky continues to neglect to take her asthma preventers and experiences an acute episode requiring hospitalisation, should she be charged for the healthcare treatment even if treated in a public hospital?

4. Considering the inequality of Indigenous Australian and Māori youth health statistics, what right does a government have to place restrictions on some indigenous communities, such as alcohol-free zones, but not on others? (See useful resource by Lohoar.)

5. Since volunteering and community connectedness are associated with better youth outcomes, should volunteering be a compulsory part of after-school 'homework' for all young people attending school?

6. As a community nurse offering a service that engages with young people living on the street, you become aware of a parent's attempt to locate one of your clients. The young person refuses to contact their family and will not discuss their decision with you. Should you inform the parents that you know where their family member is and how they are doing?

USEFUL RESOURCES

Adolescent Health Research Group NZ: http://www.fmhs.auckland.ac.nz/faculty/ahrg/

Australian Research Alliance for Children and Youth: http://www.aracy.org.au/

Centre for Adolescent Health: http://www.rch.org.au/cah/

Lohoar S 2012, *Safe and supportive Indigenous families and communities for children: A synopsis and critique of Australian research*. AIFS, Melbourne: http://www.aifs.gov.au/cfca/pubs/papers/a142302/index.html

New South Wales Centre for the Advancement of Adolescent Health: http://www.caah.chw.edu.au/

University of Nebraska – Lincoln, UNL for families: http://www.ianrpubs.unl.edu/epublic/pages/index.jsp?what=subjectAreasD&subjectAreasId=12

UNICEF *Adolescents and youth*: http://www.unicef.org/adolescence/index_3970.html

UNICEF *The state of the world's children 2011: Adolescence – An age of opportunity*: http://www.unicef.org/sowc2011/

World Health Organization *Adolescent health*: http://www.who.int/topics/adolescent_health/en/

References

Adolescent Health Research Group (2008). *Youth '07: The health and wellbeing of secondary school students in New Zealand*. Technical report. Auckland: The University of Auckland.

Agaibi, C. & Wilson, J. (2005). Trauma, PTSD, and resilience: a review of the literature. *Trauma, Violence, & Abuse, 6*(3), 195–216.

Ahern, A. (2010). Modernity. In A. J. Mills, G. Durepos, & E. Wiebe (Eds.), Encyclopaedia of case study research (vol 2, pp. 564–567). Los Angeles: Sage.

Ahern, N. R. (2006). Adolescent resilience: an evolutionary concept analysis. *Journal of Pediatric Nursing, 21*(3), 175–185.

Australian Institute of Health and Welfare (AIHW) (2011). *Young Australians: their health and wellbeing 2011* [Cat. no. PHE 140]. Canberra: AIHW.

Australian Institute of Health and Welfare (AIHW) (2012). *Social and emotional wellbeing: development of a Children's Headline Indicator* [Cat. no. PHE158]. Canberra: AIHW.

Australian Research Alliance for Children and Youth (ARACY) (2008). *The wellbeing of young Australians: Technical report*. Canberra: ARACY.

Balswick, J., King, P., & Reimer, K. (2005). *The reciprocating self. Human development in theological perspective*. Illinois: InterVarsity Press.

Blum, R. (1998). Healthy youth development as a model for youth health promotion: a review. *Journal of Adolescent Health, 22*, 368–375.

Blum, R. & Ireland, M. (2004). Reducing risk, increasing protective factors: findings from the Caribbean Youth Health Survey. *Journal of Adolescent Health, 35*, 493–500.

Blum, R., McNeely, C., & Nonnemaker, J. (2002). Vulnerability, risk and protection. *Journal of Adolescent Health, 31*(1 Suppl), 28–39.

Bronfenbrenner, U. (2001). The bioecological theory of human development. Article 1 in U. Bronfenbrenner (Ed.), *Making human beings human: biological perspectives on human development*. Thousand Oaks, California: Sage, 2005.

Bronfenbrenner, U. & Ceci, S. (1994). Nature–nurture reconceptualized in developmental perspective: a bioecological model. *Psychological Review, 101*(4), 568–586.

Bronfenbrenner, U. & Morris, P. (1998). The bioecological model of human development. In: L. Damon & R. Lerner (Eds.), *Handbook of child psychology* (6th edn., vol. 1, pp. 795–829). Lerner R (Ed.), *Theoretical models of human development*. Hoboken, New Jersey: John Wiley, 2006.

Carlisle, S., Henderson, G., & Hanlon, P. W. (2009). Wellbeing: a collateral casualty of modernity. *Social Science & Medicine, 69*(10), 1556–1560.

Carlsson, A., Bramhagen, A.-C., Jansson, A., & Dykes, A. K. (2011). Precautions taken by mothers to prevent burn and scald injuries to young children at home: an intervention study. *Scandinavian Journal of Public Health, 39*, 471–478.

Clark, T. C., Robinson, E., Crengle, S., et al. (2008). *Te Ara Whakapiki Taitamariki. Youth '07: The health and wellbeing of secondary school students in New Zealand. Results for Māori young people*. Auckland: The University of Auckland.

Cotton, S., Larkin, E., Hoopes, A., Cromer, B., & Rosenthal, S. (2005). The impact of adolescent spirituality on depressive symptoms and health risk behaviors. *Journal of Adolescent Health, 36*(6:529e), 7–14.

de Souza, M., Cartwright, P., & McGilp, J. E. (2004). The perceptions of young people who live in a regional city in Australia of their spiritual wellbeing: implications for education. *Journal of Youth Studies, 7*(2), 155–172.

Edwards, O. W., Mumford, V. E., & Serra-Roldan, R. (2007). A positive youth development model for students considered at-risk. *School Psychology International*, *28*(1), 29–45.

Fourie, C. & Theron, L. (2012). Resilience in the face of Fragile X Syndrome. *Qualitative Health Research*, *22*(10), 1355–1368.

Godin, P. (2006). *Risk and nursing practice*. Hampshire: Palgrave Macmillan.

Green, L. (2010). *Understanding the life course. Sociological and psychological perspectives*. Cambridge UK: Polity.

Hawkins, M. T., Villagonzalo, K., Sanson, A. V., et al. (2012). Associations between positive development in late adolescence and social, health, and behavioral outcomes in young adulthood. *Journal of Adult Development*, *19*(2), 88–99.

Hayes, A. (2008). Are family changes, social trends and unanticipated policy consequences making children's lives more challenging? *Family Matters*, *78*, 60–63.

Hunter, C. (2012). *Is resilience still a useful concept when working with children and young people?* CFCA paper no. 2. Melbourne: Australian Institute of Family Studies.

Johnstone, M. & Lee, C. (2012). Young Australian women and their aspirations: "It's hard enough thinking a week or two in advance at the moment". *Journal of Adolescent Research*, *27*(3), 351–376.

Keating, D. P. & Hertzman, C. (1999). *Developmental health and the wealth of nations: Social, biological, and educational dynamics*. New York: Guilford Press.

Lerner, R. (2005). Forward. In U. Bronfenbrenner (Ed.), *Making human beings human: Bioecological perspectives on human development*. Thousand Oaks: Sage.

Lerner, R. M., Alberts, A., Anderson, P. M., & Dowling, E. (2006). On making humans human: Spirituality and promotion of positive youth development. In E. C. Roehlkepartain, P. E. King, L. Wagener, & P. Benson (Eds.), *The handbook of spiritual development in childhood and adolescence* (pp. 60–72). Thousand Oaks: Sage.

Li, J., McMurray, A., & Stanley, F. (2008). Modernity's paradox and the structural determinants of child health and wellbeing. *Health Sociology Review*, *17*(1), 64–77.

Lupton, D. (1999). *Risk*. London: Routledge.

Males, M. (2009). Does the adolescent brain make risk taking inevitable? A skeptical appraisal. *Journal of Adolescent Research*, *24*(1), 3–20.

Mason, M., Singleton, A., & Webber, R. (2007). *The spirit of generation Y: Young people's spirituality in a changing Australia*. Melbourne: John Garratt Publishing.

Masten, A., Monn, A., & Supkoff, L. (2011). Resilience in children and adolescents. In S. Southwick, B. Litz, D. Charney, et al. (Eds.), *Resilience and mental health: Challenges across the lifespan* (pp. 103–119). Cambridge: Cambridge University Press.

McMurray, A. & Clendon, J. (2011). *Community health and wellness. Primary health care in practice* (4th ed.). Sydney: Elsevier.

Montgomery-Andersen, R. A. & Borup, I. (2012). Family support and the child as health promoting agent in the Arctic – "the Inuit way". *Rural and Remote Health*, *12*, 1977. Retrieved from http://www.rrh.org.au (accessed 17 January 2013).

Myers, D. (2008). Religion and human flourishing. In M. Eid & R. Larsen (Eds.), *The science of subjective well-being* (pp. 323–346). New York: Guilford Press.

O'Connor, M., Sanson, A., Hawkins, M., et al. (2011). Predictors of positive development in emerging adulthood. *Journal of Youth and Adolescence*, *40*, 860–874.

Price-Robertson, R., Smart, D., & Bromfield, L. (2010). Family is for life. Connections between childhood family experiences and wellbeing in early adulthood. *Family Matters*, *85*, 7–17.

Riesch, S., Brown, R., Anderson, L., et al. (2012). Strengthening families program (10–14): effects on the family environment. *Western Journal of Nursing Research*, *34*(3), 340–376.

Roehlkepartain, E. C., Benson, P. L., Scales, P. C., Kimball, L., & King, P. (2008). *With their own voices: A global exploration of how today's young people experience and think about spiritual development*. Minnesota: Search Institute.

Rowold, J. (2011). Effects of spiritual well-being on subsequent happiness, psychological well-being and stress. *Journal of Religion and Health*, *50*, 950–963.

Rutter, M. (2006). *Genes and behavior: Nature–nurture interplay explained*. Oxford, UK: Blackwell.

Sanders, M. R. (2008). Triple P – Positive Parenting Program as public health approach to strengthening parenting. *Journal of Family Psychology*, *22*(3), 506–517.

Semo, R. (2011). *Longitudinal Surveys of Australian Youth briefing paper 26: Social capital and young people*. Canberra: NCVER.

Sittner, B., DeFrain, J., & Hudson, D. (2005). Effects of high risk pregnancies on families. *American Journal of Maternal Child Nursing*, *30*(2), 121–126.

Smith, L. (2011). *Spiritual wellbeing and its relationship to adolescent resilience. A case study of Australian youth attending one local church*. PhD dissertation. Melbourne: Australian Catholic University.

Statistics New Zealand and Ministry of Pacific Island Affairs (2011). *Health and Pacific peoples in New Zealand*. Wellington: Statistics New Zealand and Ministry of Pacific Island Affairs.

Stoll, L., Michaelson, J., & Seaford, C. (2012). *Well-being evidence for policy: A review*. London: New Economics Foundation.

Wauchop, S. (2010). *Ten going on sixteen: A profile of young New Zealanders in the transition years*. Wellington: Ministry of Youth Development.

Wilkinson, R. & Marmot, M. (2003). *Social determinants of health: The solid facts* (2nd ed.). Copenhagen, Denmark: World Health Organization Regional Office for Europe. Retrieved from http://www.euro.who.int/__data/assets/pdf_file/0005/98438/e81384.pdf (accessed 17 January 2013).

Wright, L. & Leahey, M. (2009). *Nurses and families: A guide to family assessment and intervention* (5th ed.). Philadelphia: FA Davis.

Wyn, J. (2009). The changing context of Australian youth and its implications for social inclusion. *Youth Studies Australia*, *28*(1), 46–50.

Young, T. K. (2005). Population health. Concepts and methods (2nd ed.). New York: Oxford University Press.

Chapter 11

CHILDREN WITH CHRONIC HEALTH PROBLEMS AND THEIR FAMILIES

Jon Darvill, Kay Thomas, Pamela Henry

LEARNING OUTCOMES

Reading this chapter will help you to:

» identify common chronic health problems in Australia and New Zealand

» describe the epidemiological incidences and trends of these health problems

» recognise that children themselves have a perspective on their lives, health and nursing care

» reiterate in broad terms the best practice management approach to children with chronic health problems and their families

» identify issues around the transition from paediatric to adult-based services

» integrate current research findings into your nursing practice

» adopt a culturally sensitive approach to nursing care of children and families with differing cultural practices

» discuss the additional needs and challenges facing technology-dependent children and their families

» describe issues around the preparation for and discharge of technology-dependent children from hospitals

» identify the issues surrounding the provision of high levels of nursing care in the family home.

Introduction

Chronic diseases produce symptoms and develop over a long period of time. They are often complex and account for significant illness, disability and death in developed countries. 'A chronic condition is an ongoing impairment characterised by a physical or mental condition, functional limitation, and service use or need beyond routine care' (Australian Institute of Health and Welfare, 2007).

Chronic conditions may:

* disrupt normal growth and development
* affect social and emotional development
* place children and their families under social, psychological and economic pressure (Australian Institute of Health and Welfare, 2009; Dell'Api, Rennick & Rosmus, 2007).

The impact on the child and family depends on how severe the condition is, the effects on day-to-day living and how well it is managed or treated (Australian Institute of Health and Welfare, 2009).

This chapter focuses on Australian and New Zealand children with chronic health problems and their families. It identifies the extent of these problems and their impact on children and families and presents evidence of best practice management. The encompassed overarching assumptions begin with a comprehensive primary healthcare (PHC) approach (i.e. the philosophical basis for the wide range of activities that promote health and wellbeing using primary, secondary and tertiary prevention strategies and fostering the partnership between community members and health professionals) (McMurray & Clendon, 2011). Importantly, children and young people are considered as individuals in their own right and collaborative models of care are promoted.

After discussing aspects of chronic health in children and young people, two clinical scenarios are used to introduce specific topics. Issues that are relevant not only to the specific scenario but also to the wider population are discussed. The first scenario focuses on a young person with diabetes mellitus and the second is an infant who is dependent on technology for her survival.

Chronic health problems in children and young people

Chronic diseases in children and young people differ from those in adulthood in several ways. These include types and presentations of diseases, their risk factors and their incidence. Importantly, a chronic disease in a child affects not only the child but also their family. Although chronic disease is predominantly seen in adults, there is a significant number of children with long-term health problems. In 2006, 36.5% of New Zealand children had a chronic health problem and 2% had a psychiatric or psychological problem (Ministry of Health, 2008; Statistics New Zealand, 2007). In Australia, 41% of children suffer from a long-term problem (Australian Institute of Health and Welfare, 2009). In both countries these data include relatively minor conditions such as those associated with allergy (hay fever and allergic rhinitis) and vision.

The chronic diseases responsible for the greatest disease burden in children are outlined below. Rather than coronary artery disease, stroke and chronic obstructive pulmonary disease (COPD) seen in adulthood, in Australia childhood asthma, diabetes mellitus, cancer and mental health problems are designated national health priorities (Australian Institute of Health and Welfare, 2009, 2011). In New Zealand asthma is the most common chronic disease in children and young people, with diabetes mellitus, epilepsy and cancer also causing considerable morbidity and impacting on the healthcare system (Ministry of Health, 2008, 2011). Rheumatic fever amongst Māori and Pacific Islander children is also a national priority in New Zealand with the Ministry of Health establishing a national program in 2011 (Ministry of Health, 2012). Other children's chronic conditions include, but are not limited to, cystic fibrosis, cerebral palsy, learning disabilities, visual impairment, allergies and the consequences of injury. Psychosocial health issues include conditions such as depression/anxiety, attention deficit hyperactivity disorder (ADHD) and autism.

In an international context the World Health Organization (WHO) (2008) lists both New Zealand and Australia as high-income countries. As such the burden of disease differs from, for example, African and South-east Asian countries where there is significant mortality and morbidity amongst children from infectious diseases such as diarrhoea, pneumonia, HIV/AIDS and malaria (WHO, 2008) rather than chronic conditions.

Some trends in epidemiological data are available. Although the incidences of asthma in Australia are unchanged (trend not available for New Zealand), the incidences of both type 1 and type 2 diabetes mellitus in children and young people are rising in both countries (Australian Institute of Health and Welfare, 2009; Ministry of Health, 2010). In the past, type 2 was predominantly seen in people over 40 years of age; however, this is changing. Type 2 is associated with obesity and a sedentary lifestyle, both modifiable risk factors (Australian Institute of Health and Welfare, 2009).

Lifestyle risk factors for developing adult chronic diseases are also risk factors in children and young people. One particular concern is the proportion of children and young people whose weight is unhealthy. This has increased over the past two decades in both countries but the numbers seem to be stabilising (Bell, Curran, Byrne et al., 2011; Ministry of Health, 2010, 2011). There are no trend data for mental health disorders in Australia. In New Zealand there has been a downward trend in secondary school boys with depression but no change in girls (Fortune, Watson, Robinson et al., 2010). Tables 11.1 and 11.2 set out further information on the status of chronic diseases and the lifestyle concerns, respectively, in both Australia and New Zealand.

In addition to lifestyle risk factors for developing the classic chronic health problems of adulthood during childhood, others can occur early in life and are

TABLE 11.1 Leading chronic health problems in Australia and New Zealand for children and young people

PREVALENCE AND TRENDS	KEY POINTS
Diabetes mellitus	
Australia Type 1 (0–14 years old) 23/100,000 Increased from 19/100,000 in 2000 Type 2 is also thought to be increasing based on small reports, as national data are not collected No reliable national data for indigenous children (Australian Institute of Health and Welfare, 2009) *New Zealand* Type 1 (0–14 years old) Incidence has doubled over the past 3 decades Incidence is 5.6/100,000 for Māori and 21.7/100,000 for non-Māori (Ministry of Health, 2011) Type 2 (10–14 years old) Increasing incidence 1.8% in 1996 to 11% in 2002 in Auckland In this cohort, the mean BMI was 34.6 kg/m², 85% have dyslipidaemia and 28% have systolic hypertension Generally, incidence in Māori and Pacific Islanders > non-Māori (Māori 6.1/100,000 and 1.23/100,000 for European descent) (Ministry of Health, 2011)	Intensive control of blood glucose levels (BGL) reduces the risk of complications; HbA_{1c} is a blood test used to monitor BGL over time; it is difficult to achieve HbA_{1c} targets in children and adolescents without increasing the risk of severe hypoglycaemia Being <6 years old is also a risk factor for severe hypoglycaemia (Craig Twigg, Donaghue et al., 2011) Early signs of long-term complications in type 1: micro-albuminuria seen in 20% of children and adolescents and 50% have some degree of neuropathy; most will develop non-proliferative retinopathy (Craig et al., 2011) Other concerns are impact on cognitive function, increased prevalence of psychosocial disorders, anxiety, major depression and other psychiatric disorders (Craig et al., 2011)

TABLE 11.1 Continued

PREVALENCE AND TRENDS	KEY POINTS
Asthma	
Australia Incidence may be stabilising after increases in 1980s–1990s: in 2004–05 12% of children 0–14 years old had long-term asthma; Indigenous children 3% higher (Australian Institute of Health and Welfare, 2009) The mortality rate for children <15 years old has doubled from 2005 to 2010 (Australian Institute of Health and Welfare, 2009; National Asthma Council, 2012)	*Australia* Mortality is low in comparison to 1989 (964 deaths) but has doubled (7% to 17%), perhaps indicting parental complacency (National Asthma Council, 2012) There is a strong link between asthma and allergy; 40% of children with asthma live with smokers (National Asthma Council, 2006) Asthma hospital admissions have declined significantly over the past decade (Australian Institute of Health and Welfare, 2009)
New Zealand 25% of children aged 6–7 years and 30% of adolescents 13–14 years report asthma symptoms (Loring, 2009); 1 in 7 or 14.8% of children (2–14 years) take medication for asthma No significant difference was found on the NZ Deprivation Index, an index of socioeconomic deprivation based on geographical areas (Ministry of Health, 2008; Salmond, Crampton & Atkinson, 2007).	*New Zealand* Asthma is the most common cause of hospital admission for children and has doubled over the past 30 years Incidence is slightly higher in Māori children than non-Māori; however, Māori children suffer more frequent and severe asthma symptoms and hospitalisations and have higher mortality rates (Loring, 2009)
Cancer	
Australia Incidence of cancers in 0–14-year-olds is 14/100,000 with 55% in boys; in children 0–4 years it is 21/100,000 Most common is lymphoid leukaemia, then brain cancer and myeloid leukaemia No reliable national data for indigenous children (Australian Institute of Health and Welfare, 2009)	*Australia* Incidence is stable but the 5-year survival rate is improving Leukaemia has the highest survival rate and brain cancers are the leading cause of mortality of all childhood cancers (Australian Institute of Health and Welfare, 2009)

New Zealand Among 0–24-year-olds in 2003–2007, acute lymphoblastic leukaemia (ALL) was 5.26% of all reported cancers peaking in the 2–5-year-old group Carcinoma in-situ of the cervix was 60.4% of all reported cancers and peaked in early 20s (Ministry of Health, 2011)	*New Zealand* No significant difference in socioeconomic groups, gender or ethnicity for ALL Leading cause of cancer mortality is cancer of the brain, then ALL and bone cancers Incidence of carcinoma in-situ of the cervix is highest in Europeans, then Māori, then Pacific people and Asians; it is lowest in areas of low socioeconomic deprivation (Ministry of Health, 2011)
Mental health	
Australia In 2007, 9% of 16–24-year-olds had high or very high levels of stress and 26% experienced at least 1 mental disorder in the previous 12 months (AIHW, 2011)	*Australia* Most common conditions are anxiety and depression; no clear trend or data not available
New Zealand In 2007, 50% of secondary school students had very good–excellent emotional and mental health; 7.6% boys and 11.2% girls had some indication of a mental health problem; 6.9% boys and 14.7% girls had depression (Fortune et al., 2010)	*New Zealand* Since 2001, depression in boys has fallen but remained the same in girls
Internationally The Pediatric Cancer Genome Project data, released in 2012, provides previously unknown genetic information about childhood cancers and therefore more avenues for further research (St Jude Children's Research Hospital and Washington University, 2012)	

TABLE 11.2 Lifestyle factors of concern for children and young people in Australia and New Zealand

Unhealthy weight

Australia Over one in five (23%) children and adolescents were overweight or obese in 2007 (22% in 1995) There is little difference between genders No national data for indigenous children exist but self-reported rates for indigenous adults are higher (Australian Institute of Health and Welfare, 2005, 2009) *New Zealand* In 2002, of children aged 5–14 years, 21.3% were overweight and 9.8% were obese The prevalence is greater amongst Pacific Islander and Māori populations than New Zealand Europeans and others (Ministry of Health, 2006) Mean BMI has not changed in later trend data (Ministry of Health, 2011)	The epidemiological triad of obesity: host (the individual) environment vectors of obesity (factors that promote obesity): high-energy foods and drinks, labour-saving devices and television and computers (Lean, Lara & O'Hill, 2006) Being overweight or obese increases the risk of poor physical and psychological health; it is a risk factor for further health problems in adulthood (Australian Institute of Health and Welfare, 2009) Numbers in both countries seem to be stabilising (Bell et al., 2011; Ministry of Health, 2010, 2011)

Physical activity

Australia 74% of 9–14-year-old children met physical activity guidelines i.e. >60 minutes moderate activity daily 33% met screen time guidelines (i.e. no more than 2 hours non-educational screen time/day) (Australian Institute of Health and Welfare, 2009) *New Zealand* 47% of children 5–14 years old use an active means of transport to school (Ministry of Health, 2008)	Regular physical activity and good nutrition reduce cardiovascular risk, improve overweight, high blood pressure and type 2 diabetes; they protect against some cancers and strengthen the musculoskeletal system >2 hours of screen time/day is associated with overweight, less physical activity, fewer social interactions, consuming more sugary drinks and unhealthy snacks (Australian Institute of Health and Welfare, 2009)

Nutrition

Australia 50–60% of 4–13-year-olds meet daily requirements for fruit intake but only 2–3% consumed daily requirement for vegetables (Australian Institute of Health and Welfare, 2009) *New Zealand* 19.6% of children 2–14 years old drank >3 fizzy drinks in a week and 7.2% ate takeaway food at least 3 times in a week; percentages were higher for Māori and Pacific Islander people and in lower socioeconomic areas (Ministry of Health, 2008)	Consumption of 'fizzy' drinks and fast food (> twice/week) are associated with being overweight or obese (Ministry of Health, 2008)

TABLE 11.2 Continued

Smoking	
Australia Declining number of households where someone is smoking inside (31% in 1995 – 8% in 2007); highest amongst lower socioeconomic status and indigenous homes 5.4% of 12–14-year-olds are current smokers (Australian Institute of Health and Welfare, 2009) *New Zealand* In 2006–07, 9.6% of children were exposed to cigarette smoke in their homes; the risk of exposure was higher (2-fold) for Māori children and children in low socioeconomic areas 1 in 7 15–17-year-olds are current smokers (Ministry of Health, 2008)	Passive smoking is associated with a variety of respiratory problems, including asthma and SIDS as well as other diseases (e.g. otitis media) and slow lung growth (Australian Institute of Health and Welfare, 2009) Smoking affects most body organs and causes short-term problems such as respiratory diseases and lack of fitness; it also increases the risk of chronic diseases in adulthood (Australian Institute of Health and Welfare, 2009)
Alcohol consumption	
Australia In 2005, 2.6% of children between 12 and 14 years old engaged in risky drinking the previous week *New Zealand* In 2005–06 almost 21% of males 15–17 years old reported hazardous drinking patterns, rising to over 50% for 18–24-year-olds; female figures in equivalent age groups were 17% rising to 32% The likelihood of hazardous drinking is higher amongst Māori and Pacific people and in lower socioeconomic areas (Ministry of Health, 2008)	Alcohol health problems in children and adolescents relate to risky or 'binge' drinking (i.e. five or more drinks in one drinking session); this can lead to alcohol poisoning, accidents, violence and unprotected sex Chronic problems such as addiction, organ damage, depression and relationship problems may occur (NDARC, 2004, cited in Australian Institute of Health and Welfare, 2009) Chronic diseases, including cancers of the digestive system, cirrhosis of the liver, brain damage and fetal alcohol syndrome may occur (Australian Institute of Health and Welfare, 2009)

unique to childhood. See Table 1.1 in Chapter 1 for a summary of risk and protective factors. For example, a low birth weight (<2500 g) increases the risk of some cardiac, respiratory and renal diseases and type 2 diabetes (Australian Institute of Health and Welfare, 2009).

Chronic childhood health problems have differing patterns of presentation. Some are congenital; some develop later in life; and some the child 'grows out of'.

However, most require health care beyond the norm to enable the child to live a normal or near normal life (Australian Institute of Health and Welfare, 2009).

In summary, the key points derived from these epidemiological data are the following:

- Most children and young people are healthy in Australia and New Zealand.
- Chronic diseases exist in children, are different in several respects from those that occur in adults and impact on the whole family.
- Areas of concern relate to lifestyle risk factors and mental health issues.

The stories of Josie and Tihema and their families will personalise these data. Josie is a young person with a chronic disease.

Clinical scenario 11.1
Josie - a young person with a chronic disease

Josie has just turned 13 years old. She presents to the emergency department with her 15-year-old sister, Michelle. Josie says she is feeling really tired and has been 'vomiting'. The triage nurse begins an assessment and, during the history taking, discovers Josie has a history of type 1 diabetes mellitus. Type 1 is more common in children and young people and is characterised by the need for insulin replacement. It is an autoimmune disease, it has no known factors that prevent or delay its onset (Craig et al., 2011) and its incidence in Australasia is rising (see Table 11.1).

Josie is diagnosed with diabetic ketoacidosis (DKA) and has 5% dehydration. She is rehydrated, treated with insulin and admitted to the paediatric high dependency unit (HDU).

During her admission, a multidisciplinary team (i.e. nursing staff, the paediatric endocrinologist, diabetes educator, nutritionist and social worker) care for her.

Josie is experiencing an acute exacerbation of a chronic disease. While she requires hospitalisation and acute care now, this is a short interlude in her ongoing primary healthcare management. How Josie came to develop DKA and the fact that she presented with her sister rather than a parent are specific areas of concern for her health professionals. These may indicate she is having trouble at home. Further, there are issues facing both the individual with a chronic disease and their family, beginning with the impact of the initial diagnosis of the disease.

Diagnosis and its impact on children and their families

Josie was diagnosed with diabetes mellitus at the age of 2 years. She was living with her mother, father and sister, Michelle, who was then 4 years old. For the family, Josie's diagnosis changed their lives. The diagnosis of a chronic illness signals the end of the known world for the family and its individual members. Uncertainty and a period in which the family attempts to adapt follow. The range of responses can be conceptualised as a continuum reflecting;

- the difficulties the families have in their adaptation (Hentinen & Kyngäs, 1998; Knafl & Deatrick, 2006)

- whether individuals' experiences are similar or different (Knafl & Deatrick, 2006)
- the degree of stability within the parenting relationship (Darvill, 2003).

Families often struggle with the emotional impact, the additional stress that is encountered and the loss of important aspects of their lives. In a meta-synthesis of the literature pertaining to the impact on parents with a chronically ill child, Kepreotes, Keatinge and Stone (2010) identified a major impact as being chronic grief and sadness. The emotional impact is often ongoing with peaks of intensity at critical moments, such as if the child is not achieving a developmental milestone, transitional times including starting school and puberty or when the child is having an acute exacerbation related to their condition (Melnyk, Feinstein, Moldenhouer & Small, 2001). Barlow and Ellard (2006) found that 5 years from diagnosis, the parents can still experience a range of issues. They may be fearful and uncertain or even display symptoms of post-traumatic stress. They are also likely to worry about their child's future and health. In contrast, the authors noted positive outcomes such as good support systems, the development of new values and attitudes and increased bonding within marital relationships and families.

Parents are not the only ones who suffer. The children, both those with a chronic disease and their siblings, may also suffer. In addition to the consequences of the disease itself, 15–30% of affected children are at risk of emotional or behavioural problems (Fee & Hinton, 2011). The affected child may have difficulty adjusting to their circumstances, miss school, lose touch with friends and, therefore, risk social isolation. They may feel different, anxious and depressed, have a poor self-concept and lower self-esteem (Barlow & Ellard, 2006). Conversely some children will show resilience, which in one study was related to the degree of social support and parental adjustment rather than the severity of the disease (Fee & Hinton, 2011).

Siblings may also have psychosocial problems. The severity of the affected sibling's illness can be related to this, as can the sibling receiving less attention from their parent(s) or experiencing disruption to family plans or outings (Barlow & Ellard, 2006).

It is clear that having a chronically ill child in the family has the potential to impact on the psychosocial wellbeing of the family as a whole. An important goal of parents and children is normality and most families and children will strive to normalise and incorporate their new situations into their daily lives (Darvill, Harrington & Donovan, 2009; Knafl, Deatrick & Havill, 2012; Knafl & Deatrick, 2002).

Normalising

Normalisation is a dynamic process that changes over time. It entails two conceptual processes:

1. how individual members perceive their new situation
2. how they consequently manage the child (Deatrick, Knafl & Murphy-Moore, 1999).

Normalisation is seen in families who focus on the normal aspects of their child rather than focusing on what is different. This affects their management (Knafl & Deatrick, 2006) and enables them to eventually see their lives as normal and to manage the illness successfully (Deatrick, Thibodeaux, Mooney et al., 2006). Some families are successful in their adaptation, while others are not (Knafl, Darney, Gallo & Angst, 2010). See Table 11.3 for parental perceptions of family life in families that have normalised and those that have not.

TABLE 11.3 The parents' perceptions of normalisation

	WHEN NORMALISATION IS PRESENT	WHEN NORMALISATION IS ABSENT
Family management of the condition	'Doing a good job' (i.e. leading a normal family life)	'Living a difficult life' (i.e. condition management precludes a normal life)
Parental role	Parenting competence (i.e. leading and confident in their management); child doing well; parental effort part of normal parenting role; successful work/family balance; fleeting feelings of guilt and inadequacy; challenges diminishing over time	Parenting self-doubt (i.e. atypical nature of parenting); diminished sense of parenting competence; feelings of inadequacy, guilt, uncertainty compromise parenting; dissatisfied with parenting role; challenges unchanging and extraordinary; unchanged by child doing well
Impact on family life	Recognition of positive outcomes (i.e. identified unexpected positive aspects)	Focus on negative outcomes (i.e. focused on negative outcomes of both the individual and the family)

Adapted from Knafl et al. (2010).

Normalisation is obviously a more desirable outcome for families with a chronically ill child or adolescent and recognition of this is important. Knafl et al. (2010) propose the following interventions by nurses or other health professionals to assist in the normalising process and to help integrate the management of the child's condition into the family's daily life:

- assess parents' perception of and desire for a 'normal life'
- adapt treatment regimens to the family's circumstances, schedules and goals
- provide opportunities for the child to have a normal life
- help parents determine when a focus on condition management is appropriate
- identify strategies to reduce the burden of managing the child's condition (e.g. link struggling parents with those who have achieved normalisation).

In addition to normalising, families may adopt what Knafl, Breitmayer, Gallo and Zoeller (1996) described as a family management style (FMS). An FMS framework describes how the family incorporates managing the child's condition into family life (Knafl et al., 2012). The framework is based on a continuum of five management styles: thriving, accommodating, enduring, struggling and floundering. Examples are:

- *The 'thriving' style:* families are confident about their ability to manage both usual and unexpected demands; the treatment required is seen as proactive.
- *The 'struggling' style:* there is parental conflict based on differing views of the child's illness and their expectations of each other (Deatrick et al., 2006).

In a review of the FMS framework, further management styles have been identified, changes to the socio-cultural component have been proposed and other changes made enabling broader applications of the framework (Knafl et al., 2012).

Josie's mother and father were shocked at the diagnosis of a chronic disease requiring complex management. They watched their child suffer while undergoing medical treatment. They had to perform painful procedures such as blood glucose monitoring and injections of insulin themselves. Further, they lost a certain freedom in their lives as a new regimen was required to manage Josie's diabetes.

The child's perspective

Until recently, the point of view or voice of children with chronic illness has been ignored. Historically, children's perspectives have not been sought by qualitative researchers for two reasons. First, children are vulnerable to exploitation and, second, they have been thought of as incapable of participation. In Chapter 4, a discussion of ethical principles, guidelines and practice concerning research with children and young people is presented. Children are vulnerable, but this is not a reason to exclude them from active engagement. As helpful as developmental theories are, the division of a child's life into developmental stages has constantly forced comparisons between children and adults. It highlights what children are incapable of rather than what they can do. This could be called a deficit model of children (Woodgate, 2001).

It is increasingly recognised that children are capable of communicating thoughts and feelings on their health and that they are in the best position to do so (Darvill et al., 2009). Sartain, Clarke and Heyman (2000) explored the experiences of chronically ill children, their parents and health professionals. They found that the children (8–14 years old) were effective participants in research and their voices indicated that they were not a homogeneous group, but reacted to and coped with hospitalisation in different ways. Such findings must impact on nursing research and practice, and guide development that includes children in consultation and decision making regarding not only individual care but also potentially service planning and policy (Australian Capital Territory Government, 2010; Steinbeck & Brodie, 2006).

Adolescents: young people in transition

Josie is 13 years old. She, like other young people, is in transition. There are several aspects to her transition. Firstly, she is between childhood and adulthood physically, emotionally and mentally. Secondly, Josie will increasingly become responsible for managing her diabetes. Thirdly, over the next few years, she must also transition from the group of health professionals she knows to those in the unknown world of adult health care.

The diabetes educator speaks to Josie during her admission. The educator feels that the most likely cause of Josie's ketoacidosis is that she was not complying with her insulin administration.

COMPLIANCE WITH TREATMENT AND SELF-MANAGEMENT

Compliance (or adherence) and self-management are overlapping but separate concepts. Compliance can best be defined as how closely an individual follows medical advice

---

Box 11.1 Research highlight: Self-report measure for self-management of adolescents with type 1 diabetes mellitus

Although not the first tool developed to assess the self-management of diabetes by young people, the tool developed and tested by Schilling et al. (2009) has expanded the scope of other tools to provide a more holistic measure of an individual's self-management. The tool covers aspects of the young person's relationship with parents and healthcare providers and the goals of self-management in addition to how well they comply with treatment. The tool consists of five subscales, each focusing on an aspect of self-management. The subscales are:

» collaboration with parents
» diabetes care activities
» diabetes problems solving
» diabetes communication
» goals.

Each subscale can be used independently and a total score is not required. The study found the tool had excellent content validity and acceptable subscale reliability.

See Schilling, L. S., Dixon, J. K., Knafl, K. A. et al. (2009) A new self-report measure of self-management of type I diabetes for adolescents. *Nursing Research, 58,* 228.

(Schilling et al., 2009). Self-management refers to a more complex concept involving collaborative partnerships between the young person, their parents and health professionals as the young person moves towards independently managing their care (Schilling, Grey & Knafl, 2002; Schilling et al., 2009). Both concepts focus on the clinical control of blood glucose. A third concept, 'assuming responsibility for self-care', reflects the developmental milestone that must be achieved by the young person (i.e. to independently manage their diabetes) (Hanna & Decker, 2010). Difficulties with compliance, self-management or the developmental processes present problems that are complex and difficult to resolve. Schilling et al. (2009) have developed an assessment tool to measure the self-management of adolescents with diabetes that will assist in the evaluation of management interventions (see Box 11.1, Research highlight).

There could be many reasons why Josie was not administering enough insulin to herself. These may relate to her knowledge of diabetes and its treatment or the social context in which she lives – such things as parental support and supervision or how comfortable she feels with her peers knowing she has diabetes and needs injections. These and other factors could affect her motivation and subsequent behaviours. For example, is she exhibiting risk-taking behaviour or withholding insulin as a weight-loss scheme?

It is estimated that approximately 50% of young people with a chronic health problem do not comply with their treatment regimen at some time (Kyngäs, 2007). However, being a young person in itself is not the issue, as non-compliance figures are similar in adults. Predicting who is likely to comply, and for what reasons, is also important. In a recent Australian study using an assessment tool adapted for Australia, Wales, Crisp, Fernandes and Kyngäs (2011) found several factors that were associated with treatment compliance in an Australian group of adolescents with asthma. The factors related to compliance in this group can be seen in Box 11.2.

> **Box 11.2** Factors associated with compliant behaviours in adolescents with asthma in Australia

> » Independence
> » Support from nurses and educators
> » Support from parents
> » Experience of results
> » Motivation
> » Sense of responsibility

Adapted from Wales et al. (2011).

Wales et al. (2011) noted that there were two factors that had previously appeared in the literature (i.e. support from doctors and fear of complications) that did not appear in their study. This could be a genuine finding or reflect a weakness in the study design (Wales et al., 2011).

MOVING FROM PAEDIATRIC TO ADULT SERVICES

Regardless of Josie's compliance, self-management skills and developmental maturity, in a few years she will make the transition from the family-oriented and developmentally focused endocrinology healthcare team to more independently focused adult services. The benefits of such a change are the following:

- Developmentally appropriate care can be given.
- It may aid in maturation.
- Optimal primary health care can be given.
- It facilitates an increased sense of independence and control (Wedgwood, Llewellyn, Honey & Schneider, 2008).

The New Zealand Child and Youth Epidemiology Service (2011, p. 140) suggest 'The goal of effective transition is to provide developmentally appropriate health care services that continue uninterrupted as the individual moves from adolescence to adulthood'. Transition requires planning, on the part of the individual, their family, health professionals and policy makers. It is important that Josie, her family and her healthcare team begin planning now.

Transition can be a complex task and problems related to the pragmatic aspects of the transfer can be complicated by the developmental challenges of adolescence (Ministry of Health, 2011). Consequently, young people can remain in the care of paediatric/child health services longer than is desirable, move abruptly and, in some instances, disappear from the health services completely (Bennett, Towns & Steinbeck, 2005). Lam, Fitzgerald and Sawyer (2005) found that 2% of admissions to an Australian children's hospital were over the age of 18 years. This they described as a significant increase over the previous decade. Reasons cited related to the complexity of the conditions, a lack of planning and concerns that adult facilities lacked appropriate services (Lam et al., 2005). Although the literature is clear as to what constitutes a successful transition program (see Box 11.3) and programs are being implemented, significant shortfalls are also evident (Ministry of Health, 2011; Wedgwood et al., 2008).

Box 11.3 Principles and practices of successful transition to adult programs

» Programs are individualised to meet specific needs, holistic and nondiscriminatory
» Joint clinics with paediatric and adult teams
» Regular meetings and ongoing liaison between paediatric and adult teams
» Timing of transition is flexible and discussed in advance
» Transition occurs when health is stable
» Sufficient time allowed to help the individual familiarise themselves with the practicalities

» Services should be able to meet the needs of the individual and be appropriate for age and developmental stage
» Clear plans written and kept up to date
» Education to facilitate the process is available
» Programs able to address common concerns of young people
» Full access to medical records for the primary team
» Mechanisms in place to ensure young people are not lost to follow-up
» The programs are evaluated

Adapted from Wedgwood et al. (2008) and Ministry of Health (2011).

In summary, the key points relating to the child and adolescent with a chronic disease are the following:

• The diagnosis impacts not only the child but the parents and siblings as well.
• The impact can have positive as well as negative consequences.
• Families attempt to 'normalise' their lives with varying degrees of success.
• Children are capable of expressing their point of view, which should be considered in decision making.
• Adolescents with a chronic disease are not only in transition physically, mentally and emotionally but also face the developmental challenge of assuming responsibility for the management of their health.

Clinical scenario 11.2
Tihema – a technology-dependent infant and her family

Tihema is 7 months post-term and has tracheomalacia, chronic lung disease and hypotonia. She has associated problems of acquired subglottic stenosis and feeding difficulty. She was born at 26 weeks gestation and required prolonged mechanical ventilation, as she was difficult to extubate. Tihema has a tracheostomy. She requires continuous positive airway pressure (CPAP) with supplementary oxygen when sleeping and gastrostomy feeding via a pump with a calorie-supplemented infant formula, as she is not permitted to feed orally.

Her care is complex and a team of health professionals is working together to plan and deliver an holistic, individually designed program to support her needs and plan for her discharge.

Tihema's hospital room is crowded with equipment and she is often restricted to her cot. Some photographs of family members are taped on her wall. A greenstone (taonga) is placed on the locker – a symbol of protection left by the family. Tihema has never been home.

Tihema's mother, Moana, is Māori. She lives in an urban area with high levels of deprivation. Moana has two other young children under 5 years old, and lives with her parents and three siblings. Moana is supported by her extended family. Her partner lives nearby. There have been incidents of domestic violence.

Developmental issues

In addition to her medical conditions, Tihema has been slow in achieving growth and developmental milestones. Babies and children who have complex health issues from an early age often have delayed developmental progress. The cause of the delay (neurological and/or environmental) may not be distinguishable until the child begins to improve in health and is discharged. These children are often restricted in their movement due to the hospital environment and in the time they are held and cuddled because of physical instability and attachment to monitoring equipment. The balance between providing physical care and enhancing the achievement of milestones and family bonding is a significant challenge for both the family and the interdisciplinary health team.

A Māori model of health

For Māori, models of health are holistic. Durie's *Whare tapa wha* concept encompasses four dimensions. These include *taha wairua* (spiritual), *taha hinengaro* (mental), *taha tinana* (physical) and *taha whanau* (family). This concept of health requires an interaction of all these aspects, which represent four walls of a house. If one of these walls fails, the house will fall (Durie, 1994). The challenge for nursing is to support the physical needs of the child within a culturally acceptable environment. In Chapter 3, issues for Māori health are discussed in more detail.

Technology-dependent children and young people

Children who are 'dependent on technology' or 'medically fragile' are often defined as those '… who need both a medical device to compensate for the loss of a vital body function and substantial and ongoing nursing care to avert death or further disability' (Ministry of Health New Zealand, 2011; Wagner et al., cited in Kirk, 1998, p. 102). They are a:

> … diverse group of children who vary according to the cause of illness, age of onset ranging from birth through to adolescence, duration (months to life long dependence), incidence and severity of associated disabilities, and frequency of using technology. (Glendinning, Kirk, Guiffrida & Lawton, 2001, p. 323).

Caring for children dependent on technology in the community is now not a new concept. Countries such as The Netherlands, United Kingdom and Australia have over 30 years of experience managing children on home respiratory support programs (Paulides, Plotz & Verweij-van-den-Oudenrijn, 2012; Tibballs et al., 2010). However, it is still difficult to establish their precise number as data are not routinely collected centrally. These children are known to be significant users of health resources, disproportionately young (Glendinning et al., 2001) and increasing in numbers, particularly those requiring respiratory support (Edwards, Asher & Byrnes, 2003; Ministry of Health New Zealand, 2011).

Some indication of the prevalence in Australia and New Zealand came from a survey of Australasian hospitals. The survey showed that, of 199 children who met the inclusion criteria, 116 (58%) had a prolonged length of stay, 2 (1%) had been admitted for respite care and 10.1% were 'living in hospital' because there was no suitable alternative. Aboriginal and Torres Strait Islander and Māori populations were overrepresented in the survey (Children's Hospitals Australasia, 2005). There is a need to better identify these children in order to provide more appropriate support services and prevent further long-term inappropriate institutionalisation.

Most children dependent on technology are both chronically ill and reliant on a technological device. This suggests that there are both similarities and differences between these children and children who are chronically ill. They may be similar because of the sharing of a chronic health problem and different because of the addition of a technological device. Both groups encounter many of the same problems (see Table 11.4).

Going home

Tihema has been in hospital now for several months and discussions are in progress planning her referral to her home environment. The first transfer home with any technology-dependent child is usually the most difficult for families. Planning for the transfer home should commence early (i.e. once the child is medically stable or as soon as it is known that the child will require long-term technological support). For Māori, important decisions are often made by the *whanau* (family). Therefore, Moana and her whanau were invited to a meeting with ward staff to prepare for Tihema's transfer home. Family member meetings such as this begin a process that enables the identification and management of specific and unique family issues.

Tihema will require 24-hour care when she goes home. The idea of organising respite or in-home care is raised at the whanau meeting because respite at home is not initially welcomed by Moana. This reaction is common (Mentro & Steward, 2002; Miller, 2002). Therefore, the advantages of support should be discussed. These include a discussion of the ways to reduce the burden of stress and preventing long-term institutional care. Discussion is also needed on the prevention of potential harm, while also enhancing family coping and sibling support, and providing opportunities for social interaction (Miller, 2002; Neufeld, Query & Drummond, 2001). After some discussion within the whanau, there is agreement to access respite care.

A seven-step discharge planning process, predicated on case management, described by Boosfeld and O'Toole (2000) is useful in showing the elements of the process that is needed to successfully transfer a child like Tihema to her home. The steps are:

1. needs assessment
2. identification of key workers
3. discharge proposal
4. interdisciplinary planning meetings
5. recruitment and selection of home-care teams
6. training
7. moving home.

Despite the difficult transition, going home is important. Children have the right to grow up in the family context, as families are considered the natural environment for growth and development (United Nations, 1989). Care by families at home is

TABLE 11.4 Differentiating the impact of chronic disease and technology dependence

ISSUES	REPORTED FOR FAMILIES WITH A CHRONICALLY ILL CHILD	REPORTED FOR FAMILIES WITH A TECHNOLOGY-DEPENDENT CHILD
Shock, emotional distress and stress	Yes	Yes
Uncertainty	Yes	Yes
Social disruption	Yes	Yes
Striving for normality	Yes	Yes
Struggles for control	Yes	Yes
Fragility of control	Yes	Yes
Loss of freedom	Yes	Yes
Problematic relationships	Yes	Yes
Poor physical and mental health	Yes	Yes
Problems with the provision of support and services	Yes	Yes
Financial burden	Yes	Yes
Positive benefits	Yes	Yes
Providing 24-hour care	No	Yes
Social isolation	No	Yes
Managing a technological device	No	Yes
Requiring carers	No	Yes
Homes/rooms become like ICUs	No	Yes
Multiagency nurse-led packages of services	No	Yes

therefore preferred (Stein, 2001). The benefits are multifocal, including improved health (e.g. through fewer infections) and enhanced lifestyle through being part of a community and living in a nurturing environment with family members (Hewitt-Taylor, 2005).

As the child makes the transition through the normal stages of growth and development, they may be able to take charge and gain a sense of control regarding their care. There are already a number of young ventilator-dependent adults who, despite their challenges, are succeeding in school, university and travel and have gained independence from their immediate families (Gilgoff & Gilgoff, 2003).

Model(s) of care

The ability to access or develop a care coordination model (American Academy of Pediatrics, 2005; Tibballs et al., 2010) is essential during the discharge planning phase to ensure the child and family will be well supported in the home and community environment. Together with the child's complex medical needs there may be obstacles including housing problems and multifaceted family social issues. Funding for home care and equipment may be difficult to obtain and it may be difficult to recruit carers/nurses.

Additional complexity can arise as many of the children and young people may also require disability, education, social and other support services in both the government and the non-governmental sector (Noyes, 2006b). Involving these services helps provide holistic child and family-centred care, as family needs should not solely be defined by their child's health needs, nor should the parents be seen as nurses but rather as parents who are able to provide health care to the child as part of their overall needs (Kirk & Glendinning, 2004; Murphy, 2001). To address such complexities, coordinated services, such as the RCH @ Home Family Choice Program and Homecare Program have been developed and implemented successfully (Tibballs et al., 2010). These services are tailored to meet specific needs as outlined in Box 11.4.

The model of care should also include access to services that are flexible and responsive, including short- and long-term respite care and coordinated follow-up. These services need to be culturally appropriate and ensure the application of appropriate policies, standards and risk management (Horsburgh & Trenholme, 2002; Noyes, 2006b). The services should be planned, cost effective and avoid duplication of services while working to improve the child and family's quality of life (American Academy of Pediatrics, 2005).

The best models of care are unlikely to succeed without a partnership being established between families and professionals. Partnerships that develop concepts of team effort, sharing of knowledge, respect, support and advocacy are important (Lindeke, Leonard, Presler & Garwick, 2002). Henry (2004) identified that parents valued the care continuity provided by a key worker and the community-based specialist paediatric nursing service. Home visits by the interdisciplinary team, including a local primary paediatrician, were extremely helpful in developing these partnerships. The families also appreciated those processes that supported planning and discussions relating to boundaries and role definition.

Tihema was transferred home significantly later than had been hoped for because of the complexity of funding formulas for equipment and accessing funds for carers. Less difficult was planning her access to preexisting services covering a range of specialists, such as a paediatric specialist homecare nursing service, Well Child/child health services, Māori health services, neurodevelopmental and speech therapy services, a dietitian and a general practitioner.

The Family Choice Program and the Homecare Program are two of a range of in-home and community-based services run by Home and Community Care from the Royal Children's Hospital, Melbourne, Australia. The Family Choice program provides home-based support to families of children with high levels of complex ongoing medical care whereas the Homecare Program supports those with ongoing interventional medical care needs at home but requiring support workers to provide care. The support provided is flexible and tailored to the needs of the particular family based on a case management and individualised medical care plan approach. The key aim of these programs is to facilitate the integration of these children into their community and prevent unnecessary admissions to hospital. It is state-wide and provides services to eligible children and young people aged between 0 and 17 years.

The Victorian Department of Human Services funds the programs and it is the availability of this preexisting and coordinated funding that helps avoid the unnecessary delays in discharge commonly experienced if funding has to be sought on a case-by-case basis. The program adds to existing generic services and can be utilised to purchase respite care, carer training, medical consumables and equipment hire.

The programs support parents as the experts in the care of their child. They are based on partnerships between parents, the child's primary medical practitioner, a homecare nurse, a case manager and a diverse range of community service providers. Care is coordinated by a community case manager who links the partners. The manager undertakes an extensive, holistic assessment and works with the partners to develop a comprehensive plan of care and support based on the child's medical needs and the unique psychosocial circumstances of the child and their family.

Also pivotal is the role of the homecare nurse, a registered nurse based at the nearest hospital with a paediatric service. In collaboration with the child's parents and primary medical practitioner, the nurse is responsible for the development of a written care manual and the training, monitoring and review of care workers in the home and other community settings. The homecare nurse provides the link between the acute medical and the home setting, and it is the maintenance of this link that is vital to ensure the child can be safely cared for in their community.

Henry (2004) found that community-based paediatric services, especially within nursing, that transcend the boundaries of primary, secondary and tertiary settings help to reduce barriers encountered by families. These services are typical of what families with technology-dependent children may require in both New Zealand and Australia.

Funding home care

Tihema is discharged home with the same equipment she required in hospital. When transferring home any technology-dependent child or young person, there is the expense of purchasing equipment as well as ongoing costs such as administration, staff wages, equipment maintenance and single-use items. Care workers/professionals and family who will provide the respite care require training. Families will have individual and specific requirements. Respite staff need to be culturally aware and apply appropriate values in the home setting.

In Tihema's case, several family friends who live outside the home will be employed by an agency. In other cases, staff unknown to the family would be employed through the local health service or agency. Any respite carers should be matched with families as closely as possible, as the aim is to provide sustainable care that maintains family function.

Often tensions arise related to funding. For example, there is pressure to reduce length of stay in hospital because of the cost of admission and demand for beds. Accessing discharge funding for technology-dependent children in New Zealand is complex and revolves around eligibility criteria and government funding systems. The Ministry of Health (2011) provides a 'high and complex needs unit' for children and young people who have complex interdepartmental needs. Other government departments and the district health boards also provide support and funding (Ministry of Health, 2011). In Australia, access to funding varies from state to state and can also be dependent on eligibility criteria or be part of an overall, individual, government-funded care package.

Technology dependence and families

Families with a technology-dependent child will face unique problems, including managing the technological device. The complexity varies, with some families facing the responsibility of caring for a child on life support, whereas others manage lower levels of technology. In addition, families confront additional challenges. Four are described below.

First is the impact of needing the technology. The impact on families has been described (see Table 11.4) and is being quantified. Noyes (2007) found that ventilator-dependent children reported lower quality-of-life scores on their health and in other domains than their friends and chronically ill children. Requiring a technological device may have a number of other impacts, each one significant and needing resolution. It may: delay discharge from hospital (Noyes, 2000); increase family spending (Glendinning et al., 2001); limit school, employment and social life because of the time required to manage the technology (Heaton, Noyes, Sloper & Shah, 2005); and turn homes or rooms into intensive care areas.

A qualitative ethnographic study exploring the perceptions and experiences of Māori families caring for their technology-dependent child found that the interrelating factors that impact on the child and their families are complex and there was a significant impact on the parents' health (Henry, 2004). As with families with a chronically ill child, some families with a technology-dependent child develop strategies that maintain a functioning family and the relationships within by regularly using health and respite services and obtaining financial assistance as well as establishing a degree of privacy in their own home (Darvill, 2003; O'Brien, 2001). Other families felt their homes were taken over by strangers who became too involved in decision making (Dybwik, Nielsen & Brinchmann, 2011). Some families live in a state of chaos, experiencing constant change and extreme suffering (Darvill, 2003).

The second challenge is heeding the children's/young people's perspective. Children and young people themselves who are technology-dependent are an emerging new group creating their own novel lifestyles (Noyes, 2006a). They are able to give voice to their experiences and describe them in a way that is meaningful (Darvill et al., 2009), and describe emotional deprivation and educational and social exclusion when services provided do not meet holistic needs (Noyes, 2000).

They suffer anxiety, painful procedures, long periods of hospitalisation and being different (Darvill et al., 2009). In one unstable family, registered nurses and carers were obliged to take on a parenting role. This led to the child forming inappropriate attachments and experiencing additional emotional suffering when staff moved in and out of employment (Darvill, 2003).

Regarding their own health, children and young people may be more positive than their parents and hold more positive attitudes towards their technology. British children felt better on the ventilator (Noyes, 2006a). Canadian ventilator-dependent children described a major theme of 'It's okay. It helps me to breathe' (Earle, Rennick, Carnevale & Davis, 2006). Darvill et al. (2009) found some Australian children were growing up and doing normal things despite their health problems. They clearly understood their technology and were increasingly able to use it. Knowing the children's perspective is extremely important. It challenges professionals' understanding of the meaning of children's health and disabilities, concepts of what resources are needed to achieve a good quality of life (Noyes, 2006a) and the ability to incorporate their point of view into nursing practice (Darvill, 2009).

The third challenge focuses on incorporating technology into the family home. Families have to change to accommodate a technology-dependent child and their equipment within the home environment. Structural home modifications may be required before discharge. Other changes may include taking on an added role as administrators of complex regimens and providing highly technical clinical procedures that sometimes cause pain and suffering. The literature also includes reports of families experiencing sleep deprivation because of noisy equipment and anxiety relating to the child's condition.

With the technology often comes the need to have registered nurses or carers visiting frequently or even living with them. This is the fourth challenge. Families with a child dependent on technology are likely to share their lives with nurses and carers who can be in their homes up to 24 hours a day. This means a loss of privacy (Darvill, 2003; Kirk, 2005) and increases the potential for conflict.

The literature describes the importance of maintaining professional boundaries to protect family privacy and confidentiality (Coffman, 1995; Hewitt-Taylor, 2005; Murphy, 2001; O'Brien, 2001). Darvill (2003) found that the failure to maintain professional boundaries led to staff job losses, emotional problems and conflict. This study demonstrated the importance of good parental relationships and the support parents received from extended family members. These factors influenced the stability of the family unit, and it was the more stable family unit that established and maintained boundaries most effectively.

Establishing good working relationships with the families

The increasingly common phenomenon of in-home care has highlighted the complexity of the family unit and the importance for nurses to be acutely aware of the significance and intricacy of a working relationship in a family home. The partnerships that form with families are important (Diehl, Moffitt & Wade, 1991;

Dixon, 1996; Henry, 2004; Kirk, 2005; Lindeke et al., 2002). The use of a tool such as the family management styles framework (Deatrick et al., 2006; Knafl et al., 2012) may assist nurses to identify family management styles and subsequent support needs.

Over time, families develop expertise in caring for the child who is technology-dependent. The parents' body of knowledge may eventually equate or surpass that of the nurse and, consequently, blur the usual boundaries between the 'non-expert' layperson and the 'expert' health professional (Kirk & Glendinning, 2002). Regardless of the parents' expertise, parents must have ongoing access to nursing advice, reassurance and information. Ideally, this support should be available 24 hours a day.

Nurses working in community settings need to negotiate good working relationships with families so that there is mutual recognition of knowledge and expertise. Failure to do so can lead to anger and distress for the parents and potential harm for the child (Kirk & Glendinning, 2002). To establish and maintain good working relationships, nurses need to not only have proficient knowledge and clinical expertise but also be expert communicators, negotiating and coordinating services, engaging in education with clients and providing counselling and emotional support (Kirk & Glendinning, 2002).

The uncertainty of not knowing who is medically responsible also brings challenges for health staff working in a home (Dybwik et al., 2011). Therefore, clear role definition and procedures and plans of care are essential to healthy boundaries and relationships between families and nurses/carers.

Conclusion

Chronic illness in children and young people differs from that in adulthood and there are areas of significant concern. The diagnosis of a chronic illness means the end of life as they knew it for the child/young person, their parents and siblings. There are a wide number of issues and problems that families may encounter as they try to normalise their new situations. For the adolescent the transitions they undergo further add to the challenge to themselves, their families and health professionals.

Children/young people who are dependent on technology are both chronically ill and reliant on a technological device. They and their families face many of the same issues and problems as the family with a chronically ill child/young person; however, the degrees of difference between these two groups have not yet been researched. Technology dependence brings unique challenges, often requiring considerably more support. This can be provided through various models of care, including funded programs or care packages. Success is dependent on the adequacy of the program/package and developing a culturally appropriate partnership with the family that acknowledges their skills and expertise. Also, nurses require high levels of skill, particularly in communicating, counselling, educating and service coordination.

Children and young people are capable of expressing their perspective, which may differ from that of their parents. Their point of view should be taken into account in both nursing management and service planning.

KEY POINTS

» In New Zealand and Australia children and young people are generally well, but there are specific areas for improvement.
» Identify and use tools to assess families' responses to having a chronically ill or technology-dependent child.
» Use assessment findings to advocate for/provide individualised services.
» Develop/provide for the development of high levels of communication, teaching and planning skills.
» Begin planning discharge early with the family, child/young person and relevant services.
» Listen to the perspective of the child/young person.

CRITICAL QUESTIONS AND REFLECTION

1. Up to a quarter of children and young people in NZ and Australia are overweight or obese. What strategies do you think could improve this situation? Think about this on a variety of levels (i.e. what can governments do, what can health departments or boards do and what can individual nurses do?).

2. You are part of a team caring for a CPAP-dependent infant whose parents want to care for it at home. What community facilities and services are available in your district health board or state?

3. If you had a chronic illness and were required to take daily medications, would receiving a text message as a reminder make you more or less likely to take your meds? Take a poll amongst your friends and colleagues.

4. You're working in the emergency department when Josie presents and are looking after her. Identify your immediate nursing actions with a rationale for each action.

USEFUL RESOURCES

International Society for Pediatric & Adolescent Diabetes (ISPAD): http://www.ispad.org/

Australian Institute of Health and Welfare: www.aihw.gov.au/

Children's Healthcare Australasia: http://children.wcha.asn.au/

Ministry of Health New Zealand: http://www.health.govt.nz/

National Asthma Council Australia: http://www.nationalasthma.org.au/home

New Zealand primary health care nursing initiatives: http://www.health.govt.nz/our-work/nursing/nursing-initiatives/primary-health-care-nursing

References

American Academy of Pediatrics (2005). Policy statement: Creating a medical home: integrating health and related systems of care for children with special health care needs. *Pediatrics, 116*(5), 1238–1244.

Australian Capital Territory Government (2010). *ACT children's plan 2010–2014.* Retrieved from http://www.children.act.gov.au/default.htm (accessed 4 June 2012).

Australian Institute of Health and Welfare (AIHW) (2005). *Selected chronic diseases among Australia's children.* Bulletin No. 29 [Cat. no. AUS62]. Canberra: AIHW.

Australian Institute of Health and Welfare (AIHW) (2007). *Young Australians: their health and wellbeing 2007* [Cat. no. PHE 87]. Canberra: AIHW.

Australian Institute of Health and Welfare (AIHW) (2009). *A picture of Australia's children 2009* [Cat. no. PHE 112]. Canberra: AIHW.

Australian Institute of Health and Welfare (AIHW) (2011). *Young Australians: their health and wellbeing 2011* [Cat. no. PHE 140]. Canberra: AIHW.

Barlow, J. H., & Ellard, D. R. (2006). The psychosocial well-being of children with chronic disease, their parents and siblings: an overview of the research evidence base. *Child: Care, Health and Development, 32*(1), 19–31.

Bell, L. M., Curran, J. A., Byrne, S., et al. (2011). High incidence of obesity co-morbidities in young children: a cross-sectional study. *Journal of Paediatrics and Child Health, 47*(12), 911–917.

Bennett, D. L., Towns, S. J., & Steinbeck, K. S. (2005). Smoothing the transition to adult care. *Medical Journal of Australia, 182*(8), 373–374.

Boosfeld, B., & O'Toole, M. (2000). Discharge planning. *Paediatric Nursing, 12*(6), 20–22.

Children's Hospitals Australasia (2005). *Clinical forum: Care of children with chronic and complex healthcare needs report.* Canberra: Children's Hospitals Australasia.

Coffman, S. (1995). Crossing lines: parents' experiences with pediatric nurses in the home. *Rehabilitation Nursing Research, 4*(4), 136–143.

Craig, M. E., Twigg, S. M., Donaghue, K. C., et al. for the Australian Type 1 Diabetes Guidelines Expert Advisory Group (2011). *National evidence-based clinical care guidelines for type 1 diabetes in children, adolescents and adults.* Canberra: Australian Government Department of Health and Ageing.

Darvill, J. (2003). *Families caring for children with complex health care needs at home. Thesis.* Adelaide: Flinders University.

Darvill, J., Harrington, A., & Donovan, J. (2009). Caring for ventilated children at home – the child's perspective. *Neonatal, Paediatric & Child Health Nursing, 12*(3), 9–13.

Deatrick, J. A., Knafl, K. A., & Murphy-Moore, C. (1999). Clarifying the concept of normalization. *Image: The Journal of Nursing Scholarship, 31*(3), 209–213.

Deatrick, J. A., Thibodeaux, A. G., Mooney, K., et al. (2006). Family management style framework: a new tool with potential to assess families who have children with brain tumors. *Journal of Pediatric Oncology Nursing, 23*(1), 19–27.

Dell'Api, M., Rennick, J. E., & Rosmus, C. (2007). Childhood chronic pain and health care professional interactions: shaping the chronic pain experiences of children. *Journal of Child Health Care, 11*, 269–286.

Diehl, S., Moffitt, K., & Wade, S. (1991). Focus group interview with parents of children with medically complex needs: an intimate look at their perceptions and feelings. *Children's Health Care*, *20*(3), 170–178.

Dixon, D. (1996). Unifying concepts in parents' experiences with health care providers. *Journal of Family Nursing*, *2*, 111–132.

Durie, M. (1994). *Whaiora. Māori health development*. Auckland: Oxford University Press.

Dybwik, K., Nielsen, E. W., & Brinchmann, B. S. (2011). Ethical challenges in home mechanical ventilation: a secondary analysis. *Nursing Ethics*, *19*(2), 233–244.

Earle, R. J., Rennick, J. E., Carnevale, F. A., & Davis, M. (2006). 'It's okay, it helps me to breathe': the experience of home ventilation from a child's perspective. *Journal of Child Health Care*, *10*(4), 270–282.

Edwards, E. A., Asher, M. I., & Byrnes, C. A. (2003). Paediatric bronchiectasis in the twenty-first century: experience of a tertiary children's hospital in New Zealand. *Journal of Paediatrics and Child Health*, *39*, 111–117.

Fee, R. J., & Hinton, V. J. (2011). Resilience in children diagnosed with a chronic neuromuscular disorder. *Journal of Developmental & Behavioral Pediatrics*, *32*, 644.

Fortune, S., Watson, P., Robinson, E., et al. (2010). *Youth'07: The health and wellbeing of secondary school students in New Zealand: Suicide behaviours and mental health in 2001 and 2007*. Auckland: The University of Auckland.

Gilgoff, R. L., & Gilgoff, I. S. (2003). Long-term follow-up of home mechanical ventilation in young children with spinal cord injury and neuromuscular conditions. *Journal of Pediatrics*, *142*, 476–480.

Glendinning, C., Kirk, S., Guiffrida, A., & Lawton, D. (2001). Technology dependent children in the community: definitions, numbers and costs. *Child: Care, Health and Development*, *27*(4), 321–334.

Hanna, K. M., & Decker, C. L. (2010). A concept analysis: assuming responsibility for self-care among adolescents with type 1 diabetes. *Journal for Specialists in Pediatric Nursing*, *15*, 99–110.

Heaton, J., Noyes, J., Sloper, P., & Shah, R. (2005). Families' experiences of caring for technology dependent children: a temporal perspective. *Health and Social Care in the Community*, *13*(5), 441–450.

Henry, P. (2004). *Negotiating an unstable ladder: The experience of Māori families caring for a technology dependent child*. Thesis. Auckland: University of Auckland.

Hentinen, M., & Kyngäs, H. (1998). Factors associated with the adaptation of parents with a chronically ill child. *Journal of Clinical Nursing*, *7*, 316–324.

Hewitt-Taylor, J. (2005). Caring for children with complex needs: staff education and training. *Journal of Child Health Care*, *9*(1), 72–86.

Horsburgh, M., & Trenholme, A. (2002). *Respite and palliative care needs of families caring for a terminally ill child: a New Zealand study*. Auckland: University of Auckland.

Kepreotes, E., Keatinge, D., & Stone, T. (2010). The experience of parenting children with chronic health conditions: a new reality. *Journal of Nursing and Healthcare of Chronic Illness* doi: 10.1111/j.1752-9824.2010.01047.x

Kirk, S. (1998). Families' experiences of caring at home for a technology dependent child: a review of the literature. *Child: Care, Health and Development*, *24*(2), 101–114.

Kirk, S. (2005). Parent or nurse? The experience of being the parent of a technology-dependent child. *Journal of Advanced Nursing, 51*(5), 456–464.

Kirk, S., & Glendinning, C. (2002). Supporting 'expert' parents: professional support and families caring for a child with complex health care needs in the community. *International Journal of Nursing Studies, 39*, 625–635.

Kirk, S., & Glendinning, C. (2004). Developing services to support parents caring for a technology-dependent child at home. *Child: Care, Health and Development, 30*, 209–218.

Knafl, K., Breitmayer, B., Gallo, A., & Zoeller, L. (1996). Family response to childhood chronic illness: description of management styles. *Journal of Pediatric Nursing, 11*(5), 315–326.

Knafl, K. A., Darney, B. G., Gallo, A. M., & Angst, D. (2010). Parental perceptions of the outcome and meaning of normalization. *Research in Nursing & Health, 33*, 87–98.

Knafl, K., & Deatrick, J. A. (2002). The challenge of normalization for families of children with chronic conditions. *Pediatric Nursing, 28*(1), 49–53.

Knafl, K., & Deatrick, J. A. (2006). Family management style and the challenge of moving from conceptualization to measurement. *Journal of Pediatric Oncology Nursing, 23*(1), 12–18.

Knafl, K. A., Deatrick, J. A., & Havill, H. L. (2012). Continued development of the Family Management Style Framework. *Journal of Family Nursing, 18*(1), 1–34.

Kyngäs, H. (2007). Predictors of good adherence of adolescents with diabetes (insulin-dependent diabetes mellitus). *Chronic Illness, 3*, 20–28.

Lam, P. Y., Fitzgerald, B. B., & Sawyer, S. M. (2005). Young adults in children's hospitals: why are they there? *Medical Journal of Australia, 182*, 381–384.

Lean, M., Lara, J., & O'Hill, J. (2006). Strategies for preventing obesity. *British Medical Journal, 333*(7575), 959–962.

Lindeke, L., Leonard, B., Presler, B., & Garwick, A. (2002). Family-centered care coordination for children with special needs across multiple settings. *Journal of Pediatric Health Care, 16*(6), 290–297.

Loring, B. (2009). *Literature review respiratory health for Māori.* Asthma and Respiratory Foundation of New Zealand Te Taumatua Huango Mata Ha o Aoteoroa.

McMurray, A., & Clendon, J. (2011). *Community health and wellness; Primary health care in practice* (4th ed.). Sydney: Elsevier.

Melnyk, B. M., Feinstein, N. F., Moldenhouer, Z., & Small, L. (2001). Coping in parents of children who are chronically ill: strategies for assessment and intervention. *Pediatric Nursing, 27*(6), 548–558, 572–573.

Mentro, A., & Steward, D. (2002). Caring for medically fragile children in the home: an alternative theoretical approach. *Research and Theory for Nursing Practice, 16*(3), 161–177.

Miller, S. (2002). Respite care for children who have complex healthcare needs. *Paediatric Nursing, 14*(5), 33–37.

Ministry of Health New Zealand (MOH NZ) (2006). *An analysis of the usefulness and feasibility of a population indicator of childhood obesity.* Wellington: MOH NZ.

Ministry of Health New Zealand (MOH NZ) (2008). *A portrait of health. Key results of the 2006/07 New Zealand Health Survey.* Wellington: MOH NZ.

Ministry of Health New Zealand (MOH NZ) (2010). *About diabetes*. Retrieved from http://www.health.govt.nz/our-work/diseases-and-conditions/diabetes/about-diabetes (accessed 10 June 2012).

Ministry of Health New Zealand (MOH NZ) and Paediatric Society of New Zealand (2011). *The health of children and young people with chronic conditions and disabilities in New Zealand*. Dunedin: MOH NZ.

Ministry of Health New Zealand (MOH NZ) (2012). *Statement of intent 2012/13 to 2014/15: Ministry of Health*. Wellington: MOH NZ.

Murphy, G. (2001). The technology-dependent child at home. Part 1: in whose best interest? *Paediatric Nursing*, *13*(7), 14–18.

National Asthma Council (NAC) (2012). *April 2012 Newsletter*. Retrieved from http://www.nationalasthma.org.au/news-media/d/2012-04-26/april-2012-newsletter (accessed 4 June 2012).

National Asthma Council Australia (NAC) (2006). *Asthma management handbook 2006*. Melbourne: NAC.

Neufeld, S., Query, B., & Drummond, J. (2001). Respite care users who have children with chronic conditions: are they getting a break? *Journal of Pediatric Nursing*, *16*(4), 234–244.

New Zealand Child and Youth Epidemiology Service (NZCYES) (2011). *The health of children and young people with chronic conditions and disabilities in New Zealand*. Wellington: Ministry of Health.

Noyes, J. (2000). Enabling young ventilator dependent people to express their views and experiences of their care in hospital. *Journal of Advanced Nursing*, *31*(5), 1206–1215.

Noyes, J. (2006a). Health and quality of life of ventilator-dependent children. *Journal of Advanced Nursing*, *56*(4), 392–403.

Noyes, J. (2006b). The key to success: managing children's complex packages of community support. *Archives of Diseases in Childhood. Education and Practice*, *91*, 106–110. doi:10.1136/adc.2005.088351

Noyes, J. (2007). Comparison of ventilator-dependent child reports of health-related quality of life with parent reports and normative populations. *Journal of Advanced Nursing*, *58*(1), 1–10.

O'Brien, M. (2001). Living in a house of cards: family experiences with long term childhood technology dependence. *Journal of Pediatric Nursing*, *16*(1), 13–22.

Paulides, F. M., Plotz, F. B., & Verweij-van den Oudenrijn, L. P. (2012). Thirty years of home mechanical ventilation in children: escalating need for pediatric intensive care beds. *Intensive Care Medicine*, *38*, 847–852.

Salmond, C., Crampton, P., & Atkinson, J. (2007). *NZ Dep 2006 Index of Deprivation*. Dunedin: Department of Public Health, University of Otago.

Sartain, S. A., Clarke, C. L., & Heyman, R. (2000). Hearing the voices of children with chronic illness. *Journal of Advanced Nursing*, *32*(4), 913–921.

Schilling, L., Dixon, J., Knafl, K., et al. (2009). A new self-report measure of self-management of type 1 diabetes for adolescents. *Nursing Research*, *58*(4), 228–236.

Schilling, L., Grey, M., & Knafl, K. (2002). The concept of self-management of type 1 diabetes in children and adolescents: an evolutionary concept analysis. *Journal of Advanced Nursing, 37*(1), 87–99.

Statistics New Zealand (2007). *Hot off the press 2006 Disability Survey.* Retrieved from http://www.stats.govt.nz/browse_for_stats/health/disabilities/DisabilitySurvey2006_HOTP06/Commentary.aspx (accessed 8 June 2012).

Stein, R. E. K. (2001). Challenges in long term healthcare for children. *Ambulatory Pediatrics, 1*(5), 280–288.

Steinbeck, K., & Brodie, L. (2006). Bringing in the voices: a transition forum for young people with chronic illness or disability. *Neonatal, Paediatric and Child Health Nursing, 9*(1), 22–26.

St Jude Children's Research Hospital and Washington University (2012). Pediatric Cancer Genome Project. Retrieved from http://www.pediatriccancergenomeproject.org/site (accessed 6 June 2012).

Tibballs, J., Henning, R., Robertson, C. F., et al. (2010). A home respiratory support programme for children by parents and layperson carers. *Journal of Paediatrics and Child Health, 46*(1–2), 57–62.

United Nations (UN) (1989). *Convention on the rights of the child.* Retrieved from www.unicef.org/crc/files/Rights_overview.pdf (accessed 17 June 2012).

Wales, S., Crisp, J., Fernandes, R., & Kyngäs, H. (2011). Modification and testing of the chronic disease compliance instrument to measure treatment compliance in adolescents with asthma. *Contemporary Nurse, 39*, 147–156.

Wedgwood, N., Llewellyn, G., Honey, A., & Schneider, J. (2008). *The transition of adolescents with chronic health conditions from paediatric to adult services.* Canberra: Australian Research Alliance for Children and Youth (ARACY).

Woodgate, R. (2001). Adopting the qualitative paradigm to understanding children's perspectives of illness: barrier or facilitator. *Journal of Pediatric Nursing, 16*(3), 149–161.

World Health Organization (WHO) (2008). *The global burden of disease: 2004 update.* Geneva: WHO Press.

The authors would like to acknowledge Pamela Henry for her contributions to the previous edition on which this edition's chapter is based.

Chapter 12

PROMOTING MENTAL HEALTH

Margaret McAllister, Christine Handley

LEARNING OUTCOMES

Reading this chapter will help you to:

» understand the reasons for the need to equally emphasise prevention, treatment and promotion in mental health work

» understand how knowledge of developmental stages assists in shaping interventions that serve to promote mental health in young people and their families

» identify the range of mental health strategies clinicians use within the spectrum of interventions for mental disorders

» describe day-to-day practice activities useful in promoting a young person's mental health and wellbeing, and helping young people to flourish

» discuss issues important to organisational planning so that services in which you work can build their capacity to provide youth-centred care.

Introduction

In this chapter, we discuss the issue of youth mental health and outline strategies that emphasise prevention of distress and promotion of mental health and wellbeing. As a nurse, you may be working with children and/or adolescents in a range of settings, including: schools, general practices, community health centres, hospitals or specialised mental health services such as Child and Adolescent Mental Health Services (CAMHS) drug and alcohol recovery centres or teams working with homeless children and youth. You may be a nurse working in a mental health or youth justice residential setting. The young people with whom you work may live in urban, rural or primarily indigenous communities. The principles of mental health promotion are applicable across all of these different work settings.

We tell the story of a vulnerable adolescent whose experiences flow on to affect the health and wellbeing of his family and, without effective intervention such as systemic family work, would be likely to damage his relationships, school achievement and future. As authors we have attempted to model a *person-centred* approach to thinking about and working with the young person, as this is a key feature and aim for professional nursing practice. We have also included discussion on both *knowledge* and *practice* issues because the development of theoretical understanding and education, as well as practical skills and strategies, are essential ingredients for your work as a reflective, flexible professional.

This scenario, which we return to throughout the chapter, represents a typical referral of a young person to a mental health facility. Daniel and young people like him could be referred by a general practitioner, a paediatrician, a school guidance counsellor, a community nurse or, in this instance, a psychiatrist working in a hospital DEM. It would be easy to focus solely on the presenting problems and not see Daniel as a whole person capable of learning ways to deal more effectively with the difficulties he is experiencing. Initial energies by the nurse might be directed towards making a clinical diagnosis and treating the identified problem. However, this would be quite unproductive for both Daniel and his family. Why? How are the concepts of prevention, early intervention and mental health promotion relevant to Daniel's situation?

It is important to be clear about what mental health and mental disorder actually mean. Freud defined mental health simply as the ability to love, work and play. Almost 70 years later, the World Health Organization describes it similarly. Positive mental health is a:

> ... state of wellbeing in which the individual realises his or her own abilities, can cope with the normal stresses of life, can work productively and fruitfully, and is able to make a contribution to his or her community. (World Health Organization, 2001).

In both definitions, the emphasis is on having a rich internal, imaginative and creative life, as well as the ability to relate with others and engage competently in meaningful activities. Still more recently, the work on flourishing (Keyes, 2007; Seligman, Steen, Park & Peterson, 2005) provides an even more optimistic and proactive view of the achievement of good mental health. To flourish is to be able to enjoy life, to cope with life's difficulties, to believe in others, to feel you have a place in the world and to believe that you have something you can give to others. All of these offer a hopeful vision for a nurse's therapeutic work with Daniel and his family.

The medical model of psychiatry defines mental health problems as mental disorders or illnesses, which are classified using a diagnostic classification system such as DSM-IV-TR (Diagnostic and Statistical Manual of Mental Disorders, 4th edition, Text Revision). Daniel meets the criteria for anxiety, dissociation and Asperger's

Clinical scenario 12.1
Setting the scene

The nurse

Imagine you are a postgraduate nursing student who has only recently commenced employment for the first time in a Child and Adolescent Mental Health Centre. You are sitting in on a referral interview for the purposes of assessment. Present are a 16-year-old boy, Daniel, and his mother, Pam. Daniel appears unhappy and is mostly uncommunicative. During the interview you find out that Daniel has had a recent overnight admission to a department of emergency medicine (DEM). The notes reveal that prior to admission Daniel had become very distressed at home, was expressing a wish to die and was crying on his bed and holding a knife. His mum Pam had rung the police as Daniel refused to go to the hospital. Daniel says he does not remember any of these events. His mother appears very anxious and scared for her son. Daniel only gives monosyllabic responses to assessment questions asked and any attempt to engage is met with 'I don't know' and 'I don't remember'. The notes also state that, following a comprehensive psychiatric assessment in DEM, Daniel was diagnosed with anxiety and dissociation and has many features that meet the diagnostic criteria for Asperger's disorder.

Now try and put yourself in Daniel's shoes.

Daniel

You live with your mother, a younger brother with whom you clash often and a much younger sister. You are close to your mum, an uncle and your maternal grandparents. You have no time for your dad, who left the family when you were 7 years old. The only contact is the occasional phone call. You have always felt different from others, find it difficult to mix with others, have been bullied relentlessly both physically and verbally since primary school and have no close friends. You feel very anxious most of the time and especially if there is any change in your daily routine. It takes you longer to do homework than your mum expects because it needs to be perfect. You hate school, even though you are an A-grade student in most subjects. You desperately want to stay at home to complete your studies. You feel pretty cynical about the education system and believe yourself to be much more knowledgeable about most of your subjects than your teachers.

You have intense, almost obsessive interests in history, sharks and African butterflies and love creative writing. You feel like you just don't fit in anywhere and have thought of ending your life but wouldn't do it as you do not wish to cause your mum or grandparents any pain. Sometimes, anxiety can get so intense for you that you will go to great lengths to avoid the things that stress you and, when you cannot, your heart can race, you can't think clearly and sometimes your mind even shuts down completely. You can't remember what happens to you on these occasions and it's very confusing and upsetting for you to lose control like that. You love the family dog, music and computer gaming. Overall, you feel you have no choice or say in your life, including coming to therapy sessions.

disorder. Therefore, evidence-based approaches to treating these conditions are important to facilitate.

It is also important to search for an understanding about a client, such as Daniel, that reaches beyond a biological definition of mental disorder. Very few mental health problems can be confidently attributed to physical abnormalities, and thus they are not 'illnesses' in the true sense. So too, biological treatments are likely to treat only the symptoms of disorder and do little to promote health, wellbeing and a flourishing state in the long term. Medical treatments also do nothing to prevent disorders. As a nurse working with young people with mental health problems, it is crucial to create space for the promotion of mental health, for the individual, their family and the community in general.

Mental health issues in Australia and New Zealand

In order to be able to understand the issue of mental health promotion within Australia and New Zealand, it is important to be aware of the extent of the problem that mental disorder creates for individuals and groups. The Australian Bureau of Statistics, quoted in Slade et al. (2009), states that 7% of children under 15 have a *reported* mental health problem. The five most common diagnoses allocated to young people in child and youth mental health services are, in order of frequency: anxiety and stress, behavioural problems (including conduct disorder and aggression), mood, substance abuse and developmental disorders. Vulnerability to mental illness is at its highest during childhood and adolescence – the physical, emotional and mental development the person is undergoing is significant. This is why three-quarters of the population affected by mental disorder during their lifetime will first develop a disorder during their adolescence. Up to 2% will develop serious mental disorders, such as schizophrenia or bipolar affective disorder. This rate of mental health problems is found in all age and gender groups. Boys are slightly more likely to experience mental health problems than girls. Also, there is a higher prevalence of child and adolescent mental health problems among those living in low-income, step/blended and sole-parent families (Sawyer, Johnston, Oakley Browne, Andrews & Whiteford, 2000). This means that, each year, about half a million Australian and 100,000 New Zealand youths are affected and will suffer from at least one mental illness episode. Only a quarter of those needing help will receive it.

Mental disorders during adolescence can seriously disrupt a person's life development, interfering with their ability to make friends, develop self-confidence, complete their education, embark on a career, secure stable employment and achieve independence.

Daniel has symptoms of Asperger's disorder (he has marked impairment in social interactions and he is engaged in restricted and repetitive patterns of behaviour, without showing signs of cognitive or intellectual deficits). Daniel also experiences anxiety, particularly in social situations that he cannot avoid. When it is severe, he dissociates. Within the spectrum of autism, Asperger's disorder is considered a lifelong developmental disability. Attwood (2007) states that, over the past decade, there has been an extraordinary increase in the number of children diagnosed with Asperger's syndrome. In 2007, the estimated prevalence of autism spectrum disorders (ASD) across Australia was 62.5 per ten thousand for children aged 6–12 years. That is, there is on average one child with an ASD in every 160 children (Australian Advisory Board on Autism Spectrum Disorders and MacDermott, 2007).

In contrast with autism, with Asperger's disorder there is no significant delay in early language acquisition or in cognitive abilities. Daniel, you will remember, is an A-grade student. As a result of this, Asperger's is often detected much later than autistic disorder and sometimes not until adulthood (see http://www.autismspectrum.org.au). Daniel was being diagnosed for the first time at age 16 years, yet his family always felt he was different all his life.

The development of youth mental health services

Despite ongoing research, the causes of mental illnesses such as anxiety, schizophrenia and Asperger's remain poorly understood, and so it is still not possible to accurately predict or prevent their onset. People still lack timely access to services, and many consumers criticise healthcare providers for being patronising or stigmatising (National Mental Health Consumer and Carer Forum, 2010), which leads to feelings of isolation or discrimination. Furthermore, most services still tend to be oriented to mature adults who have disability secondary to mental health problems. This makes recovery and adaptation to illness delayed and, thus, disability and all of its associated costs are increased.

However, youth-oriented approaches are emerging. For example, in New Zealand there is now a Ministry of Youth Development, which has a vision for New Zealand to become a country 'where young people are vibrant and optimistic through being supported and encouraged to take up challenges' (http://www.myd.govt.nz/). It provides guidelines and resources for working with youth, including a code of ethics as well as access to evidence-based research, funding and policy development.

The Mental Health Foundation of New Zealand also provides a youth-service directory (www.mentalhealth.org.nz), which makes searching for information, treatment advice and support groups for Daniel and his family easy.

In Australia, the equivalent government organisation coordinating policy and service development is Youth.gov.au, an Australian Health Department initiative. Headspace, the National Youth Mental Health Foundation, is Australia's peak body for mental health services.

Importantly, in Australia and New Zealand young people now have a voice to call attention to their needs and to assert themselves more collectively when services fail to adequately communicate respect, responsiveness and action.

The Young and Well Cooperative Research Centre (YAW-CRC, http://www.yawcrc.org.au/) is an Australian research centre that established the Youth Brains Trust, a panel of young people who vet every new project or development that the YAW-CRC is planning. New Zealand has the Aotearoa Youth Voices network, which connects young people with each other and with government and community decision makers to talk about issues important to them.

The need for better mental health promotion and illness prevention

All of these initiatives have come about as a result of people voicing their unhappiness with service gaps and the perpetuation of an illness-oriented system of health care that tends to focus services only on specialised treatments. The latter approach neglects community-based and prevention-oriented programs (see Box 12.1) that can target vulnerable families, groups and individuals when they are showing signs that more could be done to promote their happiness, wellbeing, social connection and security.

Box 12.1 Research highlight: A solution-focused group program

Taking a problem-centred focus is particularly unhelpful when working with young people because, by its nature, a problem orientation tends to search for what's going wrong with a person and usually involves an expert applying solutions. This can compound loss of hope and be disempowering. The iCARE strengths program designed for school-based mental health workers to run with small groups of young people an hour a week for 6 weeks provides an innovative solution. It harnesses the power of story-telling as well as new media to engage and inspire participants (McAllister et al., 2010).

iCARE explores:

» What is going well in self and others?
» Where can we find sources of inspiration, hope, transcendence of fun?
» Resilience strategies are like skeleton keys – they can open any door and help in any situation.
» What are some obstacles that others have run into that we can appreciate and avoid?
» What strategies would be useful to share with others?
» What are the symbols that give us strength?
» And how can we share these with our friends and peers?

Pilot evaluations conducted at three schools using a pre-/post-test survey with the participants explored knowledge, coping and program expectations and found clear improvements in knowledge of mental health strategies. Gains were made across all coping domains as well as self-efficacy.

Example comments of what participants gained in the program are: 'I have learned a lot about mental health and how to care for myself and others', 'I learned new ways to deal with things' and 'I became more aware about how others could be feeling'.

Example comments of what clinicians who ran the program thought included: 'We learned a great deal about the process of respectfully collaborating with all of the key stakeholders in the school system, particularly involving the school principal as the first step of initiating the collaborative process', 'It was a joy working with the young students and witnessing their joy in being part of a process that emphasised strengths and solutions', 'Young people involved in the iCARE groups responded to the safe space provided by iCARE, with growing openness and increased confidence to speak more about the often unspoken issue of self-injury in a broader sense' and 'Young people participating in iCARE loved the use of creative media such as making their own name badges and loved the interactive use of poems, music and movie video vignettes. A great discussion about bullying, for example, followed seeing critical scenes from the movie *Muriel's Wedding*'.

McAllister M, Hasking P, Estefan A, McClenaghan K, Lowe J. A strengths-based group program on self harm: A feasibility study. Journal of School Nursing. 26, (4): 289–300, 2010. Reprinted by Permission of SAGE Publications.

The spectrum of interventions – prevention, treatment and wellbeing

Australian and New Zealand clinicians now draw on the USA-based Institute of Medicine's spectrum of interventions model of mental health service delivery (Mrazek & Haggerty, 1994). This model emphasises not just the treatment of disorders, but health promotion, prevention, rehabilitation and adaptation. In order to be systematic in this approach to mental health service coordination, it is important to understand what makes society function in a healthy way and which populations, groups and individuals may be more vulnerable to emotional or mental health breakdown than others.

The social determinants of health and mental health

According to the World Health Organization Commission on Social Determinants of Health (Irwin & Scali, 2005), the social determinants of health are the conditions in which people are born, grow, live, work and age. This includes the health system. These conditions are influenced (constrained or relieved) by the distribution of money, power and resources. The social determinants of health are mostly responsible for health inequities – the unfair and avoidable differences in health status that we see amongst groups that experience social disadvantage, such as families living in poverty, homeless people, those who lack work, migrants, refugees and people living in conflict.

In Australian and New Zealand societies there are particular populations who are considered vulnerable because they experience disproportionately higher rates of social disadvantage and who are thus more likely to develop health and mental health problems. They include: children, women, people who are ageing and those in conflict or emergency situations. A very important population that is also likely to experience higher rates of mental health breakdown is indigenous groups – not only because of social and economic disadvantage but because of longstanding cultural discrimination and marginalisation.

As a nurse, you will be required to assess a person's risk status in terms of these vulnerabilities. Importantly, you will also need to assess a person's strengths, for it is these personal and social resources that can protect an individual from health breakdown, and facilitate an early recovery or adaptation.

Vulnerability and resilience: risk and protective factors

The concepts of risk and protective factors are central to mental health promotion work with young people. Risk and protective factors can be biological, psychological, social or environmental. They can be individual, school-related and/or community and cultural factors. Recall Daniel's situation. In order to better understand his needs, it is important to consider the risk and protective factors that contribute to his psychosocial health and wellbeing and that will impact on his ability to achieve developmental tasks.

Risk factors are variables that increase the likelihood that disorder will develop and exacerbate the burden of existing disorder (Barrett & Ollendick, 2004). Not all children exposed to risk factors go on to develop a mental health disorder (Raphael, 2002). In fact, even children who experience abuse or neglect, if reconnected to a loving, nurturing and consistent family system, will recover, thrive and experience health, happiness and wellbeing (Herman, 1997). However, it does appear to be the case that, the more risk factors that exist, the greater the impact on the young person and their family (Gerard & Buehler, 2004).

In Daniel's case, there are significant risk factors. He comes from a low-income, single parent family; he has been affected by adverse life events – including his father leaving the family when Daniel was very young, relentless bullying since primary school and the complex challenges of living with Asperger's (Sawyer et al., 2000). Studies of teenage boys with Asperger's syndrome and their mothers report high degrees of stress associated with trying to complete schoolwork and meeting the social expectations of peers (Carrington & Graham, 2001).

Also being concerned with what might keep Daniel and his family strong throughout his growing years, your team assesses the family's protective factors. Protective factors are the coping resources and ways of coping that can improve a person's response to stressful life events (Stuart, 2009). Examples of protective factors include a close family, a school that expects students to be helpful and involved, social networks, productive peer activities, a community that understands and expects changeability and flux and a young person armed with optimism, hope and inner strength (resilience).

Despite the complex challenges facing Daniel, the nurse assessing him notes his strong supportive relationship with his mum and grandparents and one of the teachers at his school. She also notes his passionate interests in history, butterflies and writing and his love for his pet dog. Throughout interactions with Daniel, the nurse also appreciates that he has a caring nature and a dry sense of humour. Such protective factors, especially if noticed and developed, have the potential to reduce the impact of risk factors (Stuart, 2009). Table 12.1 sets out the risk and protective factors for young people's psychosocial health.

TABLE 12.1 Risk and protective factors influencing the development of mental health problems in children and youth

RISK FACTORS	PROTECTIVE FACTORS
Poor physical health	Physical wellbeing, good nutrition, sleep and exercise
Low self-esteem	
Insecure, inappropriate or unsafe accommodation	Secure, appropriate and safe accommodation
Exposure to physical and emotional violence	Physical and emotional security
Harmful alcohol, tobacco or other drug use	No harmful alcohol, tobacco or other drug use
Feeling disconnected from family, school and community	Positive school climate and achievement
Lack of meaningful daily activities	Supportive caring parent(s)
Lack of purpose and meaning in life	Problem-solving skills
Lack of control over one's life	Optimism
Financial hardship	Pro-social peers
Exposure to environmental stressors (e.g. school bullying)	Involvement with significant other person
Poor social skills	Availability of opportunities at critical turning points or major life transitions
Parental mental illness	Meaningful daily activities
Learning difficulties	Sense of purpose and meaning in life
Family divorce/separation	Sense of control and efficacy
Ineffective use of medication	Financial security
	Lack of exposure to environmental stressors
	Good coping skills
	Effective use of medication (when required)

Adapted from Bogenschneider, K. (1996). An ecological risk/protective theory for building prevention programs, policies, and community capacity to support youth. *Family Relations, 45*, 127–138.

Nurses working in mental health

In our view, nurses are uniquely placed within the health system to be able to straddle both the illness dimension of health care and the wellness and recovery aspects. Nurses are trained to be fluent in the language of medicine, illness, disorder and treatment, as well as in health education, health promotion, service brokerage and referral. The nurse's role is to facilitate safe transition between these positions – being able to speak the language of medicine as well as the language of wellbeing enables nurses to help individuals and families negotiate a safe passage through life's major transitions.

In addition to this philosophical approach taken by the specialist mental health nurse working in CAMHS, there are also specific techniques and strategies that support this participatory, rather than paternalistic, way of working with Daniel and his family. Importantly, the approach taken was not to exclude Daniel's family, but rather to include them in the assessment phase and in shared decision making about treatment and recovery plans. The way of working with the family was to see problems systemically – that is, how one dysfunctioning part can affect the whole system, and vice versa. There was a process to develop mutuality within the therapeutic relationship; a care plan was also collaboratively developed to addresses promotion, prevention and treatment aspects of care.

A process for working with young people

To state the obvious, there is no one right process for working with young people. However, it is helpful if your work is guided by some overarching ideas and principles. One such very practical process is provided by Slattery (2007), who describes the aims and key ideas for the beginning, middle and end stages, be it a single session or overall therapy program. See Table 12.2 for an overview of this process. The seven key ideas referred to (engagement, participation, mutuality, questioning, balancing, integration and difference) are overlapping and operate collectively throughout the process and are key to promotion, prevention and treatment aspects of the relationship as you observed with Daniel and his family.

A range of activities, which may require thinking, drawing, discussion, questions and/ or moving, will help to advance the process. Each activity has its own characteristics. For example, asking a young person to think of a time when they stood up to the bully or sought help is a quiet, reflective and introspective activity. Asking the young person to draw what they felt is an active, visual and non-verbal activity. A discussion, however, is verbal and interactive. Other activities may be physical, playful, creative, light-hearted and minimally verbal or non-verbal (Slattery, 2007). As Daniel was often verbally uncommunicative in sessions, the nurse remained present, honest and transparent in her sessions with him and drew on a range of such activities with Daniel in response to his needs at any time. As trust developed, the nurse was able to use humour at times to challenge or confront Daniel in a light-hearted way when exploring strategies to manage feelings such as depression and anxiety.

Developing a plan of care

A care plan, sometimes called an individual service plan (ISP), provides a central guide for the nurse, the young person and their family. Where possible, it should be

TABLE 12.2 Overview of Slattery's process for working with young people

STAGE OF THE PROCESS	AIM	KEY IDEA(S)
At the beginning	To catch a person's interest	**Engagement** Opening of the process where the young person's interest needs to be caught. You need to do something so the young person feels inclined to continue.
In the middle	To invite responses and then explore them	**Participation** Making sure the young person is able to have input. **Mutuality** Working together. **Integration** Combining what you are doing with how you are doing it (e.g. a playful approach combined with a serious issue to make it more approachable). Perhaps a quiet moment to reflect as part of a tense discussion.
At the end	To identify new paths	**Questioning** One powerful way to help a person explore things that concern or interest them. Can be asked and answered verbally/non-verbally. Can be asked with the intention of the person answering or privately reflecting. **Balancing** Exploring all possible outcomes of any path: the terrific and not so terrific, the pros/cons or best/worst.

The more **different** the process, from what a person expects, the more likely it is to be fresh and interesting and to invite new responses and bring into focus new options.

Adapted from Slattery, P. (2007). *Youth works: A very practical book about working with young people* (pp. 21–22). Dulwich Hill, Peter Slattery.

developed collaboratively and draw on language that has meaning for the child or young person. For example, the care plan might ask:

1. How do you and your family want things to be?
2. What are we going to do to help? What might help us get there? What might get in the way?
3. Who will be involved to help us reach your goals? When (e.g. 4 sessions, 6 weeks, 3 months) will we review your progress?

The care plan provides a map towards recovery that is defined by the young person in collaboration with a clinician. For some people, recovery may mean the ability to live a fulfilling productive life despite a disability. What matters is what the person sees as their personal goals for living a happy, connected and productive life. Some may even challenge any notion of being disabled. Research shows that having hope is central to an individual's recovery (NFCMH, 2003 in Stuart, 2009).

Daniel's care plan emphasised health promotion, prevention of ill health and access to appropriate treatment that minimised side effects. In particular, the plan included the following:

1. Create a safe place to openly discuss the clinical diagnoses. This involved ongoing discussions about stigma, stereotyping and replacing stereotyped views with accurate knowledge. Attwood (2007) provides an excellent summary of the possible advantages and disadvantages of a diagnosis of Asperger's. Daniel, his mother and grandparents were encouraged to read a book by Yuko Yoshida (2007), *How to be yourself in a world that's different*. Daniel read the entire book and returned at the next session with detailed comments in the margins of most pages, which formed the basis of many discussions. His mother and grandparents said that it really helped them to gain a much greater understanding of Daniel and that, at times, it was as if the book was about Daniel.
2. Assist Daniel to take his medication as prescribed in order to minimise anxiety and help him to think clearly. This included respectfully listening to Daniel's fears and reservations about taking too much medication and working with the team to titrate a dose that could be comfortably tolerated.
3. Assist Daniel and his mother to find meaning in his recent, frightening hospital admission and the events leading up to this. This included examining antecedent events and learning to recognise triggers that could be avoided or minimised the next time they are encountered.
4. Look for any opportunity to provide Daniel with a sense of choice in the process and thus to feel more empowered. Daniel would often say, 'I don't have a view' or 'My view does not matter'. So, instead, Daniel was involved in decisions about whether the therapy session would be with him alone or with his mum, how long the sessions would be, the activities we might use to explore issues, the choice to talk or not to talk. It is important to differentiate between a young person who is not able to speak and a young person who chooses not to speak. A person unable to speak may need help in articulating or exploring thoughts and feelings; however, we support Slattery (2007) in his claim that it would seem reasonable to respect a young person's choice not to speak.

    Daniel was also actively encouraged to have a greater say in whether he went to school. Although his mum remained anxious about his attendance or lack of it at times, the support teacher thought it was reasonable for Daniel to stay at home some days as respite, given that he was coping well academically.
5. Act as an advocate to increase and strengthen the connections between the school, Daniel and his mum. Phone calls and emails assisted with this. This included obtaining Daniel's consent to educate his support teacher about his Asperger's and how his educational and social needs could be better met and supported. Daniel, like many other young people with Asperger's, had trouble with handwriting (Attwood, 2007).

Special arrangements were made with the school to allow Daniel to use a word processor at exam times. This lessened Daniel's anxiety considerably.

6. Work with mum to help her develop more realistic expectations for Daniel. Like many parents of children with Asperger's, one of Pam's most pressing worries focused on Daniel's future as an adult. This is highlighted in research by Little and Clark (2006), who further claim that family nurses are in a unique position to assess and respond to the special adaptive needs of families of children with Asperger's syndrome. Developing realistic yet hopeful expectations for Daniel was a central aspect of his anxiety management program. Although Daniel's mum tended to have unrealistic expectations regarding Daniel's capacity to be more independent at this time in his life, one of the potential disadvantages of a diagnosis of Asperger's is that it can limit the expectations of others who incorrectly assume that the person will never be able to achieve as well as peers (Attwood, 2007). Having said this, many young adults continue to depend on their families for supportive services (Lawrence, Alleckson & Bjorklund, 2010).

7. Educate Daniel about anxiety and its management including self-care and cognitive and behavioural strategies, such as challenging anxiety-building thoughts or practising mindfulness to allow problems to simply sit and then flow away (Harris, 2009). These approaches needed to be specifically tailored to his needs, taking into account on a session-by-session basis his energy levels, motivation, interests and connectedness with the therapist.

8. Empathise with, yet challenge, Daniel's perception of himself as powerless and having no control or choice in his life. Daniel was helped to become more aware of the situations in his life where he did exert choice. For example, he made choices about when to play on the computer, walk his dog and even attend therapy sessions. Daniel was a strong, healthy boy and his tiny mum would have been powerless to get him to sessions, should he really dig his heels in and refuse to come.

9. Explore with Daniel and his mum ways to assist Daniel's transition from high school to college. The nurse as advocate and collaborator was able to strengthen useful connections between Daniel and the school, career advisors and even college. Arrangements were even made for Daniel to have an individual orientation session at the college he will be going to. This went very well.

Daniel's story is a true and an increasingly common one. His story is one of complex comorbidity and involves relationships with interactive people and systems. Daniel suffers with anxiety and dissociative responses to stress that are comorbid conditions to a diagnosis of Asperger's. There were times when Daniel felt depressed and believed that life was just too hard. Attwood (2007) notes that, over the past decade, there has been an extraordinary increase in the number of children diagnosed with Asperger's syndrome. In young people with Asperger's, the transition from school to college can be fraught with many challenges, including the need for greater independence skills and the academic and social demands of college and university. Daniel was carrying the burden of such demands and, true to Attwood's (2007) prediction, the stress and insufficient support at school and at home were contributing to the development of anxiety and depression.

We invite you to think about the above aspects of Daniel's care plan. Can you see the inextricable links between treatment, prevention and mental health promotion?

Uncaring, prescriptive implementation of even research-based interventions will not result in the promotion of mental health. The care plan is tailored to the unique needs and circumstances of each young person, and the approach needs to have an environmental as well as individual focus that reaches across the whole spectrum of interventions. The nurse works hard to maintain engagement throughout and to be honest and real; otherwise, regardless of the strategies and activities used, the client is less likely to achieve the desired goals recorded on the care plan.

A systemic approach

Children and young people learn and grow in social systems – primarily families and schools. Problems that develop, and their solutions, can be understood in terms of these social contexts (McDougall, 2006). This is why the CAMHS specialist nurse was working closely with Daniel, his mum, grandparents, his schoolteachers and even prospective teachers and guidance counsellors. The nurse was thinking about Daniel in the context of his family and social life, both in the present and the future.

Family life can be negatively impacted by a range of interpersonal and social stressors, which in turn exacerbate a young person's mental health problems. Daniel was feeling increasingly isolated and anxious in response to difficulties in meeting school assignment deadlines, trying to cope alone with the relentless bullying and feeling overwhelmed at times by his mother's expectations of him to be more independent. Even though Daniel was only in year 10, his mother was very worried about Daniel's future including employment prospects. As a full-time worker and sole parent, she too often felt overwhelmed and it did not help that she perceived the school as being unsupportive overall and not understanding of her son's needs.

Nurses using family-sensitive and systemic approaches encourage interaction between family members and do not see their work as involving only the disturbed individual client. Such an approach denies the social and cultural context contributing to problems and it delays recovery and adaptation. In a systemic way of working, it is possible for the skilled mental health nurse to include even absent family members in the therapeutic process. For example, the CAMHS nurse arranged for family meetings so that Daniel's younger brother and sister were able to describe the difficulties they experienced, and this allowed the whole family to see how Asperger's interrupted their collective wellbeing.

Family work requires multiple engagements. In contrast to working with an individual, the nurse therapist is relating to what is common and what is different within and between family members (Rhodes & Wallis, 2011). It is common for major differences to exist in how different family members come to therapy: in developmental levels, in emotional positions and in the meaning each family member gives to the presenting problem and the stories each person shares about significant family events.

Daniel was unable to remember the events leading up to his admission to the hospital emergency department, whereas his mother was extremely distressed by the events. Processing these events within a family context is central to the promotion of mental health and recovery for both Daniel and his mother.

Developmental stages and mental health promotion: What's the connection?

In relation to working therapeutically with children, young people and their families or carers, we know the following:

- Positive resolution of developmental tasks moves the adolescent towards adulthood. Assisting the child and adolescent to achieve ego competency skills (Strayhorn, 1989 in Stuart & Laraia, 1998) and developmental tasks at different stages is the role of significant adults in their lives (e.g. parents, relatives, teachers or foster carers). See Box 12.2 for a summary of the nine ego competency skills. Parents and primary caregivers often struggle with understanding expectations that are reasonable for a child and adolescent of a particular age. Sometimes, a counsellor or therapist helps the adult carer to fulfil their roles through developing a better understanding of developmental milestones, tasks and expectations.
- Normal growth and development in children requires a nurturing, supportive environment. It is important to work closely with the parent(s) or primary caregiver(s) towards achieving such an environment; otherwise, individual work done with a young person can be undermined or neutralised. With young children the focus is often on giving praise, setting limits, following logical consequences for inappropriate behaviour and reinforcing desirable behaviours.
- The young person's search for a unique, new stable identity is very challenging, as the young person is also experiencing dramatic body changes. The search will often require the young person to re-master earlier stages of development (e.g. developing trust in self and others) (Meadows & Singh, 2001). Many

---

Box 12.2 Ego competency skills

Strayhorn (1989) identified the following nine skills that all children need to become competent adults:

1. establishing closeness and trusting relationships
2. handling separation and independent decision making
3. negotiating joint decisions and interpersonal conflict
4. dealing with frustration and unfavourable events
5. celebrating good feelings and experiencing pleasure
6. working for delayed gratification
7. relaxing and playing
8. cognitive processing through words, symbols and images
9. establishing an adaptive sense of direction and purpose.

A focus on ego competency skills is an effective and culturally sensitive way of planning and implementing nursing interventions for young people, regardless of the mental health problem or setting.

Adapted from Strayhorn, J. (1988). The competent child: An Approach to Psychotherapy and Preventive Mental Health. New York: The Guilford Press.

parents struggle with understanding their adolescent child's simultaneous needs for dependence and, increasingly, for independence. The adolescent requires guidelines within which to express growing independence with safety (Meadows & Singh, 2001). You will remember that, earlier, we noted that Daniel's mum was faced with the challenge of Daniel's need to be dependent for longer than expected and that the goal of growing independence would need to be taken slowly and incrementally.

- Understanding normal developmental tasks and stages helps the nurse therapist, counsellor or youth worker to identify any marked alterations or deviations in the developmental trajectory for that particular young person. The nurse can pass this understanding on to the parent(s) or caregiver. A child or young person with a mental health illness will often have delayed physical and emotional and social development.
- Some children and young people find themselves in the situation of being the carer for their parent(s) (e.g. when the parent or caregiver has a long-term physical or mental illness or where there are severe substance abuse problems). Such children, who may have been exposed to abuse or violence, can experience a role reversal with their parent(s) and develop a pseudo-maturity (Stuart & Laraia, 1998). The child or young person may appear responsible beyond their years and may be overly compliant with adults. Although seemingly well adapted, this behaviour is developmentally inappropriate and should not be reinforced. The child in this situation needs to be encouraged to choose age-appropriate interests and play activities, and the parent or caregiver needs help to take on appropriate adult responsibilities.

Prevention strategies

Even though the direct causes of most mental disorders remain unknown, nurses can be active in modifying and reducing risks and enhancing protective influences across every stage of the lifespan (for an overview of these lifespan issues, see Raphael, [2002]). Recall the spectrum of interventions model of mental health service delivery introduced to you earlier. Notice that there are opportunities for nurses and other health professionals to take action to promote better mental health even when no disorder presently exists. Whole of community promotion activities are termed *universal prevention strategies*. Activities that are focused on groups who are at risk of mental distress are termed *selective strategies*. Activities that are focused on groups who are already showing signs of distress or who have experienced trauma are termed *indicated strategies*.

A relevant universal strategy that might be helpful for Daniel and his peers is the Inspire Foundation's National Day of Action against Bullying (www.inspire.org.au). The Inspire Foundation is an Australian organisation that provides services that aim to improve young people's mental health and let them know that they do not have to get through challenges alone. Because bullying can happen anywhere to any person, it is not a problem that only occurs in people at risk of or experiencing mental disorder. By raising awareness about bullying, how it affects people, how it can be stopped and where people who are concerned can secure help, the longer term consequences of bullying such as feelings of sadness, anger or fear or behaviours such as self-harm, aggression or suicide can be prevented.

Another example of a universal strategy that cultivates whole of community wellbeing is a New Zealand initiative, called the Porirua Community Guardians. These are people who volunteer their time patrolling the city streets to make it a friendlier place to live. Their work ranges from helping with crowd control at large public events, to stopping vandalism and thefts, to acting as ambassadors for their city and turning a rubbish tip into a garden (http://www.communityguardians.org.nz/).

Prevention also involves targeting specific interventions towards *selective* groups known to be at risk. Coping after an earthquake, particularly for vulnerable individuals such as young children, is a good example. JoJo's Place (www.jojosplace.org) is a website that provides information for very young and older aged children, as well as parents, to understand their feelings and reactions during the extraordinary experience of a disaster. People who have been directly or indirectly affected by a major disaster like this are likely to experience shock, and the symptoms of this can be quite unusual and hard to understand – intrusive nightmares, not wanting to be with people, behavioural regression such as bed wetting or clumsiness. Responding in ways that accept, tolerate and then comfort the person so that the strong emotions begin to ease are important ways to allow the body and mind to heal.

In Daniel's case, a young man who is experiencing a mental health difficulty, a selected health promotion service that may help him to develop skills to ward off the effects of bullying, find strategies to alleviate his anxiety, access a support person online or express himself openly is Reachout (www.reachout.com). The kinds of services offered by Reachout are aimed at directly helping young people early on in their disorder, helping them to restore, maintain and develop inner strengths, and treating problems early so that they are of shorter duration and lesser impact on self and others.

Indicated strategies are those that target prevention towards high-risk groups, such as those who have an established diagnosis of a mental disorder or who are experiencing a high number of risk factors known to predispose them to mental disorder. Daniel also, at some times in his life, may need interventions from this domain. In Australia, Headspace (www.headspace.org.au) is the national youth mental health foundation that provides a national directory of health services that help to facilitate early treatment for disorders like anxiety, depression or psychosis. Treatment might involve psychotropic medication, paired with well-timed education that enhances shared decision making, facilitated peer-support groups, leisure skills and carer involvement and support (Watanabe, Hunot, Omori, Churchill & Furukawa, 2007).

Treatment strategies

The specific interventions that make up mental health treatment involve a whole range of health-promoting practices, including assessment and diagnosis, application of evidence-based interventions, holistic care, collaboration and partnership and family-sensitive service delivery. In reality, 'treatment' cannot be separated from any of these elements. We have already referred to a range of activities and strategies used to help Daniel and his family.

During assessment and on an ongoing basis, a mental status examination is completed. We recommend that any nurse working with young people develop the requisite skills to complete a basic mental health status examination, even if as a result you decide to refer on to a mental health professional. An important aspect of mental health promotion is recognising personal and professional limitations with regard to treating young people who are demonstrating signs of dysfunction.

Much of the data for such an assessment will emerge spontaneously (appearance, mood/affect and thought processes), while other data will be gathered via structured questioning and activities (Meadows & Singh, 2001). For a comprehensive exploration of specific questioning styles, go to the Headspace website (www.headspace.org.au) and locate the psychosocial interview guide. Identifying the young person's positive attributes is central to taking a mental health promotion stance towards mental health assessment. For example, can the young person problem-solve? What are their strengths and interests? How do they deal with stress? How well do they understand the problem that brought them to you? What do they think caused the problem? How upset are they about the problem? What are their views about the possible solutions?

Although questions like these guided the assessment of Daniel, the process is of course ongoing, and preliminary clinical impressions may shift with time. In our experience, assessment tools are most useful in helping clinicians explore and interpret the client's behaviour and needs. When they are used rigidly or restrictively, when they close down communication between client and clinician, they function as barriers to the therapeutic relationship. Thus, it is important to use questions carefully and use tools when and only when they assist in helping you get to know the person more clearly and deeply.

Continuing care or recovery strategies

It is possible for all people to *recover* from mental health problems, even if some symptoms might recur now and then. Recovery is an important and overarching principle that underpins rehabilitation work and continuing care. It really means the development of new meaning and purpose in one's life as one grows beyond (and perhaps despite) the effects of mental illness. It means maximising wellbeing, within the constraints that might be imposed by symptoms of mental illness. Daniel, for example, was encouraged to explore a range of cognitive behavioural strategies to deal with his negative emotions and thinking, including thought records, keeping a diary and pleasant events schedules. He was also encouraged to use a punching bag and to walk the dog daily as a way of supporting his overall wellbeing.

Conclusion

It is not always easy working with children and young people who have mental health issues, but it is important to remember that it also is not easy growing up. Perhaps it is useful to remember that we were all young once, and understanding and working with children and, particularly, young people requires genuine empathy.

The art of being a good clinician, effective in promoting mental health and wellbeing, is to be knowledgeable, concerned, nurturing and ready to provide support. As Burgess (2006) said:

> Growing things are so interesting. It should be a pleasure to review a time when we were changing so much, growing, learning so much. We have a lot to learn from teenagers about how to keep on our toes, about how to be lazy, about how to be playful, and most of all, how to just grow up.

KEY POINTS

» Mental health is not simply the absence of disorder; it involves a state of happiness and fulfilment in which the person flourishes.

» Young people may be vulnerable to feelings of anxiety and depression and may need assistance from empathic, supportive, skilled clinicians who understand this life transition.

» Diagnosis of medical disorder provides only one piece of the puzzle when working with young people with mental health problems. Nurses play a critical role in being person-centred, by engaging with the young person and their family.

» Young people need to be respected as knowledgeable.

» Understanding and exploring risk and protective factors for children and young people can build resilience and protect against vulnerability.

» The spectrum of interventions in mental health is a useful model to guide a whole-of-society approach to working to promote better mental health for all.

» Mental health promotion strategies for young people are integral to effective treatment and include collaborative and family-sensitive practices.

CRITICAL QUESTIONS AND REFLECTIONS

1. In what ways did Daniel's case emphasise mental health promotion, prevention and treatment?

2. What were the risk and protective factors for Daniel and his family?

3. What day-to-day practice activities could you use as a community-centred nurse to promote a flourishing state in young people?

4. There are risks and benefits of diagnosing a young person with a mental illness. Discuss within the context of mental health promotion.

5. As a nurse working with young people in the interests of promoting their mental health you will need to make decisions about who your client is. Is it the individual, parent, carers, extended family, significant others, a combination of these? What factors will you need to consider in making your decision?

6. To what extent do the health systems with which you are familiar operate in this 'whole-of-society' approach to health promotion and illness prevention?

USEFUL RESOURCES

Australia

Australian College of Mental Health Nurses: http://www.acmhn.org/

Autism Spectrum Australia: http://www.autismspectrum.org.au

Headspace: http://www.headspace.org.au/about-headspace

Inspire Foundation: http://www.yawcrc.org.au/partners/inspire-australia

Reachout: http://www.reachout.com

The National Mental Health Commission: http://www.mentalhealthcommission.gov.au

Europe and the United Kingdom

Hands on Scotland: http://www.handsonscotland.co.uk/

National Health Service, Scotland: http://www.healthscotland.com/mental-health.aspx

National Institute for Mental Health in England: http://www.mhhe.heacademy.ac.uk/links/national-institute-for-mental-health-in-england-nimhe/

The European Commission on public health: http://ec.europa.eu/health-eu/about_en.htm

New Zealand

Health and Disability Commissioner of New Zealand: http://www.mhc.govt.nz/

Mental Health Foundation of New Zealand: http://www.mentalhealth.org.nz

Te Ao Maramatanga, New Zealand College of Mental Health Nurses: http://www.nzcmhn.org.nz/

References

Attwood, T. (2007). *The complete guide to Asperger's syndrome*. London and Philadelphia: Jessica Kingsley Publishers.

Australian Advisory Board on Autism Spectrum Disorders and MacDermott S (2007). *The prevalence of autism in Australia: Can it be established from existing data?: A report prepared for Australian Advisory Board on Autism Spectrum Disorders* (formerly known as the Autism Council of Australia). Retrieved from http://www.autismaus.com.au/uploads/pdfs/PrevalenceReport.pdf (accessed 5 February 2013).

Barrett, P., & Ollendick, T. (Eds.), (2004). *Handbook of interventions that work with children and adolescents: Prevention and treatment*. West Sussex: John Wiley & Sons.

Burgess, M. (2006). Then, thank god we grew up. *The Guardian*, 27 May. Retrieved from http://www.guardian.co.uk/lifeandstyle/2006/may/27/familyandrelationships.family (accessed 1 April 2012).

Carrington, S., & Graham, L. (2001). Perceptions of school by two teenage boys with Asperger syndrome and their mothers: a qualitative study. *Autism, 5*(1), 37–48.

Gerard, J., & Buehler, C. (2004). Cumulative environmental risk and youth problem behavior. *Journal of Marriage and Family, 66*, 702–720.

Harris, R. (2009). *ACT made simple*. Oakland CA: New Harbinger Publications, Inc.

Herman, J. (1997). *Trauma and recovery* (14th ed.). New York: Basic Books.

Irwin, A., & Scali, E. (2005). *Action on the social determinants of health: Learning from previous experiences: A background paper*. World Health Organization, Secretariat of the Commission on Social Determinants of Health.

Keyes, C. (2007). Promoting and protecting mental health as flourishing: a complementary strategy for improving national mental health. *American Psychologist, 62*(2), 95–108.

Lawrence, D. H., Alleckson, D. A., & Bjorklund, P. (2010). Beyond the roadblocks: transitioning to adulthood with Asperger's disorder. *Archives of Psychiatric Nursing, 24*(4), 227–238.

Little, L., & Clark, R. (2006). Wonders and worries of parenting a child with Asperger syndrome and nonverbal learning disorder. *American Journal of Maternal Child Nursing, 31*(1), 39–44.

McAllister, M., Hasking, P., Estefan, A., McLenaghan, K., & Lowe, J. (2010). A strengths-based group program on self harm: a feasibility study. *Journal of School Nursing, 26*(4), 289–300.

McDougall, T. (2006). *Child and adolescent mental health nursing*. Oxford: Blackwell Publishing.

Meadows, G., & Singh, B. (Eds.), (2001). *Mental health in Australia: Collaborative community practice*. Melbourne: Oxford University Press.

Mrazek, P., & Haggerty, R. (Eds.), (1994). *Reducing risks for mental disorders: Frontiers for intervention research*. Washington DC: National Academy Press.

Raphael, B. (2002). Children, young people and families: a population health approach to mental health. *Youth Studies Australia, 21*, 12–16.

Rhodes, P., & Wallis, A. (Eds.), (2011). *A practical guide to family therapy: Structured guidelines and key skills*. Melbourne: IP Communications.

National Mental Health Consumer & Carer Forum (2010). Stigma, discrimination and mental illness in Australia. Retrieved from www.nmhccf.org.au/documents/Final%20version%20Stigma%20&%20Discrimination.pdf (accessed 1 May 2012).

Sawyer, M., Arney, F., Baghurst, P., et al. (2000). *The mental health of young people in Australia*. Canberra: AGPS.

Seligman, M. E., Steen, T. A., Park, N., & Peterson, C. (2005). Positive psychology progress: empirical validation of interventions. *American Psychologist, 60*(5), 410–421.

Slade, T., Johnston, A., Oakley Browne, M., Andrews, G., & Whiteford, H. (2009). 2007 National Survey of Mental Health and Wellbeing: methods and key findings. *Australian and New Zealand Journal of Psychiatry, 43*(7), 594–605.

Slattery, P. (2007). *Youth works: A very practical book about working with young people*. Melbourne: Peter Slattery.

Stuart, G. (2009). *Principles and practice of psychiatric nursing* (9th ed.). St Louis: Mosby Elsevier.

Stuart, G., & Laraia, M. (1998). *Principles and practice of psychiatric nursing* (6th ed.). St Louis: Mosby.

Watanabe, N., Hunot, V., Omori, I., Churchill, R., & Furukawa, T. (2007). Psychotherapy for depression among children and adolescents: a systematic review. *Acta Psychiatrica Scandinavica, 116,* 84–95.

World Health Organization (WHO) (2001). *The world health report 2001 – Mental health: New understanding, new hope.* Geneva: WHO.

Yoshida, Y. (2007). *How to be yourself in a world's that different: An Asperger's syndrome study guide for adolescents.* London: Jessica Kingsley Publishers.

Chapter 13

LOSS AND GRIEF

Elizabeth Forster, Judith Murray

LEARNING OUTCOMES

Reading this chapter will help you to:

» discuss the concepts of grief and loss
» describe factors that influence grief responses
» describe differences between sudden and anticipated loss
» discuss anticipatory grief
» discuss parental grief
» discuss developmental differences in relation to children's understanding of
  death and their grief responses
» describe supportive ways to interact with parents and siblings in the
  context of loss.

Introduction

Grieving is a normal human process of healing that involves a person dealing with
the variable pain of being separated from someone or something of importance to
them and adjusting to a world in which that valued person or thing is missing. Such
adjustment involves an ability to integrate that which was lost into the ongoing life

of the person so the lost person or thing is removed from a central role in daily functioning, while its possible ongoing effect on the individual remains recognised and respected. Understanding grief and loss as concepts within the context of caring for children, young people and families is important, as appropriate responses and understanding are required at this extraordinary time.

> ### Clinical scenario 13.1
> ### Setting the scene
>
> You are working in a maternity ward where you are caring for 40-year-old Jacqui who has just given birth to a baby girl, Julie, who was stillborn. Jacqui learnt a few days ago during her antenatal appointment that her baby had died in utero when the baby's heartbeat could not be detected. She was then admitted to the labour ward and labour was induced. Jacqui is accompanied by her husband Mark and her step-children Alex, aged 4 years, and John, aged 14 years. Jacqui had been undergoing fertility treatment for 3 years prior to Julie's birth and had suffered numerous miscarriages.

Defining loss, grief and bereavement

A burgeoning theory and research base concerning grief and bereavement has arisen in the past few decades. A useful starting point in coming to understand this literature is to reflect upon definitions of grief, bereavement and loss, as well as the themes and trends in current research.

Although many definitions exist in the literature, for the purposes of this chapter, bereavement involves the loss of someone or something. The term has often been confined to the event of loss through death. However, it is also used to describe not only the event but also the internal and external processes of adaptation of individuals and family members across the many facets of the experience around death. This includes the anticipation of the loss, the loss itself and the experiences of adjustment following this loss (Genevro, Marshall & Miller, 2004, p. 498). These dual processes of bereavement that include the internal processes of adaptation to the death itself, such as dealing with separation anxiety and finding meaning, as well as the external processes of adaptation or restoration–oriented activities, which may involve relationship changes and living arrangement changes, both occur following the loss (Stroebe & Schut, 1999).

Raphael (1984) defines grief as the emotional responses to loss: the complex amalgam of painful effects, including sadness, anger, helplessness, guilt and despair. While many commonalities exist, individuals vary in their experience of grief – in its intensity, its duration and its means of expression (Genevro et al., 2004; Murray, 2005a). Some people may not experience distress or display grief responses anticipated by others. However, such responses do not necessarily indicate some problem in grieving (Wortman & Silver, 2001). In some cases, loss may represent the end of a burden and result in a lesser degree of distress for the person. In other cases, previous life experiences may have led to the person being less fearful of the grief experienced and, hence, less distressed. In fact, the experience of loss can bring forth positive emotions and changes to the affected person(s) (Calhoun & Tedeschi, 2006).

Although the term 'bereavement' refers to situations involving death, the more general term of 'loss' refers to situations over which people grieve. Loss has been defined most simply as the experience of being parted from something or someone of value. More formally, Miller and Omarzu (1998, p. 12) define loss as the experience of being separated from that of value in that loss is 'produced by an event which is perceived to be negative by the individuals involved and results in long-term changes to one's social situations, relationships, or cognitions'.

As such, it may not be confined to a single event, but may encompass an ongoing set of events. In being parted from something of value to us, complete dissociation from the lost object may never fully occur and the 'something' over which a person may grieve is defined by the person experiencing the loss, rather than others. Therefore, grief and loss are not confined to loss through the death of a loved one. They include events that are an inevitable part of life's journey, such as those associated with ageing or moving from primary to secondary school or the private, less tangible losses that human beings experience such as missing out on a job, being betrayed by a friend or unrequited love. Loss may also include deprivation or neglect, such as homelessness, disability or abuse (Murray, 2005a).

Current trends in thinking on grief and loss

Most schools of psychological thought have had something to say about grieving, with most proposing explanatory models. There have been contributions from psychodynamic theory (Freud, 1917), attachment theory (Bowlby, 1961; Kübler-Ross, 1969; Parkes, 1972; Raphael, 1984), social learning theory (Doka, 1989; Glick, Weiss & Parkes, 1974) and personal construct theory (Neimeyer & Mahoney, 1995).

Traditional models of grief, such as the phases and stages model proposed by Elisabeth Kübler-Ross (1969), have had widespread appeal, as they assist in illuminating the experience of loss. However, these models have limited empirical support, as grieving individuals demonstrate varied responses to loss rather than progressing through distinct stages or sequences of psychological states (Neimeyer, 2000). Often, these models have been seen as competing for influence in the discussions of grief when, in reality, each theory has added more to our understanding of this important human experience.

The early theorists provided the basic understandings in describing the process of mourning. In later times, others have added understanding, provided greater clarity or made corrections when empirical data or new theory contradicted accepted understandings. Some models have combined the theoretical emphases of different schools. For example, the task-based models of mourning (Rando, 1993; Worden, 1991) were a combination of the psychodynamic concepts of grief work and the phasic models of attachment theories. More recent integrated models such as the Four Components Model (Bonanno & Kaltmann, 1999) and the Dual Process Model (Stroebe & Schut, 1999) have sought to employ the knowledge of many schools of thought.

Assumptive worlds

Another perspective that offers much to the understanding of grief and loss is that of *assumptive worlds*. Parkes (1975, p. 132) defined the assumptive world as:

> The individual's view of reality as he believes it to be, i.e. a strongly held set of assumptions about the world and the self which are confidently maintained and used as a means of recognizing, planning and acting.

Assumptions are learned and confirmed through the life experiences of each individual. They are learned within the contexts of living within families, community and culture, as well as through individual life experiences. Essentially, assumptions are those understandings of the world that are reinforced over time by certain events and interactions. As such, assumptions can be both positive and negative, and become the filter through which people interpret their world and events that happen in it.

These assumptions provide the individual with the ability to make predictions about the world and so order their behaviour to conform to this world. Such predictability provides a sense of security in living everyday life. Janoff-Bulman (1992) argues that, in western civilisations, individuals hold three basic assumptions:

1. the world is benevolent (or malevolent)
2. the world is meaningful (or meaningless)
3. the self is worthy (or unworthy).

Some life events challenge the security of the world and challenge assumptions. Parkes (1988, p. 55) defined psychosocial transitions as life events:

> ... that a) require people to undertake a major revision of their assumptions of the world, b) are lasting in their implications rather than transient, and c) take place over a relatively short period of time so that there is little opportunity for preparation.

For many people, illness and death are psychosocial transitions. Parkes (1975) argues that there are different responses within the world view to psychosocial transitions. The former view of the world, or at least some aspects of it, may be abandoned, which may lead to either a satisfactory or a frightening outcome, depending on whether the event seriously threatens the sense of security. But some may refuse to abandon this world view and, hence, try to maintain it by trying to force the current world, or parts thereof, to conform to the previous assumptive world. Sometimes, the old assumptive world remains unchanged and exists alongside the new world. The individual then oscillates between the two worlds – for example, when a person maintains hope for health in the face of increasing evidence of a degenerating condition.

Certain types of deaths are more likely to shatter one's assumptive world, including deaths that are sudden or without warning or those that occur because of a deliberate act (Davis, Wortman, Lehman & Silver, 2000) and deaths that are untimely, such as the death of a child or the loss of a spouse at a young age. These deaths shatter fundamental assumptions – for example, that children should outlive their parents and that children should grow into adults and lead long and happy lives.

In response to these losses, the bereaved may embark upon a search for meaning that involves reaching a new understanding – a 'relearning' and 'reinvesting' in the world that has changed because of the loss of the loved one (Wheeler, 2001). As well as relearning or reconciling one's world from the past to the present and future in light of their loss, the bereaved person may also need to find renewed purpose and reason in living (Wheeler, 2001).

Sudden versus expected loss and anticipatory grief

Death may be expected or unexpected, the characteristics of which differ and can influence the impact on survivors. According to Iserson (2000), characteristics that may differ depending on whether the death is expected or not include the cause of death, the age of the deceased, when and where the death occurs, the involvement and reaction of the survivors, the site of last contact with health professionals, resuscitation, autopsy requirements and immediate family rituals and requirements.

The family members in the case scenario are coming to terms with the sudden and unexpected loss of their long-awaited baby. In a sudden unexpected death, the family may have only a very short time of preparation or no warning at all. The death may have occurred in a public place, at home or at work or in an emergency department or intensive care unit. Family members may or may not be present at the time of death and may be contacted and gather gradually. The family may have witnessed resuscitation procedures and may need to discuss autopsy requirements soon after their loved one's death. In some cases, coronial requirements may prevent easy and unlimited access to the person who has died or may necessitate the involvement of the police as the investigative arm of the Coroner. All this often occurs when a person is dealing with the reactions of shock that can compromise their ability to assimilate and deal with all that is required of them.

In contrast, when the death of a loved one is expected, it usually occurs following a long, chronic or life-threatening illness and may occur at home or in a hospital or aged care facility. The death usually occurs weeks, months or years following the original diagnosis, and family members may have had some time to prepare and are often present at the time of death (Iserson, 2000). However, even though a child may have been ill for a long period prior to their death, parents may still perceive the actual death as sudden, often stating that when it actually occurred they did not expect it to happen, and so they can still experience feelings of shock (Forster, 2012).

The many potential differences between sudden, unexpected and expected loss have the potential to influence the relationship between health professionals and bereaved families and the nature of support provided following loss. Paediatric death introduces additional complexities.

When the death of a child is sudden and unexpected, health professionals have a limited timeframe in which to initiate support and must provide this support to parents/families experiencing overwhelming and intense shock and grief. This may not only limit the amount and type of support health professionals can offer, but also have a negative impact on their perceived ability to provide this support. Following sudden or accidental death, many variables will influence the severity of shock that families experience: the child who died as a person, when he or she died, the relationship or degree of attachment between the parents and family and the deceased child and the coping ability of the parents and family members (Sanders, 1986). The manner in which health professionals impart the news of the death to relatives can have long-lasting and negative effects on their bereavement and leave them feeling guilty or shocked if the news was delivered in an insensitive way (Armentrout & Cates, 2011).

Perinatal death in itself is also different, to some extent, from other child death in that the whole event of pregnancy is involved. Perinatal death is defined as an unexpected death of a baby during pregnancy, labour or following birth, and encompasses miscarriage, ectopic pregnancy, loss of a twin, stillbirth and neonatal death (Clark Callister, 2006).

This experience of sudden loss may contrast with that experienced by parents and families when the child's death is expected, such as following a long-term chronic illness. Rando (1986) suggests that parents may have more time to anticipate the loss and begin their grieving, and that this may have a positive impact on their coping following the loss. When individuals are faced with the likelihood of a significant loss, they may embark upon the process of anticipatory grief (Fulton, Madden & Minichiello, 1996).

Anticipatory grief refers to commencement of the grieving process prior to the anticipated loss and may have positive outcomes, as it enables people to begin to work through the changes surrounding the loss and therefore lessens the trauma experienced when the loss occurs. However, whether anticipatory grief actually lessens the impact of the loss once it occurs is the subject of debate in bereavement literature (Walker, Pomeroy, McNeil & Franklin, 1996). It should never be assumed that, when a death was anticipated, it will be less painful than a sudden death, or that grieving will be a less difficult process. In fact, it is suggested that, in some situations where caregiving has led to other problems or a relationship is dependent or guilt-ridden, the grief can be intense (Brazil, Bedard & Willison, 2002). In addition to anticipatory grief, parents, the child and family members are likely to have been on a journey punctuated by painful procedures, therapies and surgery in an effort to cure or enhance the quality of life, periods of hope and loss of hope and cycles of relapse, remission and relapse (Rando, 1986).

The relationship between the child, their family and health professionals in the long-term care situation will also contrast with the context of sudden, unexpected death. In the former case, relationships may have developed over a long period of time and opportunities may have arisen to instigate bereavement support much earlier and offer it more constantly and consistently prior to the child's death.

Grief within the context of the family

In the context of child, youth and family nursing, it is essential to understand developmental differences in responses to loss. When loss occurs, it impacts on all members of the family. In the case scenario, the loss of baby Julie has impacted on the parents Jacqui and Mark, as well as their children, Alex and John, in unique ways. To explore your understanding so far, refer to the critical reflections and questions in Box 13.1.

Loss is both a personal and an interactional process that occurs within a social context where people grieve within personal, family and societal systems (Neimeyer, 2000).

Box 13.1 Critical reflections and questions: Responses to grief

Following your reading in the chapter so far and reflection on the case scenario, discuss how the following factors could influence the grief response for each of the family members:

1. their age and developmental stage
2. their gender
3. history of the loss/trauma
4. the nature and quality of the relationship with the deceased
5. the circumstances surrounding the loss (e.g. anticipated or sudden unexpected, traumatic and family relationships and expectations).

People's values and expectations may assert their influence on the experience of grief in subtle or overt ways. In some cases of perinatal loss, there may be powerful societal expectations concerning grieving and sometimes limited recognition of the family's need to grieve and hold rituals (Clark Callister, 2006). The manner in which family, friends and acquaintances respond to grieving families, albeit well-intentioned, can sometimes deepen rather than ease the pain experienced following the loss of a loved one (Shumaker & Brownell, 1984). In the case scenario, consider how social networks and expectations may help or hinder Jacqui, Mark, Alex and John's grief.

Debate surrounding whether it is beneficial for parents to hold their stillborn baby continues. Reynolds (2004, p. 87), in his discussion about whether parents should hold or not hold their stillborn baby, reminds us that seeing or holding the deceased baby may be confronting for parents and 'may deprive them of the much needed protection of denial'. Adverse effects among parents including post-traumatic stress disorder have been reported as being associated with seeing the deceased infant (Flenady & Wilson, 2008; Turton, Hughes, Evans & Fainman, 2001).

Reynolds (2004) and Flenady and Wilson (2008) advocate an individualised rather than 'one size fits all' approach to psychosocial care of parents following stillbirth, where options are offered to parents along with an informed discussion of the risks and benefits. Such an approach acknowledges that 'patients have the right to absorb or not absorb the full reality of their loss ... parents must face the reality of their loss on their own terms, not ours' (Reynolds, 2004, p. 87). Similarly, parents may feel that it is important for siblings to meet their deceased brother or sister. Parents in a Swedish study found that meeting the stillborn baby was a natural process for the whole family and enabled siblings to see and know the baby they were grieving for (Avelin, Erlandsson, Hildingsson & Rådestad, 2011). Parents expressed that they wanted more support from health professionals regarding how to respond to siblings' questions and reactions and sometimes appreciated some time to prepare prior to introducing their other children to the deceased baby.

Loss of a child: parental grief

According to Alam, Barrera, D'Agostino, Nicholas & Schneiderman (2012, p. 2):

> The death of a child can be a devastating experience for parents ... This event symbolizes the reversal of the natural order of life and erases the dreams and hopes that parents have for their child.

Parents who have lost a child often say that their pain is so deep that it lasts a lifetime, despite their efforts to find meaning in life and move forward (Schwab, 1997). The death of a child symbolises many social losses for parents whose focus and purpose had centred on nurturing their growth and development (Sanders, 1986). Society holds the parents of successful children in high esteem and parents love and feel responsible for their children and believe that they will outlive them, their existence ensuring that parents retain a small sense of immortality (Sanders, 1986).

When a child dies, parents can feel that they have failed their child and may become immersed in guilt and blame that may be directed towards themselves and their partners (Sanders, 1986). Regardless of whether the child is young or an adult, or the death sudden or expected, the loss of a child is devastating and shatters parental dreams, hopes, expectations, fantasies and wishes for that child (Avelin et al., 2011; deJong-Berg & Kane, 2006; Rando, 1986; Wheeler, 2001).

The grief of other children

There is considerable debate in the literature concerning the capacity of children to mourn. On one side, psychodynamic theorists, such as Wolfenstein (1966), Deutsch (1937) and Anna Freud (1960), argued that mourning was not possible until late childhood or adolescence. In contrast, John Bowlby's (1963, 1980) attachment theory argued that children as young as toddlers experienced grief reactions similar to those of adults. With respect to the attachment theory, it was argued that, once a child was able to attach to another, they would mourn when that love object was removed. Other theorists (Furman, 1964; Kliman, 1989) have suggested a middle ground, arguing that children from 3 to 4 years of age are able to mourn.

The belief that children are not affected by loss is reinforced if children manifest grief differently from adults (Dyregrov, 1990; Schwab, 1997). Adults may display constant disturbance associated with the loss, but some children do not cry or they may continue to play as if nothing has happened (Schoen, Burgoyne & Schoen, 2004).

Mourning is not only experienced; it is also learned from those around the child. The child's environment will change when adults within that environment are mourning a situation, which can make the child feel insecure and stressed. Following the death of a child, parents may gain strength and purpose from their other children, while others find their own grief can leave them so depleted of emotional energy that they have difficulties supporting their children or partner (Boerner & Silverman, 2001). The difficulty that some parents have of 'letting go' of the deceased child can lead to psychological pressure being placed on siblings to fulfil the roles of the deceased child or to take on characteristics of the deceased, a phenomenon often referred to as the 'replacement child' (Cain, Fast & Erickson, 1964; Crehan, 2004; Grout & Romanoff, 2000). This psychological pressure can undermine the sibling's opportunities to live their own life and develop an individual identity. The child may be constrained by parental overprotection and restriction, or by being viewed as replacing the lost child (Crehan, 2004; Grout & Romanoff, 2000).

Aside from adults' individual functioning following loss and its effect on children and adolescents, the family system can give children some very strong messages about loss and how it is to be handled (Silverman, Weiner & El Ad, 1995). Often these messages are given subtly and largely unconsciously. However, children learn the patterns of acceptable behaviour very quickly. Family stories and meanings reconstructed in the context of loss of a child are conveyed to all surviving family members and have a strong influence on family practices as well as child development (Grout & Romanoff, 2000).

Child development and bereavement

From conception to death, a human being is developing and changing. Innate and learned skills are used to adapt to the circumstances of our existence and the changes that are occurring around us. The major difference between adults and children is that children may be experiencing these demands on their abilities for the first time without the benefit of hindsight and the intellectual ability to 'think through' the changes, the options and their consequences in a logical manner. In addition, the intensity of change is more pronounced in the life of children than it is in the life of adults, as so many changes are occurring within a relatively short period of time from birth to adolescence.

For many children, these vast changes will occur within the security of a loving family environment. The changes will occur gradually, in line with the expectations of the supportive adults around them and in common with their peers. Children in these circumstances will likely develop positive coping skills, often mirroring the well-adjusted adults in their lives. However, many children will have to deal with the critical changes of childhood without these advantages. Into the lives of such children may come devastating loss that is out of the realm of experience of the adults around them, or that renders the adults emotionally unable to provide the necessary support and insight for the child. In other situations, the normal demands of change and the losses of life on the growing child are complicated by physical and intellectual difficulties with which the child is born, the negative physical environment in which they live and/or the maladaptive behaviours of the adults around them.

In considering the development of the child, there has been a tendency to think of physical, intellectual, emotional and social development as separate influences. However, these developmental demands occur simultaneously, with children experiencing many changes within a relatively short period of time. Difficulties in one area alone will require children to draw on their resources. Difficulties in more than one area at the same time will tax those resources – maybe even overload them.

What might a child understand about death?

Grieving is a highly emotional time in the life of a family. Hence, children with limited expressive language like Alex, who is 4 years old, may find it more difficult to verbalise their feelings or concerns about an event.

A 10-year follow-up study into children's reactions to the perinatal death of a sibling by Murray (2005b) highlighted that the stage of development of the child at the time of death is a significant factor affecting the long-term outcomes of bereavement. One of the major differences in the grieving of children and adults is that children's grieving occurs within a child's world and they lack the experiences into which to 'fit' their situation of loss.

Baker, Sedney and Gross (1992) identified two important aspects of grieving in children: the need for protection and the need to maintain an internal representation and relationship with the lost object. They argue that a failure to recognise the significance of these aspects may contribute to short-term and long-term problems in children. Burnell and Burnell (1989) suggest that there are three questions that concern children and need to be addressed in their understandings of what is happening around them:

1. 'What did I do to cause this to happen?'
2. 'Will this happen to me too? Or will something "bad" happen to me too?'
3. 'Who will take care of me?'

These questions can be linked to early childhood thinking, which is egocentric and magical and where cause and effect is poorly understood – that is, normal developmental behaviours (Hockenberry, Wilson, Winkelstein & Kline, 2003).

In relation to health and illness, young children may also be influenced by immanent justice, where they may believe they are at fault and that accidents or illness are magically caused by their own disobedience or misbehaviour, even though it was unconnected to the injury or illness (Raman & Winer, 2004). A young child's belief in immanent justice can manifest in a variety of ways. For example, if someone says 'if you keep doing that, you'll be the death of me' and then they happen to die soon after, the child may think they have caused the death of that person (Schaefer & Lyons, 1993). These cognitive distortions concerning death and their own contribution are exacerbated by lack of opportunity to talk about death and ask questions (Schwab, 1997). Infants have no concept of death or time and may be unable to form a permanent image of the object or person lost. They tend to be affected by their carer's emotional state and, if the parent or carer is grieving, this may lead to a decreased ability on the part of the carer to provide for the needs of the baby or respond to the baby's needs or actions. As a result, the baby may become more 'fussy' or 'clingy'.

The young child does not understand the irreversibility of death and may think that, if they wish hard enough, the person will return (Schaefer & Lyons, 1993). They may not understand where their playmate has gone or may wonder why their parents have changed so much. A carer may explain the situation, only to find the child asking when the situation will return to normal. Saying that, if someone is dead, they will never come back may be quickly met with the question, 'But when will … come home?' Death may only be thought of in terms of being 'not here' as opposed to being 'here'. Therefore, if someone is 'not here', you may be able to go and find them.

Young children may have difficulty distinguishing fact from fantasy. Therefore, the facts of the situation may be modified, changed or completely altered in the world of the imagination of the child. Separation anxiety and fears are common. There may be intense searching for the person who has gone or died. Children may pull away from people who remind them too much of the person they have lost.

Prelogical thinking can lead to misconceptions or misinterpretations of what is said. 'Magical', egocentric thinking can lead them to believe that they have control over the outcome of a situation or were in some way responsible for the loss by some thought or action on their part. Young children may also take adults' comments literally. For example, the comment 'your grandpa died so peacefully in his sleep' may result in the child not wanting to go to sleep for fear it will happen to them (Schaefer & Lyons, 1993).

Young children are often very curious about facts. They may not understand that, in death, the functions of life have ceased (Slaughter & Griffiths, 2007). Therefore, they may be concerned about a person being hungry, cold or breathing once buried. A lack of understanding of the consequences of a loss may result in a lack of reaction to news of the loss, which may be disconcerting to older children and adults.

Three most painful grieving emotions of the under 3s are likely to be: separation fear, where they fear that they will be abandoned by those they love; ambivalence, where they are uncertain about whether or not they should become attached to someone; and guilt and hostility, resulting from a child feeling responsible for the death or the distress in the family (Salladay & Royal, 1981).

School-aged children are beginning to understand consequences and, therefore, they may have very definite opinions about causes of a loss. They may be very sure about what caused the death and place very definite blame on a particular person, even if it is not justified. In fact, in their fantasies they can take revenge on this person. These children may also believe strongly that, if certain actions are carried out, they can avoid consequences. They may even fantasise that they can change the situation by these actions. Problems arise when the child has misconceptions concerning the causes of a loss and issues of justice and injustice begin to emerge.

School-aged children are beginning to understand that loss affects others and can understand others' perspectives to some extent. They may try to sort out their ideas through playing out a situation. Therefore, concrete expressions such as rituals and drawing can support their coping with loss.

They are gradually beginning to understand that death happens to everyone, but not themselves initially. Socialisation is also gaining importance and children's responses to loss may be influenced by their awareness of social expectations; for example, boys may begin to hide their feelings and be strong. However, isolation from peers after loss is also common. Children of this age can begin to plan and develop more coping strategies. An ability to plan may help to make a child feel more in control of their situation and their life in general.

Adolescents develop a mature understanding of death and may begin to fear death. As a result of this fear, adolescents may try to keep these thoughts at a distance; however, cognitively, they may be interrupted by thoughts and images of the lost person and this may interfere with their ability to concentrate (Balk, 2011). Adolescents may also develop a personification of death. The four main types of death personification are the macabre (decaying form), the gentle comforter (powerful force quietly employed in a kindly way), the gay deceiver (luring in the unwary and leading them to their doom) and the automaton (goes about the business of death in a bored competent fashion) (Cotter, 2003).

The need to deal with loss may be complicated by normal crises of adolescence. For example, at a time when parental support may be vital in dealing with a loss, the adolescent may be struggling with the issues and inevitable conflicts of wanting to be independent from parents.

At this stage, peer support is important. Unfortunately, many adolescents faced with a loss can feel their friends 'just don't understand', and they may hide their feelings of grief because they are reluctant to confide in their peers (Balk, Zaengle & Corr, 2011). At times, adolescents will deal with their sense of helplessness by engaging in 'risky' behaviour (e.g. experimenting with drugs, increased sexual activity, fast driving). Adolescents may also be very judgemental and can be very hard on themselves if they believe they could have done more to prevent a loss. They may also become very angry with others they perceive to have some responsibility for the loss.

Shame also plays an important part in adolescents' feelings of loss. Feelings or types of loss that an adolescent considers embarrassing or 'shameful' may be hidden. Paradoxically, the more intense the emotions an adolescent feels, the more they may try to repress them. An adolescent, particularly a boy, may be very fearful of losing control of their emotions. They may resist any attempts to get them to 'open up'. This conflict may appear in behaviour and conflicts with others in their environment.

Most researchers agree that a child needs to understand three concepts of death as they mature. These concepts are the following:

1. **Universality/inevitability**: the understanding that all things die and that there is no avoiding it.
2. **Irreversibility**: the understanding that once a living thing dies, its physical body cannot be alive again.
3. **Non-functionality**: the understanding that all life-defining functions cease at death.

A comprehensive review of studies published since the 1980s concerning the conceptions of death among children (Kenyon, 2001) led to the following conclusions:

• By 10 years of age, most children have mastered the components of irreversibility, universality, non-functionality, personal mortality and causality.
• Understanding these individual components appears to be differentiated by several factors, and appears to have different developmental trajectories.
• Abstract components such as universality appear to be affected by cognitive development, verbal ability and cultural and religious experiences.
• Physical-based components such as non-functionality and irreversibility appear to be affected by direct experience.
• Emotional factors appear to play a significant role in how children respond to questions about death and might be highly influential in the development of their understanding about death.

A child's grief reaction will depend on their developmental stage. Burnell and Burnell (1989) suggest that children under 3 in families in which death has occurred will typically exhibit loss of speech and generalised distress, whereas children under 5 may respond with disturbances in eating, sleeping and bladder and bowel control. In school-age children, school phobias, hypochondriacal concerns (fear of being 'sick' or phantom illnesses), abdominal or substernal pain or headaches without organic origin, learning problems, antisocial behaviour, aggression and withdrawal are common responses. Grief reactions among older children may be more diverse than are those among younger children whose world of experience and repertoire of behaviours is more limited.

The older sibling in the case scenario, John, is 14 years old. By the time children enter adolescence, most have developed the ability to understand loss from the perspective of adults (Geis, Whittlesey, McDonald, Smith & Pfefferbaum, 1998; Speece & Brent, 1992). They are able to understand what has occurred and the short-term and long-term implications of the situation. As intellectual and emotional development occurs, children may need to reprocess aspects of a previous experience to deepen their understanding of the event (Schoen et al., 2004). The effects of loss in the lives of children or adolescents cannot be easily segregated from normal developmental changes. Adolescents are likely to understand as adults what happens when someone dies, as they now see death as universal, inevitable and irreversible (Schaefer & Lyons, 1993).

Adolescents may express their grief through aggression, anger, withdrawal, anxiety including panic attacks, truancy, delinquency and fixation on the lost object. Bereaved adolescents may also experience work or study deterioration, problems in peer relationships, sleep disturbances, headaches and uncontrollable crying (Balk et al., 2011). They may also experience nausea and have problems maintaining their nutritional intake (Balk et al., 2011; Smith, O'Rourke, Parker et al., 1988). Consider the critical questions and reflections in Box 13.2.

Providing supportive care to families

Suffering is not a question that demands an answer;
It is not a problem that demands a solution;
It is a mystery that demands a presence. (Anonymous).

Nurses and midwives are socialised into a model of clinical decision making that includes assessment, identification of problems, planning and evaluating interventions. This clinical decision-making process underscores nurses' everyday actions and, in the context of loss and grief, may lead to a tendency to want to 'intervene' or resolve. However, this is inappropriate, as the loss is irreversible and the problem cannot be resolved. The focus shifts, therefore, to interactions with families that are helpful and do not worsen an already overwhelming and deeply sad experience.

The loss experienced cannot be understood. However, it can be acknowledged by a sincere, simple and personalised expression of sorrow. Responses to siblings are guided by an understanding of their developmental level and an understanding of death and, in the midst of parental grief, it is important to be sensitive to sibling needs, questions and reactions to seeing others around them expressing grief. It is important to be aware that children may not interpret or understand what is happening in the same way in which adults do.

Nurses and midwives are often present within the intimate family circle at the time of loss, and may be uncertain about what to say. You will at times be a supportive presence for families where no words are necessarily spoken. However, when you do speak you can verbalise your thought processes to parents simply and honestly. A useful strategy here is to listen to your thoughts at the time you are approaching or

> **Box 13.2** Critical questions and reflections: Talking to children about death
>
> When talking to children, it is important to be honest and use language to which the children can relate. It is also important to use the correct words to describe what is occurring (such as 'dead'). If children do not have information, they will often make something up to fill the gaps. This may be more damaging for them in the long term than knowing the truth if their interpretations of the event are incorrect. Tell the children that it is okay for them to feel sad, mad, angry or scared – to feel whatever it is that they need to feel or however they need to be.
>
> It is very important to hear from and listen to the children to find out what they have heard or understood. Sometimes, children will hear part of what you say and 'close down' after hearing a single word or sentence. This is where misunderstanding can occur. Hence, try to help confirm that the children have heard and understood what you have tried to tell them, and gently encourage them to tell back to you what you told them. You may need to revisit these issues a few times to confirm understanding, but do not push too hard.
>
> You are the midwife caring for Jacqui. She asks you how she should explain Julie's death to her children, particularly 4-year-old Alex. Discuss how you would suggest she explain Julie's death to her preschool-aged child.

sitting with a bereaved family. What are you thinking? Your thoughts may include: 'This is the worst experience imaginable, I can't imagine what you must be going through right now, I don't know what to say, I don't want to make things worse for you right now.'

The next step is to turn these thoughts into communication with the bereaved family: 'I was on my way here and I was thinking that this must be the most heartbreaking experience you could ever face. I can't imagine what you must be going through right now, but I want you to know that I want to do anything I can so as not to make this experience any worse for you right now.'

Lastly, nurses and midwives can personalise the child by talking to parents about their child and the memories they mention. By talking with parents you are recognising their incredible loss and acknowledging that they have lost someone so precious, along with all the hopes, dreams and future moments and milestones they wanted to share with their child.

Conclusion

In this chapter, you have considered definitions of grief and loss, reviewed current trends in thinking in relation to grief and loss and, through the critical thinking questions, have had the opportunity to reflect upon the variety of factors that impact on parents and children and their responses to loss in the realm of child health nursing practice. An understanding of the myriad factors that influence individuals and their responses to grief is invaluable in providing sensitive and supportive care in this context.

KEY POINTS

» Acknowledge and validate the person's loss.

» Verbalise your thought processes to parents simply and honestly.

» Personalise the parents' child.

» Children and young people's understanding of death and grief responses will vary according to their age and developmental stage.

» Tell children that it is okay for them to feel the way they do and find out what they have heard or understood in order to correct any misunderstandings.

CRITICAL QUESTIONS AND REFLECTIONS

When caring for a family experiencing the death of a child, it is important for health professionals to reflect upon their experiences. The following points provide a useful reflective tool for nurses:

* What was I thinking and feeling around the time the child died?

* What did the death mean to me? What meanings or personal interpretations did I make about the child's death and my communication and care provision?

* What did I do and say at the time and how does this compare to what I wanted to do or say?

* What was positive and negative about the experience?

* What else could I have done and, if a similar situation arose again, what would I do differently?

USEFUL RESOURCES

Australian Centre for Grief and Bereavement: www.grief.org.au/

Australian Child and Adolescent Trauma Loss and Grief Network (ANU) http://www.earlytraumagrief.anu.edu.au/

Australian Government Department of Health and Ageing: http://www.health.gov.au/internet/main/publishing.nsf/Content/portal-Palliative%20care

Australian Government Department of Health and Ageing (2007) Providing culturally appropriate palliative care to Aboriginal and Torres Strait Islander Peoples: Resource Kit: www.health.gov.au/internet/main/publishing.nsf/Content/palliativecare-pubs-indig-resource.htm

Compassionate Friends: http://www.compassionatefriendsqld.org.au/

GriefLink: http://grieflink.org.au/

National Association for Loss and Grief (NALAG): www.nalag.org.au

National Centre for Childhood Grief: www.childhoodgrief.org.au/

Now What, a website for young people with cancer developed by CanTeen, the Australian Organisation for Young People Living with Cancer: www.nowwhat.org.au/

Palliative Care Curriculum for Undergraduates: http://www.pcc4u.org/

SANDS Miscarriage, Stillbirth & Neonatal Death Support: www.sands.org.au

SIDS and KIDS: www.sidsandkids.org

Skylight New Zealand: www.skylight.org.nz/

References

Alam, R., Barrera, M., D'Agostino, N., Nicholas, D., & Schneiderman, G. (2012). Bereavement experiences of mothers and fathers over time after the death of a child due to cancer. *Death Studies, 36*(1), 1–22.

Armentrout, D., & Cates, L. (2011). Informing parents about the actual or impending death of their infant in a newborn intensive care unit. *The Journal of Perinatal & Neonatal Nursing, 25*(3), 261–267.

Avelin, P., Erlandsson, K., Hildingsson, I., & Rådestad, I. (2011). Swedish parents' experiences of parenthood and the need for support to siblings when a baby is stillborn. *Birth: Issues in Perinatal Care, 38*(2), 150–158.

Baker, J. E., Sedney, M. A., & Gross, E. (1992). Psychological tasks for bereaved children. *American Journal of Orthopsychiatry, 62*(1), 105–116.

Balk, D. E. (2011). Adolescent development and bereavement: an introduction. *Prevention Researcher, 18*(3), 3–9.

Balk, D. E., Zaengle, D., & Corr, C. A. (2011). Strengthening grief support for adolescents coping with a peer's death. *School Psychology International, 32*(2), 144–162.

Boerner, K., & Silverman, P. R. (2001). Gender specific coping patterns in widowed parents with dependent children. *Omega: The Journal of Death and Dying, 43*(3), 201–216.

Bonanno, G., & Kaltmann, S. (1999). Toward an integrative perspective on bereavement. *Psychological Bulletin, 125*, 760–776.

Bowlby, J. (1961). Process of mourning. *International Journal of Psychoanalysis, 42*, 317–340.

Bowlby, J. (1963). Pathological mourning and childhood mourning. *Journal of the American Psychoanalytic Association, 11*, 500–541.

Bowlby, J. (1980). *Attachment and loss: loss, sadness and depression*. New York: Basic Books.

Brazil, K., Bedard, M., & Willison, K. (2002). Correlates of health status for family caregivers in bereavement. *Journal of Palliative Medicine, 5*, 849–855.

Burnell, G. M., & Burnell, A. L. (1989). *Clinical management of bereavement: A handbook for healthcare professionals*. New York: Human Sciences Press.

Cain, A. C., Fast, I., & Erickson, M. E. (1964). Children's disturbed reactions to the death of a sibling. *American Journal of Orthopsychiatry, 34*, 741–752.

Calhoun, L. G., & Tedeschi, R. G. (2006). *Handbook of posttraumatic growth: Research and practice*. Mahwah, NJ: Lawrence Erlbaum Associates Publishers.

Clark Callister, L. (2006). Perinatal loss: a family perspective. *Journal of Perinatal and Neonatal Nursing, 20*(3), 227–234.

Cotter, R. P. (2003). High risk behaviours in adolescence and their relationship to death anxiety and death personifications. *Omega: The Journal of Death and Dying, 47*(2), 119–137.

Crehan, G. (2004). The surviving sibling: the effects of sibling death in childhood. *Psychoanalytic Psychotherapy, 18*(2), 202–219.

Davis, C. G., Wortman, C. B., Lehman, D. R., & Silver, R. (2000). Searching for meaning in loss: are clinical assumptions correct? *Death Studies, 24*, 497–540.

deJong-Berg, M. A., & Kane, L. (2006). Bereavement care for families. Part 2: evaluation of a pediatric follow-up programme. *International Journal of Palliative Nursing, 12*(10), 484–494.

Deutsch, H. (1937). Absence of grief. *Psychoanalytic Quarterly, 6*, 12–22.

Doka, K. J. (1989). *Disenfranchised grief: Recognizing hidden sorrows*. Lexington: Lexington Books.

Dyregrov, A. (1990). Children's reactions to grief and crisis situations. In A. Dyregrov (Ed.), *Grief in children: A handbook for adults* (pp. 9–28). London: Jessica Kingsley.

Flenady, V., & Wilson, T. (2008). Support for mothers, fathers and families after perinatal death. *Cochrane Database of Systematic Reviews* 2008, (Issue 1). Art. No.: CD000452. doi: 10.1002/14651858.CD000452.pub2

Forster, E. M. (2012). *Parent and staff perceptions of bereavement support surrounding loss of a child*. Brisbane: The University of Queensland.

Freud, A. (1960). Discussion of Dr John Bowlby's paper. *Psychoanalytic Study of the Child, 15*, 53–63.

Freud, S. (1917). Mourning and melancholia. In *Sigmund Freud, Collected papers*, Vol. 4. London: Hogarth Press.

Fulton, G., Madden, C., & Minichiello, V. (1996). The social construction of anticipatory grief. *Social Science and Medicine, 43*(9), 1349–1358.

Furman, R. (1964). Death and the young child: some preliminary considerations. *Psychoanalytic Study of the Child, 19*, 321–333.

Geis, H. K., Whittlesey, S. W., McDonald, N. B., Smith, K., & Pfefferbaum, B. (1998). Bereavement and loss in childhood. *Child and Adolescent Psychiatric Clinics of North America, 7*(1), 73–85.

Genevro, J. L., Marshall, T., & Miller, T. (2004). Report on bereavement and grief research. *Death Studies, 28*(6), 491–575.

Glick, I., Weiss, R. S., & Parkes, C. M. (1974). *The first year of bereavement*. New York: Wiley.

Grout, L. A., & Romanoff, B. D. (2000). The myth of the replacement child: parents' stories and practices after perinatal death. *Death Studies, 24*, 93–113.

Hockenberry, M., Wilson, D., Winkelstein, M., & Kline, N. (2003). *Wong's nursing care of infants and children* (7th ed.). St Louis: Mosby.

Iserson, K. V. (2000). Notifying survivors about sudden, unexpected deaths. *Western Journal of Medicine, 173*, 261–265.

Janoff-Bulman, R. (1992). *Shattered assumptions: Towards a new psychology of trauma.* New York: The Free Press.

Kenyon, B. (2001). Current research in children's conception of death: a critical review. *Omega: The Journal of Death and Dying, 43*(1), 69–91.

Kliman, G. (1989). Facilitation of mourning during childhood. In: S. C. Klagsbrun, G. W. Kuman, E. J. Clark, et al. (Eds.), *Preventive psychiatry* (pp. 59–82). Philadelphia: Charles Press.

Kübler-Ross, E. (1969). *On death and dying.* New York: Macmillan.

Miller, E. D., & Omarzu, J. (1998). New directions in loss research. In J. H. Harvey (Ed.), *Perspectives on loss: A sourcebook* (pp. 3–20). Philadelphia: Brunner/Mazel.

Murray, J. A. (2005a). *A psychology of loss: a potentially integrating psychology for the future study of adverse life events. Advances in Psychological Research*, Vol. 37 (pp. 15–46). New York: Nova Publishers.

Murray, J. (2005b). *Children's reactions to perinatal death of a sibling: a ten-year follow-up.* Proceedings of the 2004 Mental Health Services Inc. of Australia and New Zealand Conference, Gold Coast, 1–3 September 2004, pp. 81–86.

Neimeyer, R. A. (2000). *Lessons of loss: A guide to coping.* Victoria: Centre for Grief Education.

Neimeyer, R. A., & Mahoney, M. J. (Eds.), (1995). *Constructivism in psychotherapy.* Washington DC: American Psychological Association.

Parkes, C. M. (1972). *Bereavement: Studies of grief in adult life.* New York: International Universities Press.

Parkes, C. M. (1975). What becomes of redundant world models? A contribution to the study of adaptation to change. *British Journal of Medical Psychology, 48*, 131–137.

Parkes, C. M. (1988). Bereavement as a psychosocial transition: processes of adaptation to change. *Journal of Social Issues, 44*, 53–65.

Raman, L., & Winer, G. A. (2004). Evidence of more immanent justice responding in adults than children: a challenge to traditional developmental theories. *British Journal of Developmental Psychology, 22*, 255–274.

Rando, T. A. (1986). *Parental loss of a child.* Illinois: Research Press.

Rando, T. A. (1993). *Treatment of complicated mourning.* Illinois: Research Press.

Raphael, B. (1984). *The anatomy of bereavement: A handbook for the caring professions.* London: Hutchinson.

Reynolds, J. J. (2004). Stillbirth: to hold or not to hold. *Omega: The Journal of Death and Dying, 48*(1), 85–88.

Salladay, S. A., & Royal, M. E. (1981). Children and death: guidelines for grief work. *Child Psychiatry and Human Development, 11*(4), 203–212.

Sanders, C. M. (1986). Accidental death of a child. In T. A. Rando (Ed.), *Parental loss of a child.* Illinois: Research Press.

Schaefer, D., & Lyons, C. (1993). *How do we tell the children? A step-by-step guide for helping children two to teen cope when someone dies.* New York: Newmarket Press.

Schoen, A. A., Burgoyne, M., & Schoen, S. F. (2004). Are the developmental needs of children in America adequately addressed during the grief process? *Journal of Instructional Psychology, 31*(2), 143–148.

Schwab, R. (1997). Parental mourning and children's behaviour. *Journal of Counselling and Development*, *75*, 258–265.

Shumaker, S. A., & Brownell, A. (1984). Toward a theory of social support: closing conceptual gaps. *Journal of Social Issues*, *40*(4), 11–36.

Silverman, P. R., Weiner, A., & El Ad, N. (1995). Parent–child communication in bereaved Israeli families. *OMEGA: The Journal of Death and Dying*, *31*(4), 275–293.

Slaughter, V., & Griffiths, M. (2007). Death understanding and fear of death in young children. *Clinical Child Psychology and Psychiatry*, *12*(4), 525–535.

Smith, G. G., O'Rourke, D. F., Parker, P. E., et al. (1988). Panic and nausea instead of grief in an adolescent. *Journal of the American Academy of Child and Adolescent Psychiatry*, *27*(4), 509–513.

Speece, M. W., & Brent, S. B. (1992). The acquisition of a mature understanding of three components of the concept of death. *Death Studies*, *16*, 211–229.

Stroebe, M., & Schut, H. (1999). The dual process model of coping with bereavement: rationale and description. *Death Studies*, *23*, 197–224.

Turton, P., Hughes, P., Evans, C. D., & Fainman, D. (2001). The incidence and significance of post traumatic stress disorder in the pregnancy after stillbirth. *British Journal of Psychiatry*, *178*, 556–560.

Walker, R. J., Pomeroy, E. C., McNeil, J. S., & Franklin, C. (1996). Anticipatory grief and AIDS: strategies for intervening with caregivers. *Health and Social Work*, *21*(1), 49–64.

Wheeler, I. (2001). Parental bereavement: the crisis of meaning. *Death Studies*, *25*, 51–66.

Wolfenstein, M. (1966). How is mourning possible? *Psychoanalytic Study of the Child*, *21*, 93–123.

Worden, J. W. (1991). *Grief counseling and grief therapy: A handbook for the mental health practitioner* (2nd ed.). London: Tavistock/Routledge.

Wortman, C. B., & Silver, R. C. (2001). The myths of coping with loss revisited. In M. S. Stroebe, R. O. Hansson, W. Stroebe, & H. Schut (Eds.), *Handbook of bereavement research: Consequences, coping, and care* (pp. 405–429). Washington DC: American Psychological Association.

INDEX

Page numbers followed by 'f' indicate figures, 't' indicate tables, and 'b' indicate boxes.